HEALING
REMEDIES

HEALING REMEDIES

More Than 1,000 Natural Ways to Relieve the
Symptoms of Common Ailments, from Arthritis and
Allergies to Diabetes, Osteoporosis, and Many Others!

JOAN WILEN and LYDIA WILEN

BALLANTINE BOOKS | NEW YORK

A Ballantine Books Trade Paperback Original

Copyright © 2008 by Joan Wilen and Lydia Wilen

Published in the United States by Ballantine Books,
an imprint of The Random House Publishing Group,
a division of Random House, Inc., New York.

BALLANTINE and colophon are registered trademarks of Random House, Inc.

Some of the remedies in this book are adapted from:

Chicken Soup & Other Folk Remedies © 1984,
2000 by Joan Wilen and Lydia Wilen

More Chicken Soup & Other Folk Remedies © 1986, 2000 by Joan Wilen and Lydia Wilen

LIBRARY OF CONGRESS CATALOGING-IN-PUBLICATION DATA

Wilen, Joan.
Healing remedies : more than 1,000 natural ways to relieve the symptoms of
common ailments, from arthritis and allergies to diabetes,
osteoporosis, and many others! / Joan Wilen and Lydia Wilen.
p.   cm.
Includes index.
ISBN 978-0-345-50335-0 (pbk.)
1. Naturopathy—Popular works.   2. Alternative medicine—Popular works.
3. Herbs—Therapeutic use—Popular works.   I. Wilen, Lydia.   II. Title.
RZ440.W54 2009
615.5'35—dc22   2008035980

www.ballantinebooks.com

Book design by JoAnne Metsch

We dedicate this book to research scientists
looking for ways to improve the lives of others, and to
health care providers who really care.

CONTENTS

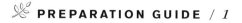

REMEDIES IN A CLASS BY THEMSELVES / *295*

HEALTHFUL HINTS, FUN FACTS, AND FOOD FOR THOUGHT / *305*

ACKNOWLEDGMENTS

Our heartfelt thank-you to:

our cousin and treasured friend, Linda Wilen, with whom we're happy to share the same last name.

Marty Edelston and his Boardroom, Inc., miracle makers.

Ballantine's Rachel Bernstein for planting the seed.

Jane von Mehren for green-lighting this project and putting us together with our wonderful editor.

Christina Duffy, an editor we didn't dread calling to say we needed the deadline extended. Christina's enthusiasm and support were a tonic we wish we could bottle.

And to the rest of the Ballantine team for helping prepare a book that makes us proud.

INTRODUCTION

When we started work on our very first folk remedy book decades ago, we went to all of our relatives, asking for their home remedies. We heard wonderful old-country stories about remarkable cures. But times and places have changed dramatically. Going to the outskirts of Lomza Gubernia in what is now eastern Poland to pick herbs is no longer a practical option.

This book *is* practical . . . and safe . . . and effective.

Yes, practical! Every herb, fruit, vegetable, vitamin, mineral, and liquid mentioned in the book can be bought at your local health food store, supermarket, or greengrocer, on the Internet, or by telephone. Be sure to check out our "Sources" section in the back of the book for worthwhile recommendations.

Our directions are easy to follow and, for the most part, specific. If exact amounts

are not indicated, it means we could not find them in our reference sources, but we thought the remedy was important enough to include anyway. With regard to dosage, please use common sense and listen to your body every step of the way, taking into consideration your size and sensitivities, and your doctor's guidance.

We Wilen sisters are not medical authorities. We're researchers and writers who are not prescribing treatment; we are reporting on what has worked for people who have shared their remedies from generation to generation, up to and including the present. We are also reporting the findings of scientific research and studies in laboratories throughout the world.

To answer our concern about the information in the book being *safe,* we did our part by carefully reviewing all of the remedies. Now you have to do your part by consulting with your health care provider before starting any self-help health treatment. Also, for your own well-being, heed the notes, cautions, and warnings throughout the book. They should make you aware that professional health care may be needed for certain ailments, especially if symptoms persist. Effective medical treatment is available for almost all conditions mentioned in this book. You can use the remedies listed here in addition to, but not as a substitute for, professional medical attention when it's really needed.

If you glance through the book, you'll see that every now and then, we have a "Noteworthy" insert. It's because we found wonderful items that we're excited about and want to share with you. We want you to know they exist, in case they can make you feel better (which is the goal of our book).

Due to our enthusiasm, it may seem as though we are doing a commercial for some of the products. Well, in a way we are, but that's because we recognize their potential for helping alleviate, eliminate, or prevent some health challenges. Please know that none of the companies we mention has paid us to be in the book. We have gotten product samples in order to use and evaluate each item. You will see only the ones that passed our scrutiny and lived up to our high standards.

Note to Internet holdouts: We made every effort to include telephone numbers in addition to Web site addresses. Truthfully, calling a company and asking questions is not the same as visiting a company online and seeing exactly what they have to offer. If, for whatever reason, you can't or won't get a computer and go on the Internet at home, do yourself a favor and take advantage of your local library's facilities. (Many senior centers also have computers.) A librarian may be able to help you go online. Computers and the Internet have become extremely user-friendly and fairly easy to learn. Don't feel left out. Get yourself in the loop, and have the world at your fingertips through the Internet.

Okay, enough introduction. We'll let you start going through the pages.

Thank you for reading our book and for your interest in our work.

Every good wish for your good health!

Joan and Lydia
THE WILEN SISTERS

PREPARATION GUIDE

Throughout the book, we refer you to this Preparation Guide when a remedy calls for using ingredients in a way in which you probably haven't used them.

The information and simple instructions included here should take out the guesswork and replace it with answers to all of your questions with regard to processing specific ingredients.

BARLEY

Hippocrates, the father of medicine, felt that everyone should drink barley water daily to maintain good health. Barley is rich in iron and B vitamins. It is said to help prevent tooth decay and hair loss, improve fingernails and toenails, and help heal ulcers, diarrhea, and bronchial spasms.

Pearl or *pearled* (also called *Scotch*) barley has been milled. During the milling process, the inedible hull and some of the bran layer are removed, which takes away some of the nutrients. Hulled barley (most often referred to as just "barley"), with only the outer, inedible hull removed, is more nutritious. It is also rich in dietary fiber and has more iron, more trace minerals, and four times the thiamine (vitamin B_1) of pearl barley. Packages of pearl barley and (hulled) barley are sold at supermarkets; packaged and loose pearl barley and (hulled) barley are sold at most health food stores.

Barley Water

Boil 2 ounces of either pearl or hulled barley in 6 cups water until there's about half the water—3 cups—left in the pot. Strain. If you find it hard to drink, add honey and lemon to taste.

Of course you can eat the barley. If it is not soft enough to eat, add just-boiled water and continue cooking it until it's the degree of softness you prefer.

BEANS

Beans! They're so good for you. If only . . .

The United States Department of Agriculture (USDA) is said to have come up with the following way to prepare beans, which should reduce the gas-producing (indigestible) sugars by about 80 percent, without sacrificing the nutrients.

Fill a pot that will easily hold three to four times the amount of beans you want to cook three-quarters full of water. Bring it to a rolling boil. Meanwhile, go through the dry beans, cleaning out the pebbles and empty bean shells, and wash the beans. Once the pot of water boils, add the beans and let it continue boiling for two minutes. Remove from the heat, cover, and let it stand for one hour. Drain and discard the water. Now use your regular recipe to cook the beans, adding fresh water or broth.

▶ If that doesn't do it for you, there's another way to de-gas beans. Soak dry beans overnight in a pot of water along with ⅛ to ¼ cup apple cider vinegar. The next morning, thoroughly rinse the beans, put fresh water and 1 or 2 tablespoons apple cider vinegar into the pot, and cook the beans as usual. Good luck!

EYEWASH

REMINDER: Always remove contact lenses before doing an eyewash.

You'll need an eye cup (available at drugstores). Carefully pour just-boiled water over the cup to clean it. Then, without contaminating the rim or inside surfaces of the cup, fill it half full with whichever eyewash you've selected. Apply the cup tightly to the eye to prevent spillage, then tilt your head backward. Open your eyelid wide and rotate your eyeball to thoroughly wash the eye. Use the same procedure with the other eye, starting with pouring just-boiled water over the cup to clean it and prevent cross contamination.

GARLIC JUICE

When a remedy calls for garlic juice, peel a few cloves of garlic, mince them finely onto a piece of cheesecloth, then squeeze the juice out of the pieces. Chances are a garlic press would make the job easier.

GINGER TEA

Peel or scrub a nub of fresh ginger and cut it into 3 to 5 quarter-size pieces. Pour just-boiled water over it, let it steep for 5 to 10 minutes, strain, and enjoy. If you want stronger ginger tea, grate a piece of ginger, then steep it in just-boiled water, strain, and drink. We keep a piece of ginger in the freezer at all times. It makes it much easier to grate and doesn't affect its healthful qualities.

HERBAL BATH

Besides offering a good, relaxing time, an herbal bath can be extremely healing. The volatile oils of the herbs are activated by the heat of the water, which also opens your pores, allowing for absorption of the herbs. As you enjoy the bath, you're inhaling the herbs (aromatherapy), which pass through the nervous system to the brain, benefiting mind, body, and soul.

Simply take a handful of one or a combination of dried or fresh herbs and place them in the center of a white handkerchief. Secure the herbs in the handkerchief by turning it into a little knapsack or closing it with a twist-tie. Toss the herb-filled bundle into the tub and let the hot water fill the tub until it reaches the level you want. When the water cools enough for you to sit comfortably, do so.

After your bath, open the handkerchief and spread the herbs out to dry. You can use them a couple of times more.

Instead of using dried or fresh herbs, you can use herbal essential oils (available at health food stores). Follow the instructions on the bottle.

CAUTION: Oils cause the tub to be slippery, so be extra careful getting out of the tub, and be sure to clean it thoroughly after you've taken the bath.

HERBAL TEA

Place a teaspoon of the herb, or an herbal tea bag, in a glass or ceramic cup and pour just-boiled water over it. (The average water-to-herb ratio is 6 to 8 ounces of water to 1 round teaspoon of herb. There are exceptions, so be sure to read the directions on the herbal tea package.)

According to many herbalists, never use water that has been reboiled. The first boiling releases oxygen dissolved in the water, and so the second boiling results in flat and lifeless tea.

Cover the cup and let the tea steep for the amount of time suggested in a specific remedy or on the tea package. The general rule of thumb is to steep about 3 minutes for flowers and soft leaves, about 5 minutes for average seeds and tougher leaves, and about 10 minutes for hard seeds, roots, and barks. Of course, the longer the tea steeps, the stronger it gets.

Strain the tea or remove the tea bag. If you need to sweeten it, use honey (preferably raw) or stevia; never use sugar, because it is said to negate the value of most herbs. When the tea is comfortably cool, drink it slowly.

ONION

The onion is in the same plant family as garlic and is almost as versatile. The ancient Egyptians looked at the onion as the symbol of the universe. It has been regarded as a universal healing food, used to treat earaches, colds, fever, wounds, diarrhea, insomnia, and warts, among other ailments. It is believed that a cut onion in a sickroom disinfects the air, as it absorbs the germs in that room. Half an onion will help absorb the smell of a just-painted room. With that in mind, you may not want to use a cut piece of onion that has been in the kitchen for more than a day, unless it was in plastic wrap and refrigerated.

Onion Juice

When a remedy calls for onion juice, grate an onion, put the gratings on a piece of cheesecloth, and squeeze out the juice into a glass bowl.

PESTICIDE REMOVAL FOR FRUITS AND VEGETABLES

Jay "the Juiceman" Kordich shared his method of removing poisonous sprays and pesticides from produce. Fill the sink with cold water, add 4 tablespoons of salt, and squeeze in the juice of half a lemon. This makes a very diluted form of hydrochloric acid.

Soak most fruits and vegetables 5 to 10 minutes; soak leafy greens 2 to 3 minutes; soak strawberries, blueberries, and all other berries 1 to 2 minutes. After soaking, rinse thoroughly with plain cold water and enjoy.

An alternative to the Juiceman's method is to soak produce in a sink or basin with ¼ cup distilled white vinegar. Then, with a vegetable brush, scrub the produce under cold water. Give them a final rinse, and they're ready to be eaten.

POTATOES

Raw, peeled, boiled, grated, and mashed potatoes; potato water; and potato poultices all help heal, according to American, English, and Irish folk medicine. In fact, a popular nineteenth-century Irish saying was, "Only two things in this world are too serious to be jested on: potatoes and matrimony."

Do not use potatoes that have a green tinge. The greenish coloring is a warning that there may be a high concentration of solanine, a toxic alkaloid that can affect nerve impulses and cause vomiting, cramps, and diarrhea. The same goes for potatoes that have started to sprout. They're a no-no.

Potato Water

The skin or peel of the potato is richer in fiber, iron, potassium, calcium, phosphorus, zinc, vitamin C, and B vitamins than the inside of the potato. Always leave the skin on when preparing potato water, but scrub it well.

Scrub two medium-size potatoes (use organic red potatoes whenever possible) and cut them in half. Put the 4 halves in a pot with four cups of water (filtered, spring, or distilled, if possible) and bring to a boil. Lower the flame a little and let it cook for 30 minutes. Take out the potatoes (eating them is optional) and save the water. Drink 1 or 2 cups of potato water—whatever the remedy calls for—and refrigerate the leftover water for next time.

POULTICES

Poultices are usually made with vegetables, fruit, or herbs that are either minced, chopped, grated, crushed, or mashed, and sometimes cooked. These ingredients are then wrapped in a clean fabric—cheesecloth, white cotton, or unbleached muslin—and applied externally to the affected area.

A poultice is most effective when moist. As soon as the poultice dries out, it should be changed—the cloth as well as the ingredients.

Whenever possible, use fresh fruits, vegetables, or herbs. If they are unavailable, then use dried herbs. To soften dried herbs, pour hot water over them. Do not let herbs steep in water that's still boiling unless the remedy specifically says to do it. Boiling most herbs will diminish their healing powers.

Comfrey, also known as knitbone, is an herb that's often used in poultice form to help heal a broken bone. For that reason, we'll use comfrey as an example of a typical poultice.

Cut a piece of cloth—a white handkerchief or two layers of cheesecloth—twice the size of the area it will cover. If you're using a fresh leaf, wash it with cool water, then crush it in your hand. Place the leaf on one half of the cloth and fold over the other half. If you are making a poultice with dried comfrey root and leaves, pour hot water over the herb, then place the softened roots and leaves down the length of the cloth, about 2 inches from the edge. Roll the cloth around the herb so that it won't spill out and place it on the affected body part. Gently wrap an Ace bandage or another piece of cloth around the poultice to hold it in place and to keep in the moisture. If the poultice is conveniently located (e.g., arm or leg), you may want to cover it with plastic wrap as a more efficient way of keeping in the moisture.

SALBA GEL

Salba (*Salvia hispanica L.*) is a registered variety of an ancient plant species belonging to the mint family and has been developed to produce white (rather than the original black) seed, with about a 60 percent more reliable omega-3 content.

So, Salba seeds are a super source of omega-3 fatty acids, plus fiber, antioxidants, vitamin C, magnesium, and a lot more good stuff (as described in "Healthful Hints, Fun Facts, and Food for Thought").

Salba can be used in cooking and baking. This simple preparation of seeds in water can be used in recipes in place of eggs. About ¼ cup of Salba gel replaces 1 egg in recipes.

To make Salba gel, pour 2 cups of warm water into a container that has a tight lid. Add ½ cup of dry Salba seeds. Put the lid on and shake vigorously for 10 seconds. Wait 1 minute, and shake it again for another 10 seconds. Let the container with the gel stay at room temperature for at least four hours, or overnight, to germinate the seeds. (Nutrients from germinated seeds are up to ten times more bioavailable.) Store the gel in the refrigerator. It will keep for up to two weeks.

REMEDIES

ALLERGIES AND HAY FEVER

There are almost as many types of allergies as there are people who have them. In addition to countless food allergies, there are insect-sting allergies, latex allergies, drug and chemical allergies, and—heading the top-ten list—seasonal allergies, including and especially hay fever (listed separately below).

Here are ways that may help pinpoint the cause, and some remedies that may give relief, protection, and possible immunization.

FOOD SENSITIVITY TEST

Known on the Internet as the "Vitamin Lady" (www.vitaminlady.com), nutritionist Lynn Hinderliter, C.N., L.D.N., uses the Coca pulse test (named for Dr. Arthur F. Coca, the renowned physician who developed it over forty years ago) as a simple, extremely effective, and inexpensive way to identify foods or substances to which a person may be allergic, sensitive, or intolerant.

Understanding and using this test as a tool can help you throughout your life to be free from the ill effects of eating foods that are not right for you.

The premise of Dr. Coca's test is that foods that are stressful to your body will reveal themselves by speeding up your pulse.

NOTE: If you are taking a medical drug to control your heart rate, such as a beta-blocker, it may distort the results.

Procedure to Ensure Accurate Results

■ For three days take your pulse fourteen times per day: once before you get out of bed, once before each meal, three times after each meal at 30-minute intervals, and finally just before going to bed.

■ Rest for 3 to 5 minutes before taking your pulse each time.

■ Your pulse should be taken sitting down, except the important one in the morning, which should be taken before getting out of bed.

■ Take a full 1-minute pulse count each time. Do not take a 15-second pulse count and multiply by 4 to save time. Accuracy is important. (See "Taking Your Pulse" in the "Healthful Hints" chapter for simple pulse-taking instructions.)

■ Write down your results, and record what you eat at each meal. For most accurate results, avoid snacks, but if you indulge, make a note of what you ate.

■ Smoking affects the results. Do *not* smoke during the three-day test.

Interpreting the Results

Make note of the highest and lowest pulse rate on each day. (The lowest daily pulse rate should be your waking rate—unless you are sleeping on something you're allergic to.)

The maximum normal range between the highest and lowest should be 16 beats. If your highest-to-lowest range is more than 16 beats, you are allergic to something. That's when the detective work begins.

To Determine the Allergen

Look at your food and pulse records. See what you've eaten when your pulse, taken after eating, was most rapid.

A routine of eliminating elements of that meal and testing again will enable you to identify the food(s) to which you may be allergic.

Once you have figured out and eliminated the edible culprits that may have compromised your health, you can cautiously reintroduce the foods into your diet, in moderation, using the pulse to monitor their acceptability.

NOTEWORTHY: Instead of taking your pulse the old-fashioned way, you may want to consider buying a digital pulse watch, the kind runners use. Visit www.CKBProducts.com for wholesale prices to the public and no minimum purchase, or call 888-CKB-BUYS for their catalog.

OTHER POSSIBLE CAUSES

The Cause May Be Right Under Your Nose

Pollen grains can get caught in your mustache, making life miserable for you during allergy season. Consider shaving it off, or at least shampoo it with liquid soap a couple of times a day.

The test subjects of a study (yes, there was actually a study done by Dr. Patricia McNally and her colleagues at the Mid-Atlantic Kaiser Permanente Medical Group in Virginia) concluded that by washing their mustaches with liquid soap twice a day, they needed fewer antihistamines and decongestants to calm their allergy symptoms.

Are You a Basket Case?

If you're a big-plant owner and you suffer from allergies, check on the planters you use. Wicker can be a wicked source of your allergies. Yes, wicker baskets look nice, but they retain moisture and are perfect breeding grounds for mold. If you insist on using wicker, first put your plants in ceramic or plastic pots and then into the baskets.

Hay Fever: Ways to Avoid Exposure

In most cases, hay fever is an allergy to pollen and mold spores in the air. In springtime, there's pollen from trees and grass. In mid-August, the pollen comes from ragweed and other weeds, along with mold spores from barley, wheat, and corn (most prevalent in the Midwest).

Since the pollen count is highest from sunrise to 10:00 A.M., if possible, stay indoors during those hours.

If you have a lawn and/or garden, keep your grass short—no taller than an inch high. That will help minimize your exposure to grass pollen.

When gardening, wear a mask (available at hardware stores) over your mouth and nose. It really prevents you from breathing in pollen. Also wear the mask when you vacuum, to avoid breathing in dust that can cause allergy problems.

ON THE ROAD

Have you noticed that your allergies seem to act up when you're driving in your car? Keep out the pollen by keeping the car windows closed. Turning on the air conditioner in the car should help you feel better.

AS SOON AS YOU GET HOME

After being outdoors, shower off and shampoo out the allergens you may have carried in with you.

WHILE AT HOME

During pollen season, keep your windows closed in your home. Filter out pollen and mold and destroy dust mites by using an air conditioner and dehumidifier in your home. Yes, it will spike your electricity bill, but think of the money you'll save on tissues.

A SICKROOM GIFT

Flowers are beautiful, but before buying that arrangement, think of something more creative and less likely to cause the recipient a stuffy nose or a sneezing fit from the pollen.

> **NOTEWORTHY:** If the patient has allergy problems—and who doesn't, to one extent or another?—consider giving a gift that makes breathing easier: Nasaline (available at pharmacies and health food stores), a self-irrigating saline rinsing system that helps decongest and drain blocked nasal passages.

Subdue the Symptoms

Having a bad hay day? Chew a bite-size chunk (a 1-inch square) of honeycomb at the start of a hay fever attack. (The honey is delicious.) The comb part turns into a ball of wax that should be chewed for 5 to 10 minutes and then thrown away. Our experience is that it gives instant, temporary relief from the sneezing, runny nose, and teary eyes of a hay fever attack.

> **NOTE:** Needless to say, but we'll say it anyway: If you're allergic to honey, do not even think about chewing honeycomb!

It's great if you have a local beekeeper and can get the honeycomb from him or her. If you go to a health food store, see if you can get honeycomb that comes from your part of the country. The closer the origin of the honeycomb is to your region's flora, the more effective it will be.

Hay Fever Prevention and Immunization

Starting about two months before hay fever season, chew a bite-size chunk of honeycomb twice a day to help you build an immunity to the pollen in your area. See details above in "Subdue the Symptoms."

ARTHRITIS

One authority in the field feels that arthritis is a catchall term that includes rheumatism (inflammation or pain in muscles, joints, or fibrous tissue), bursitis (inflammation of shoulder, elbow, or knee joints), and gout (joint inflammation caused by an excess of uric acid in the blood). Another specialist believes that arthritis is a form of rheumatism. Still another claims there is no such ailment as rheumatism, that it's an umbrella term for several diseases, including arthritis.

According to the government's National Center for Chronic Disease Prevention and Health Promotion (www.cdc.gov/arthritis), 46 million Americans have been diagnosed with arthritis, which has over a hundred different forms.

No matter what it's called, everyone agrees on two things: the pain, and that all of these conditions involve inflammation of connective tissue of one or more joints.

Knowledge is power! Check your local library, bookstores, and the Internet for information from reliable sources and learn about nonchemical treatments and low-acid (pH-balanced) diets. The following information is a good way to start your quest for a cure, or at least some comfort.

NOTE: Using common sense, you can try more than one remedy at a time. For instance, eat nine gin-soaked raisins in the morning, have sage tea later in the day, and give yourself a ginger and sesame oil rub at night. While trying these remedies, pay attention to your body so that you can learn what makes you feel better.

ANOTHER NOTE: These remedies may not be adequate substitutes for professional medical treatment.

Foods in the nightshade family—regular potatoes, eggplants, green peppers, and tomatoes being the most common ones—may be causing some of the pain. Consider being professionally tested for sensitivity to the nightshade foods (or see the "Allergies and Hay Fever" chapter for food sensitivity tests). Work with a health professional to evaluate your condition and to help you find safe, sensible methods of treatment for relief.

Here are remedies that have been said to be successful for many arthritis sufferers—that is, *former* arthritis sufferers.

THE AMAZING GIN-SOAKED RAISIN REMEDY

GIN-SOAKED RAISINS

1 pound of golden raisins
1 pint gin

Spread the golden raisins evenly on the bottom of a glass bowl and pour enough gin over the raisins to completely cover them. Let them stay that way until all the gin is absorbed by the raisins. It takes about five to seven days, depending on the humidity in your area. (You may want to lightly cover the bowl with a paper towel so that dust or flying insects don't drop in.)

To make sure that all of the raisins get

their fair share of the gin, occasionally use a spoon and bring the bottom layer of raisins to the top of the bowl, letting the raisins that were on top settle to the bottom of the bowl.

As soon as the raisins are plump as can be and can't absorb any more gin (even if there's still a little gin left on the bottom of the bowl), transfer the raisins to a glass jar, put the lid on, and keep it closed. Do not refrigerate.

Each day, eat nine raisins—exactly and only nine raisins a day. Most people eat them in the morning with breakfast.

Joe Graedon, author of *The People's Pharmacy,* had the Research Triangle Institute test the gin-soaked raisins for alcohol content. The result: Less than one drop of alcohol was left in nine raisins. So when people who take the raisins are feeling no pain, it's not because they're drunk, it's because the remedy works.

Even so, be sure to check with your health professional to make certain that this remedy will not conflict with medication you may be taking, an eating plan you may be following, or a specific condition such as iron overload.

We've demonstrated this remedy on national television, and the feedback has been incredible. One woman wrote to tell us that she had constant pain and no mo-

bility in her neck. Her doctor sent her to several specialists. She spent a fortune, and nothing helped. Her doctor finally told her, "You'll just have to learn to live with the pain." Although that was unacceptable, she didn't know what to do. And then she saw us on television, talking about a remarkable raisin remedy. We got her letter two weeks after she started the nine raisins a day. The woman had total mobility and no pain. She also had all of her friends waiting for their raisins to absorb the gin.

This is one of dozens and dozens of success stories we've received. Some people have dramatic results after eating the raisins for less than a week, while it takes others a month or two to get results. There are some people for whom this remedy does nothing.

Our feeling is that it's inexpensive, easy to do, delicious to eat, and worth a try. Be consistent; eat the raisins every day. Expect a miracle . . . but have patience!

MORE FOOD REMEDIES

Eat a portion of fresh string beans every day, or juice the string beans and drink a glassful daily. String beans contain vitamins A, B_1, B_2, and C, all of which should help overly acid conditions such as arthritis. Citrus fruits containing vitamin C—including lemons, limes, and grapefruits—are chemically acid, but when they are metabolized in the body, they actually have an alkalizing effect.

◗ Cherries are said to be effective because they seem to help prevent crystallization of uric acid and to reduce uric acid levels in the blood. It is also said that cherries have been known to help reduce or eliminate the arthritic bumps on knuckles.

Eat cherries! Any kind—sweet or sour, fresh, canned or frozen, black, Royal Anne, or Bing. Drink cherry juice, available without preservatives or sugar added and also in a concentrated form at health food stores.

One source says to eat cherries and drink the juice throughout the day for four days, then stop for four days, and then start all over again. Another source says to eat up to a dozen cherries a day in addition to drinking a glass of cherry juice. Find a happy medium as to cherry dosage, keeping your size in mind.

◗ Garlic has been used to quiet arthritis pain quickly. Rub a freshly cut clove of garlic on painful areas. Also, take a garlic supplement after breakfast and after dinner.

◗ Dice 2 cups of unpeeled potatoes and put them in a nonaluminum saucepan with 5 cups of water. Boil gently until about half the water is left. While the water is hot but not scalding, dunk a clean cloth in the potato water, wring it out, and apply it to the painful parts of the body. Repeat the procedure for as long as your patience holds out, or until the pain subsides—whichever happens first.

◗ How many times have you said, "I'll do anything to feel better"? If you really mean it, then make a drastic change in your diet. It may make a dramatic change in your painful joints, improve mobility, and, as a bonus, take off unwanted pounds. Ready? Go on a gluten-free diet.

Gluten is a mixture of plant proteins occurring in cereal grains, such as wheat, rye, barley, oats, and corn. That means no more bread, cake, crackers, pasta, beer, pastry, pancakes, oatmeal . . . and the list goes on.

NOTEWORTHY: Our thanks to Sambuca in New York City for making us aware of how good gluten-free restaurant food can be.

The diet is quite restrictive and used to be almost impossible, but now that there's a growing number of people diagnosed with celiac disease (a permanent intolerance to gluten), there are a growing number of gluten-free products on supermarket shelves. There are also many gluten-free stores on the Internet, and restaurants around the country that offer gluten-free menus in addition to their regular fare. Visit www.glutenfreerestaurants .org to find one near you.

If you're fed up with pain and immobility and serious about trying *anything,* information is available in books—go to your local library—and on the Internet. Just Google "gluten-free diet."

Commit to the diet and stick with it strictly for at least a month. By then you'll know if it's making a big difference in the way that you feel. If you feel a whole lot better, you just may want to continue on it.

It's not easy, but neither is being in pain with every step you take.

Drink to Your Health

Steep 1 cup of tightly packed parsley in 1 quart of boiling water. After 15 minutes, strain and refrigerate.

Dose: ½ cup before breakfast, ½ cup before dinner, and ½ cup anytime pain is particularly severe.

> **NOTE:** Parsley is a diuretic, so stay close to home when using this remedy.

❧ Corn silk tea has been known to reduce acid in the system and lessen pain. Put a handful of the silky strings that grow be-neath the husk of corn in 1 cup of just-boiled water. Let it steep for 10 minutes. If it's not fresh corn season, buy corn silk extract in a health food store; add 10 to 15 drops in 1 cup of water and drink daily.

❧ On a daily basis, drink ¼ teaspoon of cayenne pepper in a glass of water or fruit juice (e.g., cherry juice without sugar or preservatives), or the way we take it, in a Barlean's green drink (www.barleans .com/greens.asp).

If cayenne pepper is just too strong for you, buy cayenne capsules at a health food store and follow the dosage on the label.

❧ Each of these herbs is known as a pain reducer: sage, rosemary, nettles, and basil. Use any one, two, three, or all four of them in the form of tea (see "Preparation Guide"). Have a couple of cups a day, rotating them until you find which one or more make you feel better.

❧ Apple cider vinegar has been used in various ways to help people with an arthritis challenge. Test which of the following remedies is most palatable and convenient for you. Don't forget to have patience and give it at least three weeks to ease the twinges in your hinges.

Every morning and every evening, take 1 teaspoon of honey mixed with 1 teaspoon of apple cider vinegar. Or before each meal (three times a day) drink a glass of water containing 2 teaspoons of apple cider vinegar. Or between lunch and dinner, slowly drink a mixture of 2 ounces of apple cider vinegar added to 6 ounces of water. It may be hard to take at first, but you do get used to the taste . . . honest.

▸ Celery contains many nourishing salts and organic sulfur. Some modern herbalists believe that celery has the power to help neutralize uric acid and other excess acids in the body. Eat fresh celery daily. The leaves on top of celery stalks are also good to eat. If the roughage is rough on your digestive system, place the tops and tough parts of the stalk in a nonaluminum pan. Cover with water and slowly bring to a boil. Then simmer for 10 to 15 minutes. Strain and pour the liquid into a jar.

Dose: Drink 8 ounces three times a day, a half hour before each meal.

You can vary your celery intake by drinking celery seed tea (available at health food stores) and/or juiced celery stalks described in the next remedy.

NOTE: Celery is a diuretic, so plan your day accordingly.

▸ Vegetable juices can be particularly helpful for arthritic conditions. Use fresh carrot juice as a sweetener with either celery juice and/or kale juice. Of course you'll have to invest in a juicer, or locate a juice bar in your neighborhood.

▸ Our friend's grandfather cleared up an arthritic condition and lived out his long life pain-free, thanks to a remedy his Puerto Rican housekeeper brought with her from her home island. Squeeze the juice of a large lime into a cup of black coffee and drink it hot first thing each morning. While we're not in favor of drinking caffeinated coffee, we're *reporting,* not *prescribing* . . . and who are we to argue with success?

JOINT ANOINT

Alvaro ("Call me Al") Gallegos is the creative inventor of Z-CoiL Pain Relief Footwear. While we were interviewing him about his incredible shoes, he told us his equally incredible arthritis healing experience. Al gave us permission to share his story, with the hope that everyone who reads and follows it gets the same great results as he did.

Al has always been athletic. When he was in his forties, he expanded his passion from sprinting to distance running. That was about thirty-five years ago, of which the last ten years Al was running with some arthritis discomfort in his knees.

One day, after participating as a runner in a charity event, Al had excruciating pain, and somehow managed to limp to the hospital in town.

X-rays showed that he had a torn meniscus in his left knee. (The meniscus is cartilage that provides cushioning and helps with movement of the knee socket.) Oh, the pain!

Al was told that because of the torn meniscus, in addition to arthritis, the course of action should be orthoscopic surgery—an expensive operation. Being a veteran of the Korean War, Al thought he'd save money by going to the VA hospital. There, the doctors concurred that orthoscopic surgery was needed. But he would have to wait a month until the hospital's surgical team returned from Iraq.

Al went home to wait for the surgeons. While contemplating his dilemma, he came up with the idea of lubricating his knee joints, and started applying extra-virgin olive oil throughout the day. Using some old socks, he designed padded guards for his knees to help hold the oil in place and not drip on the floor.

For the first two days, Al didn't notice any change. On the third day, he was able to walk again with just a little pain. On the fourth day, Al was able to walk pain-free. By day six, he was up and running, doing fairly fast sprints, and couldn't believe how good his knees felt.

It is now two and a half years later and, without surgery, Al's torn meniscus has mended and the arthritis has completely disappeared. When he felt the onset of arthritis in his hands, he started applying olive oil to his finger joints, and now they're also fine.

After giving it much thought, Al decided to reap the benefits of olive oil internally as well as externally, and so he came up with a formula that seems to be answering a need. According to Al, the feedback has been great. It has done wonders to help relieve the pain of arthritic conditions for many people with whom he has shared his formula.

AL'S JOINT JUICE

$1/2$ cup of hot water
1 teaspoon of red balsamic vinegar
1 teaspoon of honey
$1^1/2$ tablespoons of extra-virgin olive oil
$1^1/2$ tablespoons of flaxseed meal
   (available at health food stores)

Combine all ingredients and drink it once a day. Make a fresh batch daily.

According to results published in the *Journal of the American Medical Association*, based on experiments by a study team at the Brusch Medical Center in Massachusetts, cod liver oil helped to reduce cholesterol levels, improve blood chemistry and complexion, increase energy, correct stomach problems, balance blood sugar, lower blood pressure, and reduce tissue inflammation.

There are several fine oils (available at health food stores) that do not have a fishy taste. Follow the recommended dosage on the label.

NOTE: Cod liver oil is a source of vitamins A and D. If you are taking A and D supplements, check the dosages carefully and consult with your health professional for the recommended dosages that are right for you.

ANTI-INFLAMMATORY HERB

The African plant devil's claw was named that because of the shape of its large fruit, which resembles a clawlike hand.

John Cammarata, M.D., author of *A Physician's Guide to Herbal Wellness*, says that this herb may be useful as an arthritis pain reliever and that "it often improves mobility and use of the affected joints, which further enhances healing."

Devil's claw has anti-inflammatory properties and acts as an analgesic (a medication that reduces or eliminates pain).

While it's hard to find dried powdered devil's claw root in local health food stores, you will find devil's claw capsules and extract. The extract may be taken orally three times a day. As for the capsules, follow the recommended dosage on the label.

For another anti-inflammatory, turn to the "Asthma" chapter and read about omega-3 fatty acids.

POULTICES

See "Preparation Guide."

Grate 3 tablespoons of horseradish and stir it into ½ cup of boiled milk. Prepare a poultice by pouring the mixture onto a doubled piece of cheesecloth, then apply it to the painful area while it's still warm (but not *burning* hot). By the time the poultice cools, you may have some relief.

Heat ½ cup of coarse (kosher) salt in a frying pan and use it to prepare a poultice in cheesecloth or a cotton handkerchief. Place it on the painful area. To keep the salt comfortably warm, put a hot-water bottle on top of it. (Chances are this old home remedy is effective with table salt, too.)

MASSAGE

Combine ½ teaspoon of eucalyptus oil (available at health food stores) with 1 tablespoon of extra-virgin olive oil and massage the mixture into your painful areas daily. You'll know within a week whether or not it's working for you.

You may want to alternate the above massage mixture with this one: Grate fresh ginger, then squeeze the juice through a piece of cheesecloth. Mix the ginger juice with an equal amount of sesame oil. Massage it on the painful areas. Ginger can be quite strong. If you are uncomfortable from the burning sensation, tone down the ginger by adding more sesame oil to the mixture.

SUPER SUPPLEMENT

An old Native American arthritis remedy is a mixture of mashed yucca root and water. Yucca contains naturally occurring saponins, a steroid derivative and a forerunner of cortisone.

In a double-blind study done at a southern California arthritis clinic, 60 percent of the patients taking yucca supplements showed dramatic improvements in their arthritic conditions. Even the side effects were good: relief from headaches as well as from gastrointestinal complaints. So while it doesn't work for everyone (then again, what does?), it works for a large enough number of people to make it worth a try.

Yucca extract capsules with 20 percent saponins are available at health food stores and vitamin shops. Follow the dosage on the label.

Aloe vera gel (available in health food stores) is an outstanding digestive tonic and stomach soother. It also may help reduce joint inflammation. You can apply the gel externally to the aching joint, and you can also take it internally—1 tablespoon in the morning before breakfast and 1 tablespoon before dinner.

Aloe vera also comes in the form of softgels. Follow the dosage on the label.

MORNING STIFFNESS PREVENTION

If you have morning stiffness caused by arthritis, try sleeping in a sleeping bag. You can sleep *on* your bed, but *in* the zipped-up bag. It's much more effective than an electric blanket because your body heat is evenly distributed and retained. Come morning, there's less pain, making it easier to get going.

ASTHMA

During an asthma attack, bronchial tubes narrow and secrete an excess of mucus, making it very hard to breathe.

In the 1800s, English athlete Peter Latham said, "You cannot be sure of the success of your remedy while you are still uncertain of the nature of the disease."

And so it is with asthma.

In some people, asthma may be attributed to emotional problems and/or allergies. At least three out of four people with asthma have one or more allergies. Be tested for common indoor allergens, and you may find the culprit(s) that cause your asthma to act up. Once you discover what triggers an attack, you can take steps to eliminate it from your home. It may mean that you have to give away a pet, stuffed animals, or plants, or do without carpeting, but breathing easier is worth it. (See "Trigger Awareness" in the "Asthma" section of the "Children's Health Challenges" chapter.)

Whatever the cause, we just hope that these remedies help alleviate the condition.

While trying to find the most effective asthma-relieving remedies, it's important that you consult with your health care provider every step of the way. These remedies are not substitutes for professional medical treatment.

AT THE FIRST SIGN . . .

The second you feel the asthma-type wheezing starting, saturate two strips of white cloth in white vinegar and wrap them around your wrists, not too tightly. For some people, this stops a full-blown attack from developing.

A relative told us that in the old country, a remedy used at the onset of an asthma attack was to inhale the steam from boiling potatoes that were cut in pieces with the skin left on them. With or without the potatoes, inhaling steam can be beneficial. Be very careful! Steam is powerful and can burn the skin if you get too close.

DURING AN ACUTE ASTHMA ATTACK WHEN MEDICATION ISN'T HELPING

According to the Heimlich Institute (www.heimlichinstitute.org), research has now proven the Heimlich maneuver to be effective for asthmatics.

Perform the Heimlich maneuver on yourself, or on a person with an acute asthma attack who hasn't responded to medication or is unable to take the medication.

The Heimlich Maneuver on Someone Else

1. Stand in back of the patient and wrap your arms around the patient's waist.

2. Make a fist and place the thumb side of your fist against the patient's upper abdomen (which is below the rib cage and above the navel).

3. Grasp your fist with your other hand and press into the patient's upper abdomen with a quick upward thrust. Do not squeeze the rib cage; confine the force of the thrust to your hands.

4. Repeat if necessary.

IN EXTREME CASES: If the patient has not recovered and you are able to do CPR, do it! But first call 911 for help.

The Heimlich Maneuver on Yourself

NOTE: If you're home alone, call 911 for help, then do the Heimlich maneuver while waiting for help to arrive.

1. Make a fist and place the thumb side of your fist against your upper abdomen (which is below the rib cage and above the navel).

2. Grasp your fist with your other hand and press into your upper abdomen with a quick upward thrust. Do not squeeze the rib cage; confine the force of the thrust to your hands.

3. Repeat if necessary.

An alternative method to use on yourself:

1. Lean over a fixed horizontal object (table edge, chair, railing) and press your upper abdomen against the edge to produce a quick upward thrust.

2. Repeat if necessary.

DURING A MILD ATTACK

After you've taken your medication and need to calm down, a prayer or affirmation is extremely helpful. Here's an affirmation that you can repeat over and over, knowing that you will be fine:

*I feel the joy of life as I breathe easily
   and freely.
I love myself as I am, and I accept
   myself as I am.*

ANTI-INFLAMMATORIES

According to information from the University of Maryland Medical Center, clinical research suggests that omega-3 fatty acids help reduce inflammation and may improve lung function in adults with asthma. By contrast, omega-6 fatty acids tend to promote inflammation, which may worsen respiratory function.

It's complicated and confusing, but the bottom line is that it's important to maintain an appropriate balance of omega-3 and omega-6 fatty acids in your diet because these two substances work together to promote good health. Here's where the complicated and confusing comes in: A healthy diet should consist of about two to four times more omega-6 fatty acids than omega-3 fatty acids. Yes, even though omega-3s can produce the anti-inflammatory results you want, the ideal balanced diet has you consuming two to four times more omega-6s than omega-3s. Keep in mind that the typical American diet consists of fourteen to twenty-five times more omega-6s than omega-3s. This imbalance is what may be causing lots of inflammatory disorders.

Processed foods are full of omega-6s; so are meat, margarine, and corn oil. Foods rich in omega-3s include leafy green vegetables, walnuts, and winter squash. Start learning to love salads, be sure to throw in flaxseed, and use an olive oil dressing. Also, start using Salba (available at health food stores), which is the richest wholefood source of omega-3 fatty acids and

fiber found in nature. Gram for gram, Salba provides eight times more omega-3s than salmon. (See the "Diabetes" chapter for more information and recipes using Salba.)

DAILY SNACKS

Eat three to six apricots a day. They're said to help promote healing of lung and bronchial conditions.

Quercetin is a bioflavonoid shown to have anti-inflammatory, antihistamine, antioxidant, and anticancer properties. Apples are rich in quercetin. Yes, an apple a day may help protect your lungs from tissue damage.

Other foods rich in quercetin are red grapes, citrus fruits, broccoli and other leafy green vegetables, cherries, and some berries, including raspberries, lingonberries, and cranberries.

Eaten daily, Jerusalem artichokes, also known as sunchokes, may be a real plus for nourishing the lungs of the asthmatic. These gnarly little tubers are low in calories, high in vitamins and minerals, and delicious. They're easy to grow and worth the effort if you have the garden space. Ask your local nursery to help you get started. Or check your local greengrocer to see if they carry them.

Eat them raw as a snack or in salads, boiled in soups, or baked in stews.

❧ We heard about a man who was able to ease off massive doses of cortisone by using garlic therapy. He started with 1 clove of garlic a day, minced, in a couple of ounces of orange juice. He gulped it down without chewing any of the little pieces of garlic. That way he didn't have garlic on his breath. As he increased the number of garlic cloves he ate each day, his doctor decreased the amount of cortisone he was taking. After several months, he was eating six to ten cloves of garlic a day, was completely off cortisone, and was not bothered by asthma.

DRINKS

We were on a radio show when a woman called in and shared her asthma remedy: cherry bark tea. (See "Sources" for herb companies that sell the tea in bulk or bags.) She drinks a cup before each meal and another cup at bedtime. The woman swore to us that it has changed her life. She hasn't had an asthma attack since she started taking it more than five years ago.

❧ This remedy requires a juicer or a nearby juice bar. Drink equal amounts of endive (also called chicory), celery, and carrot juice. A glass of the juice a day works wonders for some asthmatics.

❧ Yes, coffee has caffeine, a beneficial ingredient chemically similar to the asthma medicine theophylline. French writer, critic, and asthmatic Marcel Proust, born in 1871, wrote that caffeine was prescribed to him as a child to help him breathe.

The Coffee Science Information Centre (www.cosic.org) reports that in Scotland, caffeine has been used to treat asthma for over 150 years.

One or two cups of coffee may help open your air passages, making it easier to breathe.

We've researched caffeinated tea but couldn't find any reports or studies substantiating its benefits for asthmatics . . . only coffee.

JUST A SPOONFUL . . .

If you like garlic, you may love this garlic syrup. Separate and peel the cloves of 3 entire heads of garlic. Simmer them in a nonaluminum pan with 2 cups of water. When the garlic cloves are soft and there is about 1 cup of water left in the pan, remove the garlic and put it into a jar. Then add 1 cup of cider vinegar and ¼ cup of honey to the water that's left in the pan, boiling the mixture until it's syrupy. Pour the syrup over the garlic in the jar. Cover the jar and let it stand overnight.

Dose: Take 1 or 2 cloves of garlic with 1 teaspoon of syrup every morning on an empty stomach.

▶ Mix 1 teaspoon of grated horseradish with 1 teaspoon of honey and take it every night before bedtime.

▶ Slice 2 large raw onions into a jar and pour 2 cups of honey over it. Close the jar and let it stand overnight. Next morning you are ready to start taking the "honion" syrup.

Dose: 1 teaspoon a half hour after each meal and 1 teaspoon before bedtime.

MAGNESIUM

According to critical-care physician Michael Dacey, M.D., "Magnesium helps to improve lung function and reduce the frequency of asthma attacks." Dr. Dacey said that some emergency rooms use magnesium to treat patients having acute attacks. He also points out that asthmatics with magnesium deficiencies spend more time in the hospital than those with diets rich in magnesium.

On a daily basis, eat foods that are known to be an excellent source of magnesium, such as halibut (baked or broiled), Swiss chard (boiled), spinach (boiled), raw pumpkin seeds, broccoli (steamed), mustard greens (boiled), turnip greens (cooked), summer squash (cooked), black beans, peanuts, hazelnuts, and almonds.

For those of you interested in taking magnesium supplements, the Dietary Reference Intakes for magnesium, set in 1997 by the Institute of Medicine at the National Academy of Sciences, are as follows:

- Males and females, 1–3 years old: 80 mg
- Males and females, 4–8 years old: 130 mg
- Males and females, 9–13 years old: 240 mg
- Males, 14–18 years old: 410 mg
- Males, 19–30 years old: 400 mg
- Males, 31 years and older: 420 mg
- Females, 14–18 years old: 360 mg
- Females, 19–30 years old: 310 mg
- Females, 31 years and older: 320 mg

BREATHING

Programming yourself to breathe properly takes practice . . . a lot of practice. You may want to sign up for a meditation or yoga class to help you learn to relax and breathe. Meanwhile, here are some tips on breathing that may make a major, positive difference in your life as an asthmatic.

Start now! Sit or lie down in a quiet place and follow these instructions:

■ Breathe through your nose and let your nose hairs filter out dust and other pollutants that can trigger an attack.

■ Slow your breathing down to eight to twelve breaths per minute, the slower the better.

■ Breathe deeply. The deeper you breathe, the slower you'll breathe and the better you'll feel.

■ When you exhale, push the old air out and empty your lungs.

You really do have to work at it and keep reminding yourself to breathe properly. Most of all, be patient with yourself and be happy that you're doing this, knowing that you're going to get good results.

SALT AIR THERAPY

NOTEWORTHY: If you've been to the ocean, you probably know that breathing in the salt air is quite therapeutic for people with respiratory ailments, including asthma.

While it's not always practical to be by the ocean or to camp out in a salt mine, there is a convenient, drug-free, and noninvasive device you can use to bring salt air therapy into your home. It's the Original Himalayan Crystal Salt Inhaler. Breathing through this porcelain inhaler for 15 to 20 minutes daily can help to resolve breathing problems.

See it; read more about it; consider trying it. Visit www.americanbluegreen.com or call 877-224-4872.

VISUALIZATION

Visualization or mental imagery is a potent tool that can be used to help you heal yourself. Gerald N. Epstein, M.D., director of the American Institute for Mental Imagery in New York City, suggests that the following visualization be done to stem an asthma attack. Do it at the onset of an attack, during the first 3 to 5 minutes. Sit in a comfortable chair and close your eyes. Breathe in and out three times and see yourself in a pine forest. Stand next to a pine tree and breathe in the aromatic fragrance of the pine. As you breathe out, sense this exhalation traveling down through your body and going out through the soles of your feet; see the breath exiting as gray smoke and being buried deep in the earth. Then open your eyes, breathing easily.

NOTE: Learn this visualization and practice it when you're feeling fine so that you know exactly what to do and how to do it the second you feel a wheeze coming on.

BACK AND SCIATIC PAIN

t is estimated that eight out of ten people have, at some point in their lives, back pain that disables them. Over $5 billion is spent each year for diagnosis and treatment of back pain—making it appropriate that paper money is sometimes referred to as "greenbacks."

If you are troubled by back pain—and obviously you are, or you probably wouldn't be reading this—read through to the end of the chapter and follow your instinct as to which suggestion(s) may help your condition.

POSSIBLE CAUSES

It may come as a surprise to find out that your back pain may be caused by one leg being shorter than the other. It's hard for most people to know whether or not it's true about them. You can find out by asking a tailor to measure your legs.

If one leg is shorter than the other, a shoe insert may solve the problem, or see a podiatrist for custom-made orthotics.

We are antismoking, so much so that Lydia belongs to an organization that lobbies for nonsmokers' rights. Here's one more reason *not* to smoke—a condition called "smoker's back." According to a study done at the University of Vermont, back pains are more common and more frequent among smokers. They theorize that it has to do with the effect of nicotine on the carbon monoxide levels in the blood, which causes the smoker to cough. The cough, in turn, puts a tremendous strain on the back. One more good reason to stop smoking! (For suggestions on how to quit, see the "Smoking" chapter.)

PREVENTION POSITION

When you feel as though your back is on the verge of going out, follow the advice of our cousin Linda, who is a physical therapist. Carefully lie down on the floor, close enough to a sofa or chair so that you can bend your knees and rest your legs (knees to feet) on the seat of the sofa or chair. Your thighs should be leaning against the front of the sofa and your tush should be as close as possible to it, directly in front of it, with the rest of your body flat on the floor. In that position, you're like the start of a staircase. Your body is the lowest (or first) step, your thighs are the distance between the two steps, and your shins are the second step. (Did we just confuse you instead of painting a clear picture? Once you're on the floor, it's easy to figure out.)

Stay in that position for 15 to 30 minutes. It's a restful and healing treatment for the back. While you're there on the floor, you may want to read *Mind over Back Pain* (Berkley Trade) by John Sarno, M.D. This decades-old bestseller is still in print. And Dr. Sarno's theory, wisdom, and information still have miraculous results for many people with chronic back and sciatic pain, including conditions such as slipped and herniated discs.

MASSAGE

You need to employ the buddy system for this remedy. Get your pal to put 20 drops of eucalyptus oil (available at health food stores) in a tablespoon and warm it by carefully putting a lit match under the spoon for a few seconds. Then have that friend gently massage the warm oil on your painful area. The touch is as healing as the oil.

Have you ever had an ice rubdown? The thought of it sends chills up my spine, but it may help relieve the pain in that very same area. An easy way to do it is by freezing a polystyrene cup full of water. Then peel off about ½ inch of the cup's lip and use the rest of the cup as a sort of knob or handle, gliding the iced surface over your back.

One thing you don't want to do is strain yourself trying to reach your painful parts, so you may want to ask a friend to give you the rubdown. Say, you might want to ask a friend to give you a rubdown even if you don't have back pain.

FOOD

An Asian remedy for the relief of lower back problems is black beans, available at supermarkets and health food stores.

Soak a cupful of black beans (also called *frijoles negros*) overnight. This softens the beans and is said to remove the gas-producing compounds. Then put them in a pot with 3½ cups of water. Bring to a boil and let simmer for a half hour over a low flame. During that time, keep removing the grayish foam that forms on top. After a half hour, cover the pot and let it cook for another 2 hours. By then the beans should be soft. If there is still water in the pot, spill it out.

Eat 2 to 3 tablespoons of the black beans each day for one month, then every other day for one month. Fresh beans should be prepared as needed.

If you need to salt the beans, use a little tamari (natural soy sauce), available at health food stores and some supermarkets.

At the end of two months, if you no longer have lower back pain and you attribute it to the black beans, continue eating them every other day. If you feel your back problem would have healed anyway, stop eating the beans. At the first sign of pain in the lower back area, go back to the beans.

> **CAUTION:** Do not apply heat to acute back pain, only to chronic pain. If you have any question about whether you have chronic or acute back pain, do *not* use heat!

POULTICE

Use a flaxseed poultice for chronic back pain. Soak 1 cup of flaxseeds (available at health food stores) in cold water for 10 hours. In an enamel or glass saucepan, bring the mixture to a boil. As soon as they're cool enough to touch, but still as hot as can be without scalding yourself, make a poultice of the seeds (see "Preparation Guide") and place it on the painful area. You can keep reheating the flaxseeds and reapplying new poultices.

SUPPLEMENT

A chiropractor who specializes in helping dancers and athletes told us that he prescribes vitamin C—500 mg after each meal—to ease the pain and speed the healing of lower back conditions.

FOR MEN ONLY

Do you have back or hip pain when you sit for any length of time? Is it something you and your doctor(s) can't quite figure out and so you label it "back trouble"?

You may need a "wallet-ectomy." If you carry around a thick, bursting-at-the-seams wallet in your hip pocket, it may be putting pressure on the sciatic nerve. Keep your wallet in your jacket pocket, or carry it in a "man bag," and you'll find that sitting will no longer be a pain in the . . . anywhere.

SCIATICA

Sciatica is a painful condition affecting the sciatic nerve, which is the longest nerve in the body. It extends from the lower spine through the pelvis, thighs, and legs and ends at the heels.

We all have some nerve!

The home remedies we describe may not cure the condition, but they may help ease the pain.

▶ The juice from potatoes has been said to help sciatica sufferers. So has celery juice. If you don't have a juicer, find a neighborhood health food store that has a juice bar and ask them to accommodate you. Have them juice a 10-ounce combination of potato and celery juice. Add carrots and/or beets to improve the taste. In addition to the juice, drink a couple of cups of celery tea throughout the day.

▶ Stimulate the nerve by applying a poultice of fresh minced horseradish (see "Preparation Guide") to the painful area. Keep it on for an hour. If it offers relief, reapply a fresh poultice every couple of hours.

▶ We heard about a man who went from doctor to doctor for help with his sciatica. Nothing they prescribed worked for him. As a last resort, the man followed the advice of a folk medicine practitioner who recommended garlic milk. The man minced 2 cloves of garlic, put them in ½ cup of milk, and drank it down without chewing the pieces of garlic. He had the garlic milk each morning and each evening. Within a few days, he felt some relief.

Within two weeks, all the pain had completely disappeared.

▶ Water has tremendous therapeutic value for a sciatic condition. It can reduce pain and improve circulation. Take a long, hot bath or shower and follow it with a short, cold shower. If you can't stand the thought of a cold shower, then follow up the hot bath with ice-cold compresses on the painful areas.

PREVENTION

According to the Germans, eating a portion of raw sauerkraut every day helps prevent sciatica.

BLOOD PRESSURE

When blood pressure is measured, there are two numbers reported. The first and higher number is the systolic pressure. It measures the pressure inside the arteries while the heart is contracting. The diastolic pressure is the second, lower number and measures the pressure in the arteries when the heart is at rest.

There are many reasonably priced home

blood pressure monitors. It's a good idea to get one, as long as you promise not to drive yourself crazy with it. The two main advantages of having a home monitor are that you can check your progress (to see if whatever you're doing is working) and you get used to having your pressure taken so that when you go to the doctor, you're an old hand at having your arm cuffed.

NOTEWORTHY: Omron has a selection of blood pressure monitors (available at pharmacies and health food stores). Visit www.omronhealthcare.com and go to "Blood Pressure FAQs" to find out how to select the most appropriate home monitor for you.

More than 20 million Americans have high blood pressure (hypertension). We saw a woman wearing a T-shirt that said: "Anybody with normal blood pressure these days just isn't paying attention." If you're one of those 20 million, now is the time to do something about it.

We urge you to take a look at your lifestyle, review the basics below, and start making the changes necessary to help you lower your blood pressure numbers. You know you can do it, so do it!

■ If you're overweight, diet sensibly.

■ Cut down on or cut out meat.

■ To reduce the stress from your everyday life, try meditation, biofeedback, and/or yoga.

■ Exercise, even if it's just a daily walk, is a great stress reducer and goes a long way in lowering blood pressure.

■ If you smoke, stop! (See the "Stop Smoking" chapter.)

■ If you drink, stop! At least cut down . . . all the way down.

■ Eliminate salt. (However, see "High-Quality Energy and Balance" in the "Remedies in a Class by Themselves" section, and learn about Himalayan Crystal Salt, which may actually be good for people with high blood pressure.)

Read on for additional high and low blood pressure health hints.

HIGH BLOOD PRESSURE (HYPERTENSION)

The most important dietary recommendation for lowering blood pressure is to increase the amount of plant foods in the diet, according to Jade Beutler, R.R.T., R.C.P., San Diego–based CEO of Lignan Research LLC and a licensed health care practitioner. A primarily vegetarian diet typically contains less saturated fat and refined carbohydrates and more potassium, complex carbohydrates, fiber, calcium, magnesium, vitamin C, and essential fatty acids.

Double-blind studies have demonstrated that fish oil supplements, flaxseed oil, and Salba—all rich in omega-3 fatty acids—are very effective in lowering blood pressure. (All are available at health food stores.)

Food

Eat 2 apples a day. The pectin in apples may help lower high blood pressure.

Eat garlic raw in salads and use it in cooking. Also take garlic supplements daily. Follow the recommended dosage on the label.

Cucumbers are rich in potassium, phosphorus, and calcium. They're also a good diuretic and calming agent. To help bring down blood pressure, eat a cucumber every day. If you have a juicer, drink ½ cup of fresh cucumber juice. You can also include carrot and another diuretic, parsley, in the juice.

In a blender, or with a mortar and pestle, crush 2 teaspoons of dried watermelon seeds. Put them in a cup of just-boiled water and let them steep for 1 hour. Stir, strain, and drink that cupful of watermelon-seed tea a half hour before a meal. Repeat the procedure before each meal, three times a day. After taking the tea for a few days, check your pressure and see if the tea works for you, or if this watermelon remedy is the pits.

Incidentally, watermelon seeds are known to tone up kidney function. Be prepared to use bathroom facilities often while drinking this tea. Also, watermelon-seed tea can be bought at health food stores.

A Pet Project

According to a university study, blood pressure can be reduced by staring at fish in a fish tank. The relaxation benefits of fish watching are equal to biofeedback and meditation. If caring for a tank of fish isn't for you, check your local video store for tapes and DVDs of fish swimming in aquariums or in their natural habitats. If you have a computer, consider downloading the popular swimming-fish screensaver.

According to published scientific research, having a companion pet—a cat or a dog in particular—helps lower blood pressure by keeping the owner's anxiety level lower.

Speak Slowly

The faster you talk, the less oxygen you have coming in. The less oxygen, the harder the blood has to work to maintain the supply of oxygen. The harder the blood has to work, the higher the blood pressure seems to go. The bottom line here is that if you talk slower, theoretically you will take bigger and better breaths, giving you more oxygen and preventing your blood pressure from climbing.

Let a Machine Guide You

> **NOTEWORTHY:** If you have high blood pressure, you should know about RES-PeRATE, the only nondrug medical device clinically proven to lower blood pressure.

This portable electronic device, which is smaller than the size of this book, adapts to your unique breathing rate and pattern, and interactively guides you to reduce your breathing rate.

Put a sensor belt around your abdomen (over your clothes) and put on the headphones. Sit back and relax for about 15 minutes. Follow the musical tones that guide your breathing to the therapeutic zone.

Your blood pressure is lowered by gently relaxing constricted blood vessels through the power of paced breathing. It's easy. It's pleasant. It works!

Do this at least four times a week, and expect the same results reported in clinical trials—significant reduction in blood pressure without any side effects.

If someone else in your household also has high blood pressure, consider the RESPeRATE Duo, which allows two users to store their performance records in two separate memories with one machine.

Visit www.resperate.com to see a demonstration of the device, or if you have questions, call 877-988-9388.

LOW BLOOD PRESSURE

We heard from a Russian folk healer who recommends drinking ½ cup of raw beet juice when a person feels that his or her blood pressure may be a little too low. This healer also told us that a person with low blood pressure *knows* that feeling.

◗ Deep breathing may bring blood pressure levels up to normal. First thing in the morning and last thing at night, do this breathing exercise: Let all the air out of your lungs—exhale, squeezing all the old air out—then slowly let the air in through your nostrils to a count of seven. When no more air will fit in your lungs, hold tight for a count of fourteen. Next, gently let the air out through your mouth to a count of seven—all the way out. Inhale and exhale this way ten times, twice a day.

Even when your blood pressure is normal, continue this breathing exercise for all kinds of physical benefits.

BLOOD PRESSURE STABILIZER

Just as there are people with high blood pressure, there are people (though not nearly as many) with low blood pressure.

Scientific studies have shown that 5 to 10 minutes of laughter first thing in the morning improves blood pressure levels. The problem is, what's there to laugh at first thing in the morning? There's usually a funny local disc jockey on the radio, or go to an Internet search engine (e.g., Google, Yahoo, Dogpile) and type in "jokes." You'll have tons of jokes and lots of laughs.

Cayenne pepper is a wonderful blood pressure stabilizer. If some kind of trauma (even a minor one) happens that may cause your blood pressure to spike or drop, mix some cayenne pepper in water and drink it down. Cayenne is strong. Start with ⅛ teaspoon in water and gradually work your way up.

BODY ODOR

DEODORANTS

If you have a problem with bad-smelling armpits, raise your hand. Oops—better not. Instead, take a shower, dry off, then apply any one of the following on your armpits:

- Green tea extract (available at health food stores)

- Witch hazel (an antiseptic)

- Apple cider vinegar (which should change the pH level, making it harder for bacteria to grow)

- Tea tree oil (this strong-smelling antimicrobial is available at health food stores)

- Turnip juice (grate a turnip into cheesecloth, squeeze out the juice, and vigorously massage 1 teaspoon turnip juice into each armpit)

While the solutions above will not keep you from perspiring, they can kill the bacteria that cause the unpleasant smell.

INTERNAL DEODORANTS

"Think zinc—don't stink!" Credit for that slogan goes to a Pennsylvania man who rid himself of body odor by taking 30 mg of zinc every day. Within two weeks, he was smelling like a rose. Correction: Within two weeks, he had no body odor.

> **CAUTION:** High doses of zinc give some people stomachaches. Continued use of high doses of zinc may increase a man's risk of developing prostate cancer. Before taking this supplement, consult your health professional.

◗ A vegetarian friend's sense of smell is so keen, she can stand next to someone and tell whether that person is a meat-eater. If you are a heavy meat-eater and are troubled by body odor, change your diet. Ease off meat and poultry and force yourself to fill up on green leafy vegetables. There will be a big difference in a short time. You may lose weight and perspire less. Even if you continue to perspire a lot, the smell won't be as strong. That change of diet will be healthier for you in so many ways. And it will be appreciated by all the people in all the crowded elevators you ride.

◗ In addition to eating green leafy vegetables (mentioned above), take a daily 500 mg capsule of wheat grass (available at health food stores). Or if your local health food store sells fresh wheat grass juice, have an ounce first thing each morning. Be sure to take it on an empty stomach and drink it down with water. The chlorophyll in wheat grass juice can reduce body odor dramatically or eliminate it completely.

◗ If tension causes you to perspire excessively, which then causes unpleasant body odors, drink sage tea. Use 1½ teaspoons of dried sage, or 2 sage tea bags in 1 cup of just-boiled water. Let it steep for 10 minutes. Drink it in small doses throughout the day. The tea should help you to relax, so don't sweat it.

SKUNK SPRAY

When you've gotten in the path of a frightened skunk, add 1 cup of tomato juice to 1 gallon of water and wash your body with it. Do the same with your clothes.

BRUISES, CUTS, BLACK EYES, AND MORE

BLACK AND BLUE MARK PREVENTION

If you seem to bruise easily, you may need to increase your vitamin K intake. One portion of cooked broccoli has almost double the amount of the daily recommended intake of 150 mcg of vitamin K. Other foods rich in vitamin K are olives, Brussels sprouts, potatoes, green leafy vegetables, soybeans, cauliflower, and green tea.

By eating these foods on a regular basis, the additional vitamin K in your diet may help strengthen your blood-vessel walls, preventing them from breaking easily, and so averting the bruising. Until then, here are some on-the-spot preventive suggestions:

■ Place ice on a fresh bruise to help prevent the area from turning black and blue, and to reduce the swelling.

■ Make a poultice (see "Preparation Guide") with grated turnip or daikon (Japanese radish, available at greengrocers and Asian markets). Put the poultice on the fresh bruise and leave it there for 15 to 30 minutes. These roots have been known to help clean up the internal bleeding of a bruise, preventing it from turning black and blue.

■ Peel a banana and rub the inside of the peel across the fresh bruise, then leave the peel on the area, binding it in place with a handkerchief or Ace bandage. The peel will lessen the pain, speed healing, and reduce discoloration.

■ As soon as you bruise yourself, press a knife (flat side only) or a spoon on the bruise for 5 to 10 minutes.

■ Prepare a salve by mashing pieces of parsley into a teaspoon of butter. Gently rub the salve on the fresh bruise.

DOOR, DRAWER, OR HAMMER BASH

If you close a door or drawer on your finger or hit it with a hammer, grate an onion, mix some salt into the grated onion, then stick your finger into the mixture. The pain will disappear within seconds.

▶ Once you've caught your breath after slamming a door, drawer, or hammer on your finger, dunk your finger in ice water for a minute. Then pinch the injured fingertip while keeping it raised over your head. After a minute of pinching and raising, plunge it into ice water again for another minute. Repeat this dunking-pinching-raising procedure about ten times. By then the throbbing will have stopped, and with any luck your fingernail will not turn black and blue.

SCRATCHES, SMALL CUTS, AND GRAZES

The first thing to do when you get a scratch, small cut, or graze is to rinse it with cold water. Then put honey on the injured skin. Honey's antibacterial properties will protect the skin from almost all strains of common wound-infecting bacteria, and its enzymes will help the healing process. You may want to put a Band-Aid lightly over it.

GASHES—BLEEDING WOUNDS

If the wound is bleeding quite profusely, apply direct pressure, preferably with a sterile dressing, and seek medical attention immediately.

If the bleeding is not severe, the following remedies may help.

▶ Sprinkle on some cayenne pepper to stop the flow of blood. Pour it directly on the cut. Yes, it will sting. It will also stop the bleeding. If you don't have cayenne handy, use black pepper. If you do have cayenne, it's a good idea to also mix ¼ teaspoon in a cup of water and drink it down. It will help stabilize your blood pressure while you're going through this bloody trauma.

▶ Lemon is an effective disinfectant and also stops a cut from bleeding. Squeeze some lemon juice on the cut and get ready for the sting.

▶ If you cut yourself outdoors, away from pepper and lemon, find a smoker who will give you a cigarette, and apply a clump of wet tobacco, or even the wet cigarette paper, on the cut to stop the bleeding.

▶ If there's a geranium plant around, grab and crush a few leaves, then apply them to the cut. The leaves will act like a styptic pencil and stop the bleeding.

SPLINTERS

Boil water, then carefully fill a wide-mouthed bottle to within ½ inch of the top. Place the part of the finger with the splinter over the top of the bottle and lightly press down. The pressing should allow the heat to draw out the splinter.

▶ If the finger with the splinter is puffy and sore, tape a slice of raw onion around it, cover it with a bandage, and leave it on overnight. The swelling and the splinter should be gone by morning.

▶ For real tough splinters, sprinkle salt on the splintered area, then put half a cherry tomato on it. Bind the tomato on the salted skin with a bandage or a plastic covering to keep from messing up the bed linen, and sleep with the tomato overnight. (Now, now, fellas!) The next morning, the splinter should come right out.

Also see the "Children's Health Challenges" chapter for more splinter remedies.

PAPER CUTS

Clean the cut with the juice of a lemon. Ow! Then, to ease the pain, wet the cut finger with water and dip it into powdered cloves. Since cloves act as a mild anesthetic, the pain should be gone in a matter of seconds.

Put a dab of petroleum jelly on the paper cut. It will keep it closed. If possible, cover it with a Band-Aid.

BLACK EYE

A black eye—a shiner—is caused by injury to the face and will usually heal itself within a week or two. These suggestions can speed the healing process.

Pour witch hazel on a cotton pad and apply it to the bruised, closed eye. Lie down with your feet slightly higher than your head for a half hour while the witch hazel stays in place.

Walk into a door, did you? I hope it was the door to the kitchen. If you're there now, peel and grate a potato (red potato is best). Make a poultice out of it (see "Preparation Guide") and keep it on the black eye for 20 minutes. Potassium chloride is one of the most effective healing compounds, and potatoes are the best source of potassium chloride. (This remedy is also beneficial for bloodshot eyes.)

Eat ripe pineapple and ripe papaya—lots of it—for two or three days, and let the enzymes in those fruits help eliminate the discoloration around the eye. Both fruits are rich in vitamin C, which also promotes healing.

If you can't get fresh pineapple or papaya, take papaya pills (available at health food stores). Take one after every meal.

If you were a character in a movie and you got a black eye, in the following scene you would be nursing it with a piece of steak. Cut! The steak may have bacteria that you don't want on your eye, and since the only reason it's being used is because it's cold, retake the scene with a flexible package of frozen vegetables or a cold wet cloth. Leave it on the bruised area for about 20 minutes, off for 10 minutes, on for 20, off for 10. Get the picture?

BROKEN ARM BONE

If you think you have a broken arm bone, make an impromptu, temporary splint by gently placing the injured area—palm down—on top of a thick magazine. Chances are you'll need someone to help you roll the magazine into a U-shape, supporting the arm. Then keep the arm in place by tying an Ace bandage, duct tape, or a man's tie around the magazine that you've turned into a cradle-like cast.

Once that's done, seek professional medical help immediately.

BURNS

Burns are classified by degrees. A first-degree burn involves painful, red, unbroken skin. A second-degree burn involves painful blisters and broken skin. A third-degree burn destroys underlying tissue as well as surface skin. It may be painless because nerve endings may have also been destroyed. A fourth-degree burn involves deeply charred and blackened areas of the skin.

Second-degree burns that cover an extensive area of skin and *all* third- and fourth-degree burns require immediate medical attention. Any kind of burn on the face should also receive immediate medical attention as a precaution against swollen breathing passages.

As for first-degree burns—grabbing a hot pot handle, grasping the iron side of an iron, the oven door closing on your forearm, a splatter of boiling oil—here are first-aid suggestions, using mostly handy household items.

FIRST-DEGREE BURNS

Apply cold water or a cold compress first. Then try one of these treatments.

▶ Draw out the heat and pain by applying a slice of raw potato, a piece of fresh pumpkin pulp, or a slice of raw onion. Keep the potato, pumpkin, or onion on the burn for 15 minutes. Leave it off for 5 minutes, and then put a fresh piece on for another 15 minutes.

▶ If you burn yourself while baking and happen to have salt-free unbaked pie crust around, roll it thin and place it on the entire surface of the burn. Let it stay on until it dries up and falls off by itself.

▶ If you have vitamin E or garlic oil gels, puncture either one of them and squeeze the contents directly on the burn.

▶ Uncooked chicken fat placed directly on burns and scalds is said to be quite soothing.

▶ If you have a smooth piece of charcoal, put it on the burn and keep it there for an hour. Within minutes, the pain may begin to subside.

⟩ Plain honey on the burn may ease the pain and help the healing process.

⟩ Spread apple butter over the burned area. As it dries, add another coat to it. Keep adding coats for a day or two, until the burn is just about butter—uh, better.

⟩ People have had remarkable results with apple cider vinegar. Gently pour it on the burned or scalded area.

⟩ Keep an aloe vera plant in your home. It's like growing a tube of fine ointment. Break off about a ½-inch piece of stem. Squeeze it so that the juice oozes out onto the burned area. The juice is most effective if the plant is at least two to three years old and the stems have little bumps on the edges.

FIRST-DEGREE BURNS WHEN OUTDOORS

If you're outdoors, without access to a kitchen, pack mud on the burn to draw out the heat.

Better yet, and probably more accessible, put your own urine on the burn. The warmth of the fluid will make the burn radiate with pain for a few seconds, but it will stop soon, and the burn should heal without blistering.

SECOND-DEGREE BURNS

While waiting for professional medical attention, dip the burned area in cold water, or apply a towel that's been drenched in ice-cold water and keep it that way for at least half an hour. Do not use lard, butter, aloe vera, or salve on the burn! You don't want to seal in the heat, and you don't want the doctor to have to wipe off the goo to see the condition of the skin.

If the burn is on an arm or leg, keep the limb raised to help prevent swelling.

CHEMICAL AND ACID BURNS

Until you get medical attention, immediately get the affected area under the closest running cold water—a sink, a garden hose, or the shower. The running water will help wash the chemicals off the skin. Keep the water running on the burned skin for at least 20 minutes, or until medical help arrives.

BURNED TONGUE

Keep rinsing your mouth with cold water. A few drops of vanilla extract may relieve the pain.

⟩ Ease the pain of a burned tongue with a mouthful of plain yogurt.

▶ Some white sugar on a burned tongue is known to relieve the pain.

ROPE BURNS

Soak the hands in salt water. If salt and water are not available, do what they do in Italy for rope burns: Soak the hands in urine.

CARPAL TUNNEL SYNDROME

This problem results from swollen tendons that compress the median nerve within the carpal tunnel in the wrist. It's usually accompanied by odd sensations, numbness, swelling, soreness, stiffness, weakness, tingling, discomfort, and pain . . . a lot of pain. It's usually caused by continual, rapid use of your fingers, wrists, and/or arms, and many people feel the requirements of their job contribute to the onset of carpal tunnel syndrome (CTS). People who spend their workday at a computer aren't the only ones doing repetitious work: Musicians, supermarket checkers, factory workers, hair stylists, bus drivers, seamstresses, tailors, and countless others are plagued by this repetitive-motion injury.

If you believe that you may become a candidate for CTS because of your job requirements, doctors are recommending vitamin B_6 as a preventative. It's also being used successfully as a treatment. But too much B_6 can be toxic and harmful to the nervous system. Therefore, it is important to work with a health professional, such as a supplement-savvy nutritionist, to determine a safe dosage of B_6 specifically for you.

If you have CTS and are taking B_6 but don't notice any improvement after three weeks, you may want to switch to pyridoxal-5-phosphate (P-5-P), a form of B_6 that has been found more effective for some people.

WARNING: High doses of B_6 taken daily over a long period of time can cause nerve damage. Again, we repeat: It is important to work with a health professional who will monitor you.

CARPAL TUNNEL CHECKLIST

You may be predisposed to CTS if you are hypothyroid, have diabetes, are pregnant, or are on birth control pills. The following items on the checklist are things you can do something about immediately:

■ *Do you smoke?* Smoking worsens the condition because nicotine constricts the blood vessels and carbon monoxide replaces oxygen, reducing the blood flow to your tissues.

■ *Are you overweight?* Being overweight can present that blood-flow-to-your-tissues problem again. Also, the more weight you're carrying, the more the muscles must support to move your hand and arm.

■ *Do you exercise?* Aerobic exercise—30 minutes, four times a week—can increase the flow of oxygenated blood to your hands and help remove waste products from inflammation.

SELF-TEST

If you're not sure that the symptoms you're feeling are, in fact, carpal tunnel, try this self-test. It may be inconclusive, but it also may be a wake-up call.

Bend your wrist forward and, with your other hand, gently apply pressure on your bent wrist, pushing it toward your palm. Hold it that way for 2 to 3 minutes. If it brings on or aggravates the numbness, chances are you have CTS. The next step is to verify it with your health care provider.

SLEEPING WITH CARPAL TUNNEL

The pain may be more severe while sleeping because of the way you fold your wrist. You may find it more comfortable to wear a splint or wrist brace to bed. Now that the problem is so common, you can get a selection of splints and wrist braces at most drugstores. You may want to wear the splint or brace during the day, too.

If your problem is computer-related, visit your local computer store and see what they have in the way of ergonomic products to support your wrists while at the computer.

Also, you may want to look into a speech recognition program. Newer computers often have the software built in—you supply the headset and microphone. After going through the program's tutorial, you talk into the mike and the computer types it out for you. Theoretically, it's great. Realistically, it takes time until you learn the commands and until the program gets your voice and speech patterns down correctly. It is entertaining in the beginning to see how your words are misinterpreted.

EXERCISE FOR CTS PREVENTION

A team of doctors from the American Academy of Orthopaedic Surgeons has developed special exercises that can help prevent carpal tunnel syndrome. The exercises, which decrease the median nerve pressure responsible for CTS, should be done at the start of each work shift, as a warm-up exercise, and again after each break.

Stand straight, feet a foot apart, arms outstretched in front of you, palms down. Bring your fingers up, pointing toward the sky. Hold for a count of five. Straighten both wrists and relax the fingers. Make a tight fist with both hands. Then bend both wrists down while keeping the fists. Hold for a count of five. Straighten both wrists and relax the fingers for a count of five. The exercise should be repeated ten times. Then let your arms hang loosely at your sides and shake them for a couple of seconds. *Don't rush through the exercise.* Let the ten cycles take about 5 minutes.

Dr. James A. Duke, author and one of the world's leading authorities on herbal healing traditions, confesses that he uses a computer sometimes as much as fourteen hours a day, but he hasn't developed CTS. He gives some of the credit to the fact that he's a man. "Women develop carpal tunnel problems more than men do," explains Dr. Duke, "because the cyclical hormone fluctuations of the menstrual cycle, pregnancy and menopause can con-

tribute to swelling of the tissues that surround the carpal tunnel."

Another reason he thinks he's been spared the discomfort of CTS is hand exercises. "Adopting a Chinese technique that improves flexibility," says Dr. Duke, "I hold two steel balls in one hand and roll them around when I'm not typing. The Chinese balls provide a gentle form of exercise, and the rolling motion massages the tiny muscles and ligaments of the hands and wrists." When he's at the computer, he takes frequent breaks to twirl the Chinese balls in each hand.

Chinese balls are inexpensive and readily available at Chinese markets. Some health food stores also carry them.

HERBS FOR CTS

Dr. Duke, in his book *The Green Pharmacy* (Rodale Press), reports on quite a few herbs that can help alleviate CTS. With his permission, we share some of them with you.

"Willow bark, the original source of aspirin, contains chemicals (salicylates) that both relieve pain and reduce inflammation. You might also try other herbs rich in salicylates, notably meadowsweet and wintergreen." With any of these herbs, Dr. Duke steeps 1 to 2 teaspoons of dried, powdered bark, or 5 teaspoons of fresh bark, for 10 minutes or so, then strains out the plant material. You can add lemonade to mask the bitter taste. Dr. Duke says to drink 3 cups of this tea a day. He cautions that if you're allergic to aspirin, you shouldn't take aspirin-like herbs.

Chamomile's active compounds (bisabolol, chamazulene, and cyclic esters) also have potent anti-inflammatory action. Dr. Duke says, "If I had CTS, I'd drink several cups of chamomile tea a day."

Dr. Ray Wunderlich Jr. adds devil's claw and burdock (both available at herb shops) to the list of herbs that often help.

❧ Another way to duke it out is with bromelain, the protein-dissolving (proteolytic) enzyme found in pineapple. According to Dr. Duke, "Naturopaths suggest taking 250 to 1,500 milligrams of pure bromelain a day, between meals, to treat inflammatory conditions such as CTS. Bromelain is available at many health food stores."

Since ginger and papaya also contain helpful enzymes, Dr. Duke, who favors food sources to store-bought supplements, suggests, "You might enjoy a Proteolytic CTS Fruit Salad composed of pineapple and papaya and spiced with grated ginger."

❧ One more suggestion from Dr. Duke: "Also known as cayenne, red pepper contains six pain-relieving compounds and seven that are anti-inflammatory. Especially noteworthy is capsaicin. . . . You might add several teaspoons of powdered cayenne to a quarter-cup of skin lotion and rub it on your wrists. Or you could make a capsaicin lotion by steeping five to ten red peppers in two pints of rubbing alcohol for a few days. Just wash your hands thoroughly after using any topical capsaicin treatment, as you don't want to get it in your eyes. Also, since some people are quite sensitive to this compound, you should test it on a small area of skin before using it on a larger area. If it seems to irritate you, discontinue use." (Well, yeah.)

IF YOU WORK AT A COMPUTER . . .

The National Institute of Occupational Safety and Health recommends the following:

■ Position the screen at eye level, about 22 to 26 inches away.

■ Sit about arm's length from the terminal or tower. At that distance, the electrical field is almost zero.

■ Face forward and keep your neck relaxed.

■ Position the keyboard so that your elbows are bent at least 90 degrees and you can work without bending your wrists.

■ Use a chair that supports your back, lets your feet rest on the floor or on a footrest, and keeps thighs parallel to the floor.

■ If you can step away from the computer for 15 minutes every hour, it can help prevent eyestrain. When you're working at the computer, make a conscious effort to blink often. Frequent blinking will help prevent eye irritation, burning, and/or dry eyes.

CHILDREN'S HEALTH CHALLENGES

Every baby care book tells you to childproof your home. Make a crawling tour of each room in your house in order to see things from a child's-eye view. Once you're aware of the danger zones, you can eliminate them by covering wires, anchoring furniture, and so on. Do this every four to six months as the child grows and is able to reach more things.

Still, no matter how childproof a place is, a mishap can happen. We suggest that parents have a first-aid book handy and/or take a first-aid course through the local American Red Cross.

It's also very important to keep a list of the following emergency numbers near every telephone in the house:

■ Pediatrician
■ Poison control center
■ Police
■ Fire department
■ Hospital
■ Pharmacy
■ Dentist
■ Neighbors and close relatives (preferably with cars)

In terms of home remedies for common conditions, we caution you that children's systems are much more delicate than ours. So while lots of the remedies throughout the book can certainly be applied to youngsters, use good common sense in adjusting doses and strengths. In all cases, check with the pediatrician first.

ONE MAJOR CAUTION: Never give honey to a child under one year old! Spores found in honey have been linked to botulism in babies.

Here are some remedies specifically for children's ailments. Again, in all cases, check with the pediatrician first.

APPETITE STIMULANT

Prepare a cup of chamomile tea and add ⅛ teaspoon of ground ginger. An herbalist recommends 1 teaspoon of the warm tea half an hour before meals to stimulate a child's appetite.

ASTHMA

See the "Asthma" chapter for helpful hints, keeping in mind that children's systems require children's doses. *Always* check with your child's health care provider before administering any new treatment.

Trigger Awareness

FIREWORKS

If you've been near a fireworks display, remember that peculiar smell in the air? It comes from the emission of chemicals, including sulfur dioxide, following each explosion. Keep your asthmatic child far away from those lung-irritating chemicals. The good thing about fireworks is that they can be seen from a distance. Better yet, watch them on television instead of exposing your child to that bad air.

GAS STOVE

Does your child seem to start wheezing while you're preparing food in the kitchen? Do you have a gas stove? The nitrogen dioxide emitted by the gas may be the chemical that's causing the coughing. Consider changing to an electric stove. Meanwhile, keep your child out of the kitchen when you're cooking.

SWIMMING POOLS

Water treated with chlorine may trigger breathing problems. Watch your child carefully when he or she goes into a pool. If you notice any wheezing or shortness of breath, get him out of the pool immediately.

ATTENTION DEFICIT DISORDER (ADD) AND ATTENTION DEFICIT HYPERACTIVITY DISORDER (ADHD)

If your child has been diagnosed with ADD or ADHD, chances are you are looking for an answer so that he or she doesn't have to start taking Ritalin or can be taken off that drug.

Have you checked out possible causes, including the following?

- Toxic metal excess (lead from toys made in China)
- Pesticides in the home
- Malnutrition (to see if your child is digesting his food, check his stools for pieces of undigested food)

- Allergies (including sweets, milk, and cheese)
- Gluten intolerance (be sure to read "Immune Function Strengthener" later in this chapter)

While your child's diet may play a major part in causing and overcoming this condition, you may not know that several studies point to a connection between children with ADHD and an omega-3 fatty acid deficiency. According to a paper published in *Physiology and Behavior* by a research team from the Department of Foods and Nutrition at Purdue University, boys with lower levels of omega-3 fatty acids in their blood showed more problems with behavior, learning, and health than those with higher total levels of omega-3 fatty acids.

You may want to find out more about this, and then consider adding Salba (available at health food stores), one of the richest sources of omega-3 essential fatty acids, to your child's daily diet. (Learn more about Salba in the "Diabetes" chapter.)

Your Karate Kid

Consider enrolling your child in a martial arts class. There are karate courses specifically designed for children with ADD and ADHD. Karate encourages these children to focus, reinforcing their ability to concentrate and learn discipline, while boosting their self-esteem, all without over-stimulation.

Parents, contact local and national ADD/ADHD support groups for recommendations of martial arts schools in your area. You want a school that teaches the nonviolence-above-all philosophy, like that of Mr. Miyagi in the *Karate Kid* movies.

When checking each school, interview the owner and instructors to determine which one is most prepared to work with an ADD or ADHD child. There may even be a school with specially trained ADD/ADHD instructors.

NOTEWORTHY: While working with children for thirty years, Janet Tubbs developed a teaching technique, along with fun activities, designed to reduce hyperactivity, increase and prolong focus, decrease anger, develop fine motor skills, improve social and verbal skills, and help these children relate to their environment without fear, anxiety, or discomfort. It's all in the book, *Creative Therapy for Children with Autism, ADD, and Asperger's* (Square One).

AUTISM AND ASPERGER'S SYNDROME

Autism is a complex condition. The diagnosis most often is based on observation of social interaction when a child is two or three years old. While we have no quick-fix remedies, we do have a recommendation—a book by a dedicated husband-and-wife team who have developed a prescreening program based on physical movement. *Does Your Baby Have Autism?* by Philip Teitelbaum, Ph.D., and Osnat Teitelbaum (Square One) provides a key for parents to detect autism or Asperger's syndrome within the first six months of their baby's life.

Early diagnosis can make a major difference in the treatment of both conditions.

BEDWETTING

Give the bedwetter a few pieces of cinnamon bark to chew on throughout the day. For some unknown reason, it seems to control bedwetting for some kids.

This exercise strengthens the muscles that control urination. Starting with the first urination of the day, have the child start and stop urinating as many times as possible until she has finished. If you turn it into a game, counting the number of starts and stops, the child might look forward to breaking her own record each time. It's important, however, not to pressure the child into feeling inadequate if she finds this exercise difficult. Be pa-

tient and supportive . . . as if we had to tell you.

Prepare a cup of corn silk tea by adding 10 to 15 drops of corn silk extract to 1 cup of boiled water. Stir, let cool, and have the bedwetter slowly sip the tea at least 3 hours before bedtime.

NOTE: Chronic bedwetters should be treated by a health professional.

BRUISING: A BONDING OPPORTUNITY

Psychiatrist Paul C. Holinger, M.D., M.P.H., and author of *What Babies Say Before They Can Talk* (Simon and Schuster), offers great advice on how to deal with your child when he falls or bruises himself in some way but is not seriously hurt.

Dismissing the child's feelings or experience by saying "That didn't hurt" and encouraging him to have a "be brave" attitude can cause a toddler to have a tantrum, and may send a teenager out the door. No matter how old the child is, get in tune with him by telling him you can imagine how that must hurt, and how scary it was to fall like that, or to be hit by the branch when you didn't see it coming. And yes, by all means, kiss the boo-boo!

Your empathy and caring about your child in this way help you bond with him and allows him to develop those qualities for others.

CHICKEN POX

Of course a child with chicken pox should be in bed, kept warm, and on a light diet, including lots of pure fruit juices. According to herbalists, yarrow tea (available at some health food stores, or check our "Sources" chapter for herb shops) seems to be the thing for children's eruptive ailments. Add 1 tablespoon of dried yarrow to 2 cups of just-boiled water and let it steep for 10 minutes. Strain, then add 1 tablespoon of raw honey.

> **CAUTION:** Never give honey to a child under one year old!

Give the child ½ cup of yarrow tea three or four times a day.

To relieve the itching, a pediatrician recommends a spritz of ordinary spray starch on the itch areas.

COLD

See "Ear Infection," below.

COLIC

A popular European colic calmer is fennel tea. Add a fennel tea bag (available at health food stores) or ½ teaspoon of fennel seeds (available in the supermarket spice section) to 1 cup of just-boiled water and let it steep for 10 minutes. Strain the liquid tea into the baby's bottle. When it's cool enough to drink, give it to the baby. If he's not thrilled with the taste of fennel, try dill seeds instead. If neither fennel nor dill is his cup of tea, use 1 tablespoon of bruised caraway seeds in 1 cup of just-boiled water. Steep, strain, then put 2 teaspoons of the tea into the baby's bottle and, when it's cool enough, let him drink it.

If you are breast-feeding your baby and she is colicky, try eliminating milk from your diet. There's a 50/50 chance that if you no longer drink milk, the baby will no longer have colic. Be sure, however, to eat calcium-rich foods such as canned salmon, canned sardines, sunflower and sesame seeds, almonds, whole grains, green leafy vegetables, soy products including tofu, and molasses. Salba, available at health food stores, has six times more calcium than whole milk. (See the "Diabetes" chapter to learn more about Salba.)

Milk isn't the only thing to eliminate

from your diet while nursing a colicky baby. Avoid foods that may be hard for you and baby to digest: bell peppers, beans, cucumbers, eggs, chocolate, onions, leeks, garlic, eggplant, lentils, zucchini, tomatoes, sugar, coffee, and alcoholic beverages. Go easy on the amount of fruit you eat. Remember, it's not forever . . . the diet restrictions *or* the colic!

For 15 minutes, boil a cup of water with ⅓ of a bay leaf in the water. Let it cool, then pour it into the baby's bottle and let the baby drink it. This old Sicilian remedy has cured many colicky bambinos.

Also see "Indigestion and Gas" (below) for remedies to help calm down a colicky child.

COUGH

When a child has a hacking cough—you know, the kind that usually acts up at bedtime—lightly spray the pillow with wine vinegar. Both you and the child may sleep better for it.

Right before bedtime, smear a thin layer of Vicks VapoRub on the soles of the child's feet, then cover the feet with a pair of white socks. This remedy is reported to help clear up a bronchial cough, as well as calming the nighttime cough and allowing everyone in the family to sleep.

In 2007, after news broke that some over-the-counter cough medicines for children could be harmful rather than helpful, an old folk remedy was revisited. The results of a study concluded that 1 teaspoon of honey a half hour before bedtime calmed a child's cough, soothed an irritated throat, and helped the child sleep better.

CAUTION: Never give honey to a child under one year old.

A woman from Oklahoma called to tell us that whenever her child gets a cough that gets worse at night, she *loosely* ties a black cotton thread around the child's neck. It must be black. This woman said she tried other colors and nothing but black works.

We were intrigued with this remedy and tested it on our friend's child. Much to our surprise, it worked like magic. We researched it and found a printed source that credited it to shamans in ancient Egypt.

CROUP

Scottish folk healers treat croup by wrapping a piece of bacon (uncooked, of course) around the child's neck, bundling him up in a blanket, and taking him into a steamy bathroom for a few minutes. Steam without the bacon works too.

Well, it's something to do till the doctor arrives.

DIAPER RASH

Let the baby's bottom be exposed to the air. If weather permits, the sun (no more than 10 to 15 minutes at a time) can do wonders for clearing up diaper rash.

Gently apply raw honey to the rash. It helps promote healing.

CAUTION: Never let a baby under one year old eat honey.

DIARRHEA

Give baby pure blackberry juice, 2 or 3 tablespoons four times a day.

Another way of treating diarrhea in infants is to give them barley water throughout the day. (See "Preparation Guide" for the barley water recipe.)

Carrot soup not only soothes the inflamed small bowel, it also replaces lost body fluids and minerals. Also, carrots have an antidiarrheal substance called pectin. You can prepare the soup by mixing a jar of strained carrots with a jar of water. Feed the child carrot soup as long as the diarrhea persists.

From the Pennsylvania Dutch comes this children's remedy for diarrhea. In a warmed cup of milk, add ⅛ teaspoon of cinnamon. The child should drink as much as possible.

DIGESTION

If a baby can't seem to keep his food down, you may want to try putting a teaspoon of carob powder (available at health food stores) in his formula. In some instances, it may make the difference.

EAR INFECTION

"Children who get recurring ear infections, or nose and throat infections, or colds during cold season, should be taken off dairy products," advises pediatric neurologist Dr. Sharon Herzfeld (www.holistic neuro.com).

Dr. Herzfeld says that dairy interferes with iron absorption and other things that impede the immune function. "There are wonderful substitutes for cow's milk. If the child isn't allergic to nuts, use almond milk, or use rice milk, or soy milk. There are many ways for children to get calcium in their diet. Broccoli and green leafy vegetables are rich in calcium. These are foods the whole family should be eating."

So eliminate dairy products and you may eliminate your child's recurrent ear infections.

> NOTEWORTHY: Salba, available at health food stores, has six times more calcium than whole milk. (See the "Diabetes" chapter to learn more about Salba.)

FEVER

To help pull down a child's fever, put sliced raw potatoes on the soles of the feet and keep them in place with an Ace bandage or man's-size handkerchief. Let the novelty of this remedy provide a few laughs for you and your child. Isn't laughter the best medicine?

▶ Give your child a long, soothing bath in tepid water. Then, when you put your child to bed, be sure the blanket is not tucked in too tightly. Leave it loose so that the heat can escape into the air.

FOREIGN BODY IN THE EYE

Irrigate the eye with water, or peel an onion near the child so that tears wash away the foreign body.

FOREIGN SUBSTANCE IN THE NOSE

When Lydia was about three years old, our father saw her sitting still for more than 30 seconds at a time, and so he knew that something was very wrong. Of course he questioned her, and when she answered in a peculiarly nasal voice, he figured out the problem. Lydia had stuck something up her nose . . . a Yankee bean, to be exact.

If your child sticks something up his nose, open his mouth, place your mouth over it, and briskly blow once. Your gust of breath may dislodge the object from the child's nostril. If it's still there after that first try, take that rotten kid to a doctor!

In case you're wondering about Lydia, by the time the bean was extracted from her nostril, it had actually begun to take root. Not a pretty picture, but a helluva way to grow a plant.

HICCUPS

While it's cute to see an infant with hiccups, it's not fun for her to have them. Forget "Boo!" This is a gentle remedy that doesn't involve scaring the baby. Just take a piece of red (must be red) cotton thread, wad it up in your mouth with your spittle, then put the red wad on the baby's forehead. Hiccups? All gone!

⟫ When a child about age six or over has the hiccups, promise to double the week's allowance if she can hiccup once more after you say "Go!" Chances are there will not be another *real* hiccup after you say "Go!" We don't know why, but it works . . . most of the time. Don't try this unless you're willing to pay up if it doesn't work.

⟫ See the general "Hiccups" chapter for many more suggestions.

IMMUNE FUNCTION STRENGTHENER

Sharon Herzfeld, M.D. (www.holistic neuro.com) has a pediatric and adult practice in which she takes an integrative approach, prescribing alternative treatments, including homeopathic remedies (which are FDA-approved and, unlike most traditional medications, have no side effects).

The initial consultation typically takes two hours. It is no wonder, then, that when we asked Dr. Herzfeld for remedies, she explained, "General guidelines may be helpful, but I treat every patient as an indi-

vidual, and what works for one may not work for another." Here are Dr. Herzfeld's general guidelines, which we hope will inspire you to make changes to help boost the immune function for your children and the entire family.

"There is no one medication for immune function, but there are many homeopathic remedies that can help improve it, along with nourishment," says Dr. Herzfeld. "In terms of nourishment, don't think of what you *can't* have; focus on what you *should* and *can* have.

"Embrace whole foods. Our bodies reflect what we're eating. I teach my children that if there's a chemical on a label, we shouldn't be eating it. The best things are foods that come without labels on them, such as fruits and vegetables.

"If you buy food with labels, you have to be cautious. If it says 'natural strawberry flavor,' it has dozens of unpronounceable chemicals in it. No one should be eating strawberry-flavored anything. People tell me they're feeding their children Pop-Tarts for breakfast. No wonder those children can't sit still in class.

"For maximum immune function, I repeat, go back to whole foods. Also, consider eliminating dairy and gluten. Gluten is the protein in wheat, barley, spelt, and rye. Casein is the protein in dairy. On a molecular level, structurally they are very similar. Both impact our immune system, digestive tract, and serotonin levels in the brain. Children who have sensory integration dysfunction, attention issues (ADD, ADHD), or autistic spectrum disorder do much better without gluten and casein in their diet.

"People think it's hard to do, but it's really doable. It's one of the first things you should think of doing to help your child, especially one who's having symptoms of the challenges I just mentioned."

> **NOTE:** Before you present the argument that there are not enough hours in the day for all that you already have to do, we would like to tell you that Dr. Herzfeld has a busy full-time practice and two young children for whom she prepares all of their homemade meals, including baked goods, that are chemical-free, dairy-free, gluten-free, sugar-free, and white-carb-free (e.g., no white flour), all while adhering to strict religious dietary principles.

If Dr. Herzfeld's words have impacted your thinking about the foods your children are eating, this is a good start. Go to your local library or bookstore, or check the Internet, and do some research about feeding your family whole foods. Books on celiac disease will educate you about cutting out gluten. If you're serious about making dietary changes, one source will lead you to another as you gradually eliminate some foods and replace them with healthful alternatives. Before long, you will become an expert, eating healthfully will be manageable, and you and your family will be better off for it.

> **NOTEWORTHY:** If you're looking for products made with integrity (unlike the chemical-laden "strawberry" items referred to above by Dr. Herzfeld), visit Kozlowski Farms in Forestville, California, or on the Internet at www.kozlowskifarms.com, or call them at 800-473-2767. They have an exceptionally delicious line of chemical-free jams and preserves, some organic, and all made with the finest fruits.

INDIGESTION AND GAS

To help relieve indigestion and dispel gas, give your infant mild ginger tea. Steep 1 or 2 quarter-size pieces of fresh ginger in just-boiled water for 5 minutes. As soon as it's cool, let your baby drink it.

Mild chamomile tea will soothe an upset stomach and calm down a colicky kid. Steep a chamomile tea bag in just-boiled water for 5 minutes. Let it cool, then give it to your baby.

If your child seems to have a minor digestion problem, try 2 teaspoons of apple juice concentrate (available at health food stores) in half a glass of water before meals. Make sure the liquid mixture is room temperature, not chilled.

LICE

It's estimated that at any given time, 10 million Americans have head lice. Lice are transmitted from child to child via common objects, such as a mat in the school gymnasium, or a seat at the movies. Just about the only way you could prevent a child from ever being exposed to lice is by keeping the child in a bubble. Since the bubble is not an option, if your child comes home with head lice, there's no need to panic. There are over-the-counter shampoos that are safe and somewhat effective, unlike some prescription shampoos that can be dangerous to young children, pregnant or nursing women, and anyone with a cut on her hand or arm.

If you use commercial lice shampoo and get rid of the lice, you must also get rid of any remaining nits (eggs or young lice) by thoroughly rinsing with equal parts of distilled white vinegar and water. Or use a fine-tooth comb to comb tea tree oil (available at health food stores) through the hair, and then rinse with vinegar and water.

CAUTION: Do not use your fingers to hunt down these critters; they can burrow their way under your fingernails. Yuck!

If the nits move down to the eyelashes, *do not use tea tree oil*! It's much too strong and dangerous near the eyes. Instead, before breakfast and after supper, carefully put a thin layer of petroleum jelly on the lashes. Do this for eight days. By then, the jelly will have smothered the nits and you will be able to simply remove them.

NOTEWORTHY: LiceMD (clinically proven and pediatrician-tested) eliminates lice and nits. This nontoxic, odorless, and safe treatment is available at pharmacies. A lice comb is included. Visit LiceMD.com or call 800-431-2610.

MEASLES

Yarrow tea is good for calming eruptive ailments (see "Chicken Pox," above).

To strengthen the child's eyes, which are usually affected when one has the measles, and to ease the discomfort in them, make sure the child gets food rich in vitamin A—carrot juice, cantaloupe, and green and yellow fruit.

MOLLUSCUM CONTAGIOSUM VIRUS

We first heard about molluscum contagiosum virus (MCV) when a friend called to ask if we had any home remedies for the ailment. Once we started researching, we were surprised how widespread MCV is among children as well as adults. According to medical research, up to 17 percent of American children will contract MCV, a skin infection with disfiguring lesions that can spread to any part of the body. It's highly contagious and passes easily from person to person by direct skin-to-skin contact, from contact with contaminated objects such as toys, towels, toilets, faucet handles, or doorknobs, and in pools, lockers, and gymnasiums.

> **NOTEWORTHY:** While looking for a remedy or two for this condition, we quickly discovered that there is no quick fix. We also discovered and interviewed David B. Phillips, Ph.D., a brilliant man whose products offer hope and help when the rest of the medical community can't and doesn't.

To give you an idea of this man's creativity and motivation, Dr. Phillips was given the Inventor of the Year Award for developing the first infrared ear thermometer when his children were small, because he did not like the danger of mercury and glass rectal thermometers, or the indignity of them. (Not only brilliant but a class act!)

Years later, when Dr. Phillips' four-year-old granddaughter contracted MCV, the family doctor said that it would go away on its own—perhaps in two or three years—and that the options for treatment (not cure) were limited to cutting, freezing, or using acid and chemicals to burn off the lesions.

Once again, Dr. Phillips sprang into action, and after intensive research he created the SilverCure System.

Dr. Phillips and his team at ReBuilder Medical Technologies invent, develop, and make all of their amazing products in their U.S. factory, where they know firsthand the quality of the ingredients that are used and the cleanliness of the manufacturing process, and can test each batch themselves.

Dr. Phillips says, "Children's skin is very sensitive, and everything we make is hypoallergenic and made without any animal products."

Visit www.molluscum.com and learn more about the treatment kit, or call 866-725-2202. They have full-time, licensed medical professionals on staff to answer your questions.

PIMPLY-FACED INFANTS

It's common to see infants with an outbreak of pimples. According to a folk remedy from the 1600s, gently dab the premature case of acne with mother's milk. If you're not nursing the baby, use a few drops of whole (not skim) milk. Or gently dab the outbreak with the baby's own wet diaper. The urine has healing antibodies.

PRICKLY HEAT

Gently rub the afflicted area with the red side of a piece of watermelon rind. It should stop the itching and help dry out the rash.

SPITTING UP

Warm a little heavy syrup from canned peaches and give it to your baby to stop nausea.

SPLINTERS

To pinpoint the exact location of a splinter, pat some iodine on the area. The sliver of wood will absorb it and turn dark, enabling you to see it.

Once you've located the splinter, soak the area in vegetable oil for a couple of minutes. The oil should allow the splinter to glide right out. It may be necessary to help it along with tweezers.

If the child has a sliver of glass, numb the area with an ice cube or some teething lotion before you start the painful squeezing and scraping.

SUNBURN: PROTECTION AND PREVENTION

See "Sunburn" chapter.

TANTRUM TAMERS

Put a drop of lavender oil (available at health food stores) on your shoulder and let your baby's head rest on that shoulder as you comfort him. In fact, use lavender oil often, so that it becomes Mommy's scent. When you have to leave your child with a babysitter, give her a tissue with a drop or two of lavender oil on it to keep in her pocket. The scent will make your baby feel secure even though Mommy is not around.

TEETHING

Gently massage sore little gums with extra-virgin olive oil to help relieve the pain.

TONSILLITIS

We've been told about lots of cases of swollen tonsils because of an intolerance for milk. That's easy enough to test. Simply eliminate milk and milk products (including ice cream and cheese) from the child's diet and check the results within a day or two. If the child does not assimilate milk properly, there are many other wonderful sources of calcium and it is no big deal for a child not to have milk.

Sunflower and sesame seeds are rich in calcium. So are almonds, green leafy vegetables, canned salmon, sardines, molasses, and whole grains, including Salba, which has six times more calcium than whole milk. (See the "Diabetes" chapter to learn more about Salba.) There are also delicious soy products, soy milks, and calcium supplements. You may want to consider a consultation with a nutritionist who can best advise your child on a personal level.

Master herbalist Dr. John R. Christopher says that puberty will be easier to go through if teenagers still have their tonsils. Girls will have easier menstrual periods and boys will have less chance for prostate malfunction. The reason is that the tonsils are the filtering system for the reproductive organs and are needed by the body.

WARTS

The power of the mind and creative imagery are very effective when it comes to making a child's wart disappear.

We met a woman whose daughter had a wart on her hand. A dermatologist tried all kinds of removal tactics, including burning it off with acid, but the stubborn wart kept returning. When the woman told the child's pediatrician about it, he suggested the following remedy: Take a piece of tracing or tissue paper, put it on the child's wart, and with a pencil, trace the wart. Take your child and the paper with the traced-on wart into the bathroom. Then be sure to impress upon the child, "Only Mommy or Daddy can do this!" While the child watches, burn the tracing paper and flush away the ashes. In about a week, the wart should be gone. Really!

We received a letter from a woman who read this remedy in our previous book. She said, "A little over a week ago, I used this remedy on my daughter. As I write this letter, there is a fading pink spot where the wart used to be, and it gets lighter every day."

CHOLESTEROL

The only foods that have cholesterol are animal products—meat, poultry, fish, and dairy. Yes, dairy—cheese, butter, milk.

There is a harmful cholesterol component (LDL) and a protective cholesterol component (HDL).

If you have high cholesterol, start a heart-smart diet immediately by cutting down or cutting out animal products. There are foods that can help lower your LDL and raise your HDL.

There have been a variety of cholesterol studies with impressive results. So start getting that heart-smart diet in place, incorporating the foods and supplements listed below.

⟩ Eating 2 large apples a day caused cholesterol levels to drop 16 percent. That may be because apples are rich in flavonoids and pectin. Pectin may form a gel in the stomach that keeps fats in food from being totally absorbed.

⟩ Eating half an avocado a day may lower cholesterol by 8 to 42 percent. Yes, they're high in fat, but it's monounsaturated fat, which does good things for the system. Avocado also contains thirteen essential minerals, including iron, copper, and magnesium, and is rich in potassium. It tastes great, too.

⟩ Eating 2 raw carrots a day for three weeks reduced serum cholesterol levels by 11 percent, according to the *American Journal of Clinical Nutrition.*

You may want to scrub the carrots you eat instead of peeling them. If you can get organic carrots, do so. The peel is rich in vitamins B_1 (thiamine), B_2 (riboflavin), and B_3 (niacin).

⟩ People who consumed about ¾ cup of fenugreek seeds daily for twenty days cut their LDL (bad cholesterol) levels by 33 percent; their HDL (good cholesterol) levels, happily, stayed the same. Instead of having to eat tablespoons of ground fenugreek seeds, take fenugreek capsules—580 mg (available at health food stores)—and follow suggested dosage.

⟩ Eating 4 cloves of garlic a day can cut total cholesterol by about 7 percent. (While fresh garlic is best, garlic supplements are next best.)

⟩ Kiwi has what it takes to help keep cholesterol down: magnesium, potassium, and fiber. It makes a satisfying, energy-boosting afternoon snack.

Omega-3 fatty acids have the ability to break down cholesterol in the lining of blood vessels, as well as serving as a solvent for saturated fats in the diet. The end result is less cholesterol in the body and bloodstream, and a reduced likelihood of high-cholesterol-related problems. Flaxseed oil and Salba are both rich in omega-3 fatty acids. For more details, see the "Food for Thought" chapter.

Test results build a good case for the effectiveness of lecithin in lowering LDL levels and raising HDL levels. Health food stores have liquid lecithin, softgels, and granules. Once you decide which form you prefer, follow the dosage on the label.

Eating oats can improve blood flow and help remove cholesterol from the body, bringing down your cholesterol number, just like the TV commercials say it does. Reap this benefit by eating oatmeal or any other form of oats at least two or three times a week. One portion is about ½ cup of dry oats. Don't overdo it.

SUPPLEMENTS

Dr. Ray C. Wunderlich Jr. of the Wunderlich Center for Nutritional Medicine in St. Petersburg, Florida, recommends grapeseed oil (available at health food stores) as a reliable HDL (good cholesterol) increaser. Follow the dosage on the label.

It seems that very small amounts of chromium are vital for good health. A deficiency in chromium may be linked to coronary artery disease. Take 1 to 2 tablespoons of brewer's yeast daily (read labels before buying, and select the brewer's yeast with the highest chromium content), or eat a handful of raw sunflower seeds. The chromium is said to lower the LDL and raise the HDL.

According to Dr. James W. Anderson, professor and researcher at the University of Kentucky College of Medicine, eating 1½ cups of legumes daily lowers cholesterol an average of 19 percent after three weeks. Beans contain fiber and at least five other cholesterol cutters. This benefit can be attributed to dry beans, such as pinto beans, rather than green beans.

COLDS, FLU, SORE THROAT, ETC.

f you're out there with a red, runny nose, chest congestion, and that achy flu feeling, instead of making much achoo about nothing, keep reading for some simple cold-helping hints.

COLDS

The first round of ammunition for fighting the cold war is chicken soup (Jewish penicillin). According to *Medical World News,* the director of medical services at Mount Sinai Medical Center in Miami Beach, Dr. Marvin A. Sackner, proved that chicken soup can help cure a cold.

Using a bronchofiberscope and cineroentgenograms and measurements of mucus velocity, Dr. Sackner tested the effectiveness of hot chicken soup and hot and cold water. Cold water lowered nasal clearance and hot water improved it, but it was nothing compared to the improvement after hot chicken soup. Then, to negate the effects of the steam from the hot water and hot chicken soup, the fluids were sipped through straws from covered containers. Hot water had very little effect this way. The hot chicken soup still had some benefit.

Chicken Soup, the Medicine, and More Proof

Soon after we completed our first *Chicken Soup* folk remedy book, the respected Mayo Clinic printed the following in its *Health Letter:*

There is now evidence that our ancestors may have known more about how to treat sniffles than we do. And that should not be surprising. Indeed, scientific study of folk medicines and cures often has proved to be remarkably rewarding.

Moses Maimonides, a twelfth-century Jewish physician and philosopher, reported that chicken soup is an effective medication as well as a tasty food.

Next time you come down with a head cold, try hot homemade chicken soup before heading for the pharmacy. Chicken soup can be an excellent treatment for uncomplicated head colds and other viral respiratory infections for which antibiotics ordinarily are not helpful.

Soup is less expensive, and it carries little if any risk of allergic reactions or other undesirable side effects.

> **CAUTION**: This chicken soup is a *medicine* and is *not* to be eaten as one would eat a portion of soup. Please follow the dosage instructions at the end of the recipe.

Irwin Ziment, M.D., professor of medicine at the University of California, Los Angeles, and chief of medicine and director of respiratory therapy at Olive View Medical

Center in Los Angeles, is also an authority on pulmonary drugs. Considering the research, experience, and expertise it took to earn his credentials, we believe Dr. Ziment's chicken soup recipe, which he generously shared with us, should be taken seriously for colds, coughs, and chest congestion.

DR. ZIMENT'S CHICKEN SOUP

1 quart of homemade chicken broth, or low-fat, low-sodium canned chicken broth
1 head of garlic (about 15 cloves), peeled
5 parsley sprigs, minced
6 cilantro sprigs, minced
1 teaspoon of lemon pepper
1 teaspoon of dried basil, crushed, or 1 tablespoon chopped fresh basil
1 teaspoon of curry powder
Optional: hot red pepper flakes to taste, sliced carrots, a bay leaf or two

Place all ingredients in a pot without a lid. Bring to a boil, then simmer for about 30 minutes. (If the soup is for your own personal use, carefully inhale the fumes during preparation as an additional decongesting treatment.)

Remove the garlic cloves and herbs and, along with a little broth, puree them in a blender or food processor. Return the puree to the broth and stir.

Serve hot.

Dose: Take 2 tablespoons of Dr. Ziment's Chicken Soup at the beginning of a meal, one to three times a day. (If you feel you want a little more than 2 tablespoons, fine, but do not exceed more than ½ cup at a time.)

More Cold-Fighting Food

In the former USSR, garlic was known as "Russian penicillin." It has been reported that colds have actually disappeared within hours—a day at most—after taking garlic. Keep a peeled clove of garlic in your mouth, between the cheek and teeth. Do not chew it. Occasionally release a little garlic juice by digging your teeth into the clove. Replace the clove every 3 to 4 hours.

The allicin in garlic is an excellent mucus thinner and bacteria killer. It's no wonder many cold remedies include garlic.

If taking garlic by mouth is not for you, then peel and crush 6 cloves of garlic. Mix them into ½ cup of petroleum jelly or vegetable shortening. Spread the mush on the soles of your feet and cover them with a (preferably warmed) towel or flannel cloth. Put plastic wrap or cut up a plastic tablecloth and put it on the sheet, under the feet, to protect the bedding. Garlic is so powerful that even though it's applied to one's feet, it will be on one's breath, too.

Apply a fresh batch of the mixture every 5 hours until the cold is gone.

The onion, a close relative of garlic, is also a popular folk medicine for colds. Here are some ways in which the onion is used:

■ Dip a slice of raw onion in a glass of hot water. After a few minutes, remove the onion and, when the water cools, start sipping it. Continue to do so throughout the day.

■ If you like your onions fried, take the hot fried onions, put them in a flannel or woolen cloth, and bind them on your chest overnight.

■ Put slices of raw onion on the soles of your feet and hold the slices in place with woolen socks. Leave them that way overnight to draw out infection and fever by morning.

Beverages

It's good to keep flushing out your system by drinking nondairy liquids, including water, unsweetened fruit juice, and any of the following drinks.

Prepare tea with equal parts of cinnamon, sage, and bay leaves (about ½ teaspoon of each) in 8 to 10 ounces of just-boiled water. Let it steep for about 5 minutes. Strain. Before drinking the tea, add 1 tablespoon of lemon juice. If you want to sweeten the tea, use honey.

SWEAT-IT-OUT DRINKS

When our friend the contessa from the Italian hills has a cold, she makes a mug of very strong black or green tea and adds 1 tablespoon of honey, 1 tablespoon of cognac, 1 teaspoon of butter, and ¼ teaspoon of cinnamon. She drinks it as hot as she can and goes to bed between cotton sheets. If she wakes up during the night and is all sweaty, she changes her nightclothes and sheets and goes back to bed. By morning, she feels *molto bene!*

"What doesn't kill you will make you stronger." That's the way we felt about the drink our grandmother, whom we called

Bubbie, made the second someone in our family came down with a cold. The dreaded drink was called a "guggle-muggle." We thought it was a cute name that Bubbie made up. Imagine our surprise when Edward Koch, during his last term in office as mayor of New York, talked about an ancient cure: his family's recipe for a guggle-muggle.

It sounds like a magic potion from the Harry Potter books, but it seems that many Jewish families have their own healing guggle-muggle recipes—some more palatable than others. Our family's is the worst; Mr. Koch's is one of the best. As Ed Koch said to us, "It is not only medically superb, it is delicious!" With his permission, we share with you the Koch family for-adults-only guggle-muggle recipe.

CAUTION: If you're taking medication, check with your doctor or pharmacist about negative grapefruit-drug interaction.

In a saucepan, combine the juice of 1 grapefruit, 1 lemon, 1 orange (preferably a Temple orange, because of its taste), and 1 tablespoon of honey. Stir while bringing it to a boil. Take it off the heat, pour it into a glass, then add at least 1 ounce of your favorite liquor. (Brandy is Ed Koch's.) As

with most guggle-muggles, drink it down, then get under the covers, go to sleep, and sweat it out. Next morning, no cold.

Sweat-It-Out Bath

Before bedtime, take a ginger bath and sweat away your cold overnight. Put 3 tablespoons of grated fresh ginger into a stocking and knot the stocking closed.

TIP: Ginger is fibrous and hard to grate. Keep a piece of ginger in the freezer. It doesn't lose its value, and frozen ginger is easier to grate. Also, you'll always have it when you need it.

Toss the grated ginger into a hot bath along with 4 tablespoons of powdered ginger. Stir the bathwater with a wooden spoon. Then get in and soak for 10 to 15 minutes. Once you're out of the tub, dry yourself thoroughly, preferably with a rough towel. Put on warm sleep clothes and cover your head with a towel or woolen scarf, leaving just your face exposed. Get in bed under the covers and go to sleep. If, during the night, you perspire enough to feel uncomfortably wet, change into dry sleepwear and go back to bed. You should feel a lot better in the morning.

A Gem of an Idea

Talk about sweating it out—a gem therapist said that wearing a topaz activates body heat and, therefore, helps cure ailments that may benefit from increased perspiration.

Herbs

Herbalist Angela Harris says that the combination of echinacea and goldenseal is effective in either stopping a cold from blossoming or cutting short the duration and minimizing the severity of a cold. The secret is to combine 1 dropper of each herb extract (available at health food stores) in a few ounces of water every hour for the first 4 hours of the day that you feel a cold coming on. After that, take 1 dropper of each in water every 4 hours. (Do not take echinacea for more than two weeks at a time.)

Acupuncture Points

To stimulate appropriate acupuncture points that can help cure a cold, place an ice cube on the bottom of both big toes. Keep them in place with an Ace bandage or piece of cloth. Place feet in a basin, in two plastic shoe boxes, or on plastic to avoid a mess from the melting ice. Do this procedure three times a day—morning, noon, and night.

Chest Cold

Mix the white of 1 raw egg with 4 teaspoons of prepared mustard and rub it on the chest. Take a (preferably white) towel and dip it in hot water, then wring it out and place it on top of the mixture already on the chest. As soon as the towel is cool, redip it in hot water, wring it out, and again put it back on the chest. Reapply the towel four or five times. After the last application of the towel, wash the chest clean, dry thoroughly, bundle up, and go to bed.

Cold Prevention

The natural sulfur in broccoli and parsley is supposed to help us resist colds. Eat broccoli and/or parsley once a day.

An apple a day . . . A university study showed that the students who ate apples regularly had fewer colds.

Pomegranate juice has been getting lots of press, and just about all of it is good. It seems to be due to a Pace University biology professor, Milton Schiffenbauer, Ph.D., who designed an exploratory study that was conducted by his students, proving that pure pomegranate juice and pomegranate liquid extract are effective in fighting viruses and bacteria. The juice and the extract could significantly reduce microbes found in the mouth that commonly cause colds, cavities, staph infections, and food poisoning.

Even though the study was funded, in part, by POM Wonderful pomegranate products, in conjunction with Pace University, the results are impressive. Drinking 100 percent pomegranate juice (available at most supermarkets) or taking POMx liquid extract (available at health food stores) daily may help prevent a cold.

NOTE: If you drink too much pomegranate juice (sorry, but we don't know how much too much would be for you), it can cause constipation.

CAUTION: If you are taking any prescription medication, especially to help bring down your cholesterol, do *not* have pomegranate juice or extract. It may interact with the medication, similar to the way grapefruit interacts. (Then again, it may not, but the jury is still out, and better safe than lawsuit.)

By drinking raw sauerkraut juice once a day, you should avoid getting the flu. (It's also a good way to avoid constipation.)

Move to the North Pole for the winter. None of the standard cold- and flu-causing microorganisms can survive there. The problem is, you might not be able to, either.

FLU: TREATMENT AND PREVENTION

The second you feel like you're coming down with the flu, take 1 tablespoon of liquid lecithin (available at health food stores). Continue to take 1 tablespoon every 8 hours for the next two days. Some naturopaths believe that these large doses of lecithin may prevent the flu virus from flourishing.

This formula was handed down from generation to generation by a family who tells of the many lives it saved in Stuttgart, Germany, during the 1918 flu epidemic.

Fever

Thomas Sydenham, a seventeenth-century English physician, said, "Fever is Nature's engine which she brings into the field to remove her enemy."

It seems as though research scientists are agreeing with Dr. Sydenham with regard to fevers below 104 degrees Fahrenheit.

Dr. Matthew J. Kluger, author of *Molecular Mechanics of Fever* and one of the leading researchers of fever therapy, recommends that fever be allowed to run its course and that it may actually shorten the duration of an illness. Studies at the University of Texas Health Science Center in Dallas showed that fever supports antibiotic therapy. And researchers at the Yale University School of Medicine proved that patients with fever are less contagious than those with the same infection but who have suppressed their fever with medication.

Now then, you decide whether or not fever is friend or foe. If you're intent on lowering the fever, you may want to try one or more of the following:

Place an ice pack under your arm or on your groin area. When either spot is iced, your body will cool down in no time.

After coating the bottoms of the feet with a thin layer of petroleum jelly, bind sliced onions or peeled garlic cloves to the bottoms of the feet, using an Ace bandage or handkerchief to keep them in place. Don't be surprised if you have onion or garlic on your breath. And don't be surprised if it brings down your temperature.

Eat grapes (in season) throughout the day. Also, dilute pure grape juice and sip some of it throughout the day. Drink it at room temperature, never chilled.

Boil 4 cups (1 quart) of water with 1 teaspoon of cayenne pepper. As you're ready to drink each of these 4 cups throughout the day, add to each cup 1 teaspoon of honey and ¼ cup of orange juice. Heat it up just a little and then drink it slowly.

Stuffed Nose

Since this remedy is less than attractive, we suggest that you do it in the privacy of your bathroom and spare those around you.

Cut four thin-as-can-be strips of orange rind. Put two strips back-to-back with the white spongy part (the pith) on the outside, and stick it in your nostril. Be sure to leave orange rind sticking out of your nose so you can easily dislodge them. Do the same with the other two strips. Stay that way for 5 to 10 minutes, then gently remove the rind. It should feel and have a mentholatum effect, clearing up your nasal congestion.

Runny Nose

The first of our five senses to develop is our sense of smell. Eventually, the average human nose can recognize ten thousand different odors, but not when we have a head cold.

While cold weather, spicy food, and hormonal changes can trigger a runny nose, mostly it's the body stepping up mucus production in an effort to clear cold or flu viruses or allergens from your nasal passages.

Glands in your nose and sinuses continually produce mucus—as much as 1 to 2 quarts a day. The mucus cleans and moisturizes your nasal membranes and helps fight infection.

Here's a strange remedy that may help stop your runny nose and clear up your cold. Begin by cutting the crust off a piece of bread. Turn your iron to "hot"—the wool or cotton setting. Iron the bread crust. (You read that correctly.) When the crust begins to burn, lift the iron off the crust and carefully—very carefully—inhale the smoke through your nostrils for a couple of minutes. Repeat the procedure three times throughout the day. We've been told that the runny nose stops and the head cold clears up in a short time—one or two days. What we weren't told is how in the world someone discovered this remedy!

SORE THROAT

The trouble with sore throats is that each swallow is a painful reminder that you have a sore throat.

Some sore throats are caused by allergies, smoking, postnasal drip, yeast overgrowth, or a mild viral infection that attacks when your resistance is low.

If you have a sore throat right now, think about your schedule. Chances are you've been pushing yourself like crazy, multitasking, running around, and sleep-

ing a lot less than the recommended 8 hours a night.

If you take it easy, get lots of rest, flush your system by drinking nondairy liquids throughout the day, and stay away from heavy meals, the remedies we suggest will be much more effective.

NOTE: If there's fever and the presence of enlarged lymph nodes below the angles of the jaw, as well as the continuation of throat soreness, you may need medical attention. Call your health professional immediately, report your symptoms, and set up an appointment.

Sore Throat Gargles and Drinks

When it comes to getting rid of a sore throat, this remedy is our first line of defense. Add 2 teaspoons of apple cider vinegar to 1 cup of warm water. Gargle a mouthful, spit it out, then swallow a mouthful. Gargle a mouthful, spit it out, then swallow a mouthful. (Notice a pattern forming here?) Keep this up until the liquid is all gone. An hour later, start all over.

Chances are you may not have to do it for more than a couple of hours. Yes, that's how quickly this remedy may work. And trust us, you will get used to the taste of apple cider vinegar.

A singer we know says this works for her every time she has a sore throat. Steep 3 tea bags—black or green—in a cup of just-boiled water. Leave them there until the water is as dark as it can get.

While the water is still quite hot but bearable, gargle with the tea. *Do not swallow any of it.* No one needs all that caffeine. Repeat every hour until you feel relief.

Next time you wake up with that sore throat feeling, add 1 teaspoon of sage to 1 cup of just-boiled water. Steep for 3 to 5 minutes and strain.

Gargle in the morning and at bedtime. It would be wise to swallow the sage tea while gargling, instead of spitting it out.

When we were growing up, the words that would follow "Ma, my throat hurts" were "I'll get the honey and lemon." Mom would add the juice of 1 lemon to a glass of hot water (our family was very big on having hot drinks in a glass) and then sweeten to taste with honey—about 1½ tablespoons. We'd have one of these brews every 4 hours. It usually worked . . . and it tastes good with toast and jam.

Syrups and Elixirs

Mix ¼ cup of apple cider vinegar with an equal amount of honey. Take 1 tablespoon six to eight times a day.

This elixir is particularly effective for a sore throat that's part of a cold.

External Sore Throat Treatments

For this classic folk remedy, warm ½ cup of coarse (kosher) salt in a frying pan. Then carefully pour the warm salt into a large, clean white sock or handkerchief. If you use a handkerchief, fold it so that none of the salt can seep out. Wrap the salt-filled sock or hanky around your neck and wear it that way for an hour.

This was one of our great-aunt's favorite remedies. The only problem was she would get laryngitis explaining to everyone why she was wearing a sock around her neck.

Prepare chamomile tea. As soon as it cools enough for you to handle, soak a towel, preferably white, in the tea, wring it out, and apply it to the throat. As soon as it gets cold, reheat the tea, redip the towel, and reapply it.

The chamomile will help draw out the soreness; the heat will relax some of the tension built up in that area.

Exercise

We came across a beneficial exercise to do when you have a sore throat. Stick out your tongue for 30 seconds, put it back in, and relax for a couple of seconds. Then stick out your tongue again for another 30 seconds. Do it five times in a row and it will increase blood circulation, help the healing process, and make you the center of attention at the supermarket.

A Gem of an Idea

According to a gem therapist, wearing yellow amber around your neck will help heal a sore throat. The electromagnetic powers of this fossilized golden resin are also said to help prevent a sore throat if you wear it daily.

Strep Throat: Do You Have It?

Strep throat is caused by streptococcal bacteria, some causing more serious conditions than others. If your sore throat is part of a cold, with coughing, sneezing, and a runny or stuffy nose, chances are it is not strep throat.

The common symptoms of strep are a sudden, severe sore throat, swollen tonsils and lymph nodes, pain when you swallow, fever, and white or yellow spots on the back of a bright red throat.

For a proper diagnosis, go to a doctor. Chances are you will be given antibiotics. They shorten the duration of it, reduce the severity of symptoms and the risk of complications, and decrease the length of contagion time.

POSSIBLE CAUSES

Do you have a dog or a cat? If you do and you're troubled by frequent bouts of strep throat, have a veterinarian examine the animal for streptococci. Once your pet is free of the bacteria, chances are you will be, too, after treatment by your health professional.

Are we all grown-ups here? Okay: If you participate in oral sex, have your partner's *part* checked. It may help you find out why you keep getting strep throat.

LARYNGITIS (HOARSENESS)

Rest your vocal cords as much as possible. If you have to talk, talk in a normal voice, letting the sound come from your diaphragm instead of your throat. *Do not whisper!* Whispering tightens the muscles of your voice box and puts more stress on your vocal cords than does talking in your normal voice.

Drink a cup of hot, strong peppermint tea with a teaspoon of honey. It's relaxing for the entire body as well as for the throat. It also will help with digestion.

In 1 cup of water, simmer ½ cup of raisins for 20 minutes. Let it cool, then eat and drink it all. This is a Tibetan remedy. It must work—we've never met anyone from Tibet with laryngitis.

When you're hoarse and hungry, eat baked apples. To prepare them, core 4 apples and peel them about halfway down from the top. Place them in a greased dish with about ½-inch of water. Drop 1 teaspoon of raisins into each apple core, then drizzle 1 teaspoon of honey into each core and over the tops of the apples. Cover and bake in a 350-degree oven for 40 minutes, basting a few times with the pan juices.

Eat the apple while it's still warm, or at room temperature. An apple a day . . . you know the rest.

Grate radishes or daikon and squeeze them through cheesecloth to get radish juice. Let 1 teaspoon of the juice slide down your throat every half hour.

If your cold seems to have settled in your throat in the form of hoarseness and congestion, peel and mince an entire head of garlic. Cover all the little pieces with raw honey and let it stand for 2 hours. Take a teaspoon of the honey/garlic mixture every hour. Just swallow it down without chewing the garlic. That way you won't have garlic on your breath. In case you're wondering, the honey-garlic combination actually tastes good . . . if you like honey and garlic.

See the apple cider vinegar remedy above under "Sore Throat Gargles and Drinks." After 7 hours and seven doses of the vinegar and water, and a good night's sleep (although with all that vinegar and water, your sleep may be interrupted with trips to the bathroom), there should be a major improvement by morning.

TONSILLITIS

Tonsils: Good

The holistic health professionals we talked to believe that tonsils should not be removed unless it's absolutely necessary. They function as armed guards, destroying harmful bacteria that enter through the nose and mouth. Asian medical practitioners feel that when tonsils are unable to fulfill this function, it's not that the tonsils should be taken out; it's that the body's immune system needs to be strengthened.

> **NOTE:** If you keep getting tonsillitis, have your immune system evaluated and treated. Be aware that untreated bacterial tonsillitis may have serious consequences, including rheumatic fever, scarlet fever, or even kidney disease (nephritis).

Tonsillitis: Bad

When your tonsils are swollen, with or without white patches on them, juice garlic cloves (see "Preparation Guide") so that you have 1 tablespoon of fresh garlic juice. Add the juice and 2 ounces of dried sage to 1 quart of water in a glass or enamel pot. Cover the pot and bring the mixture to a boil. As soon as it starts to boil, turn off the heat and let it stand until it's lukewarm. Strain the solution. Drink ½ cup of this sage-garlic tea every 2 hours. Gargle ½ cup every hour until swelling and pain disappear.

⟩ Bake a medium-size banana in its skin for 30 minutes at 350 degrees. Peel and mash the banana, adding 1 tablespoon of extra-virgin olive oil. Spread the mush on a clean white cloth and apply it to the neck. Leave it on for a half hour in the morning and a half hour in the evening. You may want to take a warm shower right after you remove the oily banana.

THROAT TICKLE

Take your pick: throat tickle or numb tongue? Chewing a couple of whole cloves will relieve throat tickle, but it will also leave you with a numb tongue for a little while.

⟩ Eat a piece of well-done whole-wheat toast to put an end to that throat tickle.

SCALDED THROAT

Swallow 2 teaspoons of extra-virgin olive oil to soothe and coat the throat.

CONSTIPATION

You are most likely reading this page because you're seeking a natural laxative. Therefore, you may already know that some of the commercial chemical laxatives can kill friendly bacteria, lessen the absorption of nutrients and get rid of necessary vitamins, stuff up the intestinal walls, habituate your intestines to need the laxatives, and eventually *cause* constipation.

We offer easy-to-take, inexpensive, non-chemical constipation relievers that should not present any problematic side effects if taken in moderation, using good common sense.

NOTE: If, after trying these remedies, you still have a persisting problem, check it out with your health professional to prevent it from becoming a major health problem.

ELIMINATING POSSIBLE CAUSES

If you take a daily multivitamin, check the ingredients on the label. If it contains iron, find a new multivitamin. Not only can it cause constipation, but the unneeded extra iron may increase the risk of colorectal (colon and rectum) problems. If you're a woman of childbearing age, check with your doctor before eliminating a multivitamin with iron.

Are you taking calcium carbonate supplements? If you are, good. If you're taking them all at once, not so good. To be sure they do not cause you to be constipated, take half the amount with lunch and the other half with dinner. Yes, always with meals. It may also help your body better absorb the calcium. And remember not to eat chocolate right before, with, or after the calcium supplements. Chocolate can prevent the proper absorption of calcium.

START THE DAY

The most natural time to move your bowels is within a few hours of arising. Drinking water on an empty stomach stimulates peristalsis—the wave-like action that carries food and waste products through the gastrointestinal tract to the rectum—and makes you feel like you gotta go.

Before breakfast, drink the juice of half a lemon in 1 cup of warm water. While it may help cleanse your system, it may also make you pucker a lot. If you find it hard to drink, sweeten it with honey.

If lemon and water are not for you, try any one of the following at room temperature (not chilled).

- Drink prune juice or eat stewed prunes.

- Eat a portion of papaya.

- Soak 6 to 8 dried figs or dates overnight in a glass of water. In the morning, drink the water, then eat the figs or dates.

- Scrub and eat 2 small beets in the morning. You should have a bowel movement 12 hours later.

- Mix 1 teaspoon of blackstrap molasses in ½ cup of warm water and drink an hour before lunch.

MORE EDIBLE MILD LAXATIVES

Flaxseed is a popular folk treatment for constipation. Sprinkle 1 to 2 tablespoons on your cereal or oatmeal, or mix it in a glass of water and drink it down right after lunch or dinner.

Salba (available at health food stores) can also be sprinkled on food, or mixed in a beverage for healthful, fast, and effective relief. (Learn more about the benefits of Salba in the "Food for Thought" chapter.)

🌿 Eat at least three raw fruits a day. One of the three, preferably an apple, should be eaten 2 hours after dinner.

🌿 The findings of recent studies say that monounsaturated fatty acids—the kind found in olive oil—are best for lowering cholesterol levels. Olive oil is also a help when a laxative is needed. Take 1 tablespoon of extra-virgin olive oil in the morning and 1 tablespoon an hour after eating dinner.

🌿 For some people, brewer's yeast and wheat germ do the trick. (Both are available at health food stores.) Gradually work your way up to a maximum of 1 heaping teaspoon of brewer's yeast and 1 heaping teaspoon of wheat germ with each meal. Stop increasing the amount when what you're taking gets results.

🌿 Hippocrates, the father of medicine, recommended eating garlic every day to relieve constipation. Cook with it and/or eat it raw in salads whenever possible.

🌿 Two natural laxatives available at your greengrocer are escarole (eat it raw, or boil it in water and drink the water as well as eating the escarole) and Spanish onion (roast it and eat it at bedtime). The cellulose in escarole and onions as well as cabbage and broccoli gives intestinal momentum.

🌿 Raw spinach makes a delicious salad, has lots of vitamins and minerals, and is a mild laxative, too. Be sure to wash the spinach thoroughly, even if it's organic (see "Pesticide Removal for Fruits and Vegetables" in "Preparation Guide").

ACUPRESSURE

We were told about an acupressure technique that is hard to believe but worth a try. It is supposed to encourage a complete evacuation in 15 minutes. For 3 to 5 minutes, massage the area underneath your lower lip, in the middle of your chin.

BEDTIME

Just as you're falling asleep, when your mind is most open to autohypnotic suggestion, say to yourself, "In the morning, I will have a good bowel movement." Keep repeating the sentence until you doze off. Pleasant dreams!

COLON CLEANSING

For those of you who feel you need a good colon cleansing and are not planning to go out for a while, drink 8 ounces of raw sauerkraut juice (available with sauerkraut at health food stores). Follow the sauerkraut juice with 8 ounces of unsweetened grapefruit juice, one right after the other. It should do the job. Okay, so it may rip your throat out in the process.

CAUTION: If you're taking medication, check with your doctor or pharmacist about negative grapefruit-drug interaction.

STOOL SOFTENER

Every night, before eating dinner, eat 1 tablespoon of raisins or 3 prunes that have been soaking in water for a couple of hours.

COUGHS

n the morning, when the doctor examined her patient, she remarked, "I'm happy to say your cough sounds much better."

The patient answered, "Well, it should. I had a whole night of practice."

This may be a joke, but it's not funny if you're the one who's coughing, especially at night, when coughs seem to act up.

We all have a cough center in our brain. It's generally stimulated by an irritation in the respiratory tract. In other words, a cough is nature's way of helping us loosen and get rid of mucus that's congesting our system.

Read on for remedies that may quell the cough and help you (and everyone around you) sleep through the night.

NOTE: If the cough persists, have it checked by a health professional.

SYRUPS

Combine the juice of 1 lemon, 1 cup of honey, and ½ cup extra-virgin olive oil and cook for 5 minutes over medium heat. Then stir vigorously for a couple of minutes and bottle the mixture. Take 1 teaspoon every 2 hours.

Peel and finely chop 6 medium onions. Put them and ½ cup of honey into the top of a double boiler or in a pan over a pot of boiling water. Cover the mixture and let it simmer for 2 hours. Strain this concoction, which we call "honion" syrup, and pour it into a jar with a cover. Take 1 tablespoon every 2 to 3 hours.

A similar but different enough syrup: Preheat the oven to 400 degrees. Take a couple of large beets. Do not wash them because moisture will cause the beets to steam and you don't want that. Just wipe off the dirt with a paper towel. Cut a deep hole in the middle of each beet and put the beets in a foil-lined casserole dish. Fill the holes with honey or brown sugar. Cover the beets completely with foil and bake them until they're soft (an hour or two, depending on their size and the efficiency of your oven). Once the beets are tender, it's easy to peel away the skin, and a treat to eat the beet, along with the syrup, whenever you feel a cough coming on.

Grate 1 teaspoon of horseradish and mix it with 2 teaspoons of honey. (In place of horseradish, you can use 1 finely chopped clove of garlic.) Take 1 teaspoon every 2 to 3 hours.

Combine ½ cup of apple cider vinegar with 1 cup of water. Add 1 teaspoon of cayenne pepper and sweeten to taste with honey. Bottle it. When the cough starts acting up, take 1 tablespoon of this mixture. Take another tablespoon at bedtime.

BEAN PUREE

This remedy seems to work on those mean, down-deep coughs that are hard to reach. Put 1 cup of kidney beans in a strainer and rinse them with water. Then put them in water and let them soak overnight (while you probably cough your head off). Next morning, drain the beans, tie them up in a clean cloth, and bruise them by pounding them with a blunt object such as a rolling pin, frying pan, or hammer. Place the bruised beans in an enamel or glass saucepan with 3 cloves of garlic, peeled and minced, and 3 cups of water. Bring the mixture to a boil, then simmer for 1½ to 2 hours, until beans are tender. Puree, adding more water if necessary. If, by the time you prepare this puree, your cough isn't gone, take 1 tablespoon of it the second your cough acts up.

DRINKS

For a delicious, thirst-quenching, and soothing drink, squeeze the juice of 1 lemon into a big mug or glass. Add hot water, 2 tablespoons of honey, 3 whole cloves, and/or ½ piece of stick cinnamon. Cover, let it steep for about 15 minutes, and drink the entire glassful. Repeat every 3 hours.

Cook 1 cup of barley according to the directions on the package. Add the juice of 1 fresh lemon and some water to the cooked barley. Then liquefy the mixture in a blender. Add honey if you want it sweetened. Drink it slowly—1 cup every 4 hours.

ACUPRESSURE

An acupressure joint that has been known to stop a cough is the one near the end of the middle finger. With the fingers of your right hand, squeeze the top joint of the left hand's middle finger. Keep squeezing until you stop coughing.

FOOTBATH

Right before going to bed, add 1 teaspoon of dry mustard powder to a half-filled bathtub of hot water.

Prepare a hot drink—peppermint or chamomile tea, or any good old lemon and honey combination.

Wear nightclothes that leave your chest accessible. Have two rough terrycloth towels and a comfortable chair or stool in the bathroom.

Sit down and dip your feet in the bathtub water. Keep them there as you slowly sip the tea. When the water cools, add more hot water and keep sipping the tea. After about 15 minutes of dipping and sip-

ping, dunk the towel in the bathwater, wring it out, and place it on your bare chest. Once the towel cools off, dunk it again, wring it out, and place it back on the chest. After dunking and wringing three times, thoroughly dry your feet and chest, bundle up, and go to bed.

PHLEGMY COUGH

To help loosen phlegm, fry 2 finely chopped medium onions in coconut oil or vegetable shortening. As soon as it's cool enough to touch, rub the mixture on the cougher's chest and wrap the chest with a clean (preferably white) cloth. Do this procedure in the evening. This may help the congestion break up during the night while the cougher is enjoying a good night's sleep.

BRONCHIAL COUGH

Add 3 drops of oil of fennel and 3 drops of oil of anise (both available at health food stores) to 6 tablespoons of honey. Shake vigorously and bottle it. Take 1 teaspoon when you start to cough.

If you haven't prepared the syrup in advance of your cough and don't have the necessary ingredients but do have the liqueur called anisette, you may want to settle for second best. Take 1 teaspoon of anisette in 1 tablespoon of hot water every 3 hours.

The polyunsaturated fatty acids in whole-grain oats have been said to soothe bronchial inflammation and relieve coughing spasms.

Make a mash from the oats by following the directions on the oats box, but reduce the amount of water by ¼ cup. Add honey to taste.

Eat 1 cup at a time, four times a day, and whenever a coughing spell starts. Be sure the oat mash is eaten warm.

Take a piece of brown grocery-bag paper, about the size of your chest, and soak it in distilled white vinegar. When it stops dripping, sprinkle black pepper on one side of the paper. Then place the peppered side on your bare chest. To keep it in place overnight, wrap a wide Ace bandage or cloth around your chest. By morning, don't be surprised if the bronchial cough is just about gone.

Also see the "Children's Health Challenges" chapter under "Coughs."

OVER-THE-COUNTER COUGH MEDICINE

If you insist on using commercial cough medicine, steer clear of suppressants that contain dextromethorphan. It will prevent you from coughing up stuff your body should get rid of. You don't want the phlegm to stay in your lungs where it can cause a bad secondary infection. So if you're going the over-the-counter route, look for an expectorant with the ingredient guaifenesin, a chemical that will make it easier for you to cough up and get rid of the yucky stuff you don't want.

NERVOUS COUGH

We know a stage manager who wants to give remedies to each audience member before the curtain goes up. If the producer let him, he would announce: "To stop nervous-type coughs, apply pressure to the area between your lip and your nose. If that doesn't work, press hard on the roof of your mouth. If neither works, please wait till intermission, then go outside and cough."

SMOKER'S COUGH

This remedy is updated from the 1888 *Universal Cookery Book*. Pour 1 quart of just-boiled water over 4 tablespoons of whole flaxseed and steep for 3 hours. Strain, then add the juice of 2 lemons and sweeten with honey (which replaces the crystals of rock candy used in the original remedy). Take 1 tablespoon of the syrupy mixture when the cough acts up.

An even better remedy for smoker's cough: Stop smoking! (See the "Smoking" chapter.)

TICKLING COUGH

Many people are bothered by a tickling-type cough, usually at night in their sleep. Put 2 teaspoons of apple cider vinegar in a glass of water and keep it by your bedside. When the tickling wakes you up, swallow 1 or 2 mouthfuls of the vinegar water and go back to a restful sleep.

DEPRESSION

Just about everyone goes through less-than-happy times, ranging from short-term blue moods to extended periods of depression. Why?

Maybe it's the weather, or a change of season. For women, it could be that time of month. It's depressing to have a job you don't like. It's more depressing to be out of work. What about failed relationships? Talk about depressing! Then there are additives in foods and side effects from medications that can cause chemical imbalances that can lead to depression.

Whatever the reason, when you're going through a bad time and you reach the point where you say to yourself, "I'm sick and tired of feeling sick and tired," good for you. You're ready to do something about it.

CAUTION: For cases of deep depression, we suggest you seek professional assistance to help pinpoint the cause and recommend treatment.

Start by taking better care of yourself, and know that you're worth it. Cut down on your sugar intake. Excessive sugar can fuel your depression by giving you spurts of energy followed by extreme fatigue and that let-down feeling of depression. Cigarettes, alcoholic beverages, and excessive caffeine in coffee and cola may also contribute to depression by producing unnerving highs and lows. Take them out of your life. They may be taking the life out of you!

We're sure you already know this, but as a reminder, eat a sensible diet of whole grains, steamed green vegetables, lean meat and fish, and raw garlic in big salads with onion and lots of celery. (Celery has phthalide, a chemical known to have sedative properties good for healing a broken heart.) Have sunflower seeds, raisins, sauerkraut, whole-wheat pasta, and beans. What could be bad?

For cases of deep depression, seek professional assistance to help pinpoint the cause.

Meanwhile, here are some suggestions that may lift you out of your (temporary) funk.

FOOD AND DRINK

To lighten a heavy heart, drink a cup of thyme tea, sweetened with honey.

Have a pizza with lots of oregano. If you don't have the oregano, forget the pizza. In fact, forget the pizza and just have the oregano. Stir some of the herb into a glass of water and drink it down. It has a way of lifting one's spirits.

SUPPLEMENT

SAM-e (S-adenosyl-L-methionine) is a natural substance produced by the body and seems to be one of the best-documented natural antidepressants available in supplement form. It is fast-acting and is said to be a safe, effective alternative to Prozac.

Researchers' information that we've read seems to agree that no serious negative side effects have ever been reported with SAM-e. In fact, many say that the side effects are all beneficial, such as promoting healthy joint function, helping relieve joint pain, strengthening the liver, and aiding the cardiovascular system.

SAM-e is available at health food and vitamin stores. Follow the recommended dosage on the label. Take it and expect to notice a boost in your mood and emotional well-being.

BATH TIME RITUAL

While running a warm bath, prepare a cup of chamomile tea. Add the used tea bag to the bath, along with a new one. If you use loose chamomile, wrap the herb in cheesecloth before putting it in the tub to avoid messy cleanup. Once the bath is ready, take pen and paper along with your cup of tea. As you relax in the warm water, sipping your tea, make a list of a dozen wishes. Be specific and detailed . . . and be careful. Know that by preparing the list, you are setting things in motion, and the things you wish for may come true.

IT'S UP TO YOU!

Abraham Lincoln said, "Most folks are as happy as they make up their minds to be." Not that he was a barrel of laughs, but his words are wise and true.

If you're mildly depressed and don't want to be, simply change your physiology and your emotions will follow suit. In other words, do the physical things you do when you're happy and you'll get happy. Smile! Laugh! Jump up and down! Sing! Dance! Get dressed up!

If you're not willing to go along with this suggestion, then you're not willing to let go of your depression. There's nothing wrong with staying in a funk as long as you understand that it is your choice.

◗ Cheer yourself up by wearing rose colors—pinks and scarlets. Colors in the orange family are also pick-me-ups.

DIABETES

While I (Joan) was growing up, my father always said to me, "Joany, you're one in a million!" Now, having been diagnosed with type 2 diabetes, it turns out that I'm one of 20.8 million.

Diabetes is a disease in which the blood glucose (sugar) levels are too high. Glucose comes from the foods you eat. Insulin is a hormone that helps the glucose get into your cells to give them energy.

The two most common types of diabetes are type 1 (insulin-dependent) diabetes mellitus, when the body does not make any insulin, and type 2 (non-insulin-dependent) diabetes mellitus, when the body does not make enough insulin or doesn't use insulin well. Without enough insulin being properly used, the glucose stays in the blood. Having too much glucose in the blood is what can cause serious problems.

Anyone can get any type of diabetes at any age. It is for that reason the American Diabetes Association (ADA) changed the name from "juvenile-onset" to "type 1," and from "adult-onset" to "type 2."

According to the ADA (www.diabetes .org), 7 percent of the U.S. population, including children, have diabetes. Nearly one-third of those people (6.2 million) have not yet been diagnosed, which means they are probably not taking appropriate and proper care of themselves, and are at risk for serious problems, often referred to as complications, related to diabetes.

NOTE: If diabetes runs in your family, or if anyone you know has one or more symptoms—unusual thirst, frequent urination, blurred vision, unexplained weight loss, constant fatigue—tell them to make the phone call for an appointment to be tested. All it takes is a simple blood test to be diagnosed.

Through the years, since being diagnosed, I've done so much reading, researching, interviewing, experimenting, and participating in diabetes groups, desperately wanting to eliminate or at least completely control this condition. No one said it was going to be easy. And it isn't! But each new day brings new ways to make diabetes more manageable.

Ideal is to have an endocrinologist, diabetes educator and/or nutritionist, and physical trainer who will help you discover the treatment plans that work best for you. Then you keep careful records of your daily diet, blood sugar numbers (with the help of a glucometer—available through your health insurance company and at pharmacies), food intake, and exercise routine. Have your health care providers monitor your results on a regular basis (about every three months) and make the necessary adjustments to fine-tune it all.

If you don't have that kind of health care support system (and who does?), it is up to you to do the right thing for yourself. Remember, information is knowledge, and knowledge is power! Learn about your choices of eating plans by having a session with a diabetes educator or nutritionist (ask your insurance company for names in your area). Go to your local library or bookstore and browse through the books in the health/diabetes section. To give you a head start, there's a book list at the very end of this chapter.

After reading the brief descriptions of some books we've listed, it should be clear that to control diabetes, you need a food plan, weight control, exercise, and possibly prescribed medicine. Our plan is to steer you in the right direction in terms of ways to find all of the above.

Meanwhile, for the rest of this chapter, Lydia and I would like to share with you the helpful tips and treats and things we've discovered along the way.

Please know that we've checked out everything included here as thoroughly as possible, and we're being as discerning as possible, reporting only the information and items we truly believe might help. Keep in mind that both of us are researchers and writers who are reporting, not prescribing. Please proceed with caution, and with the approval of your health care provider.

> **NOTE:** What works for one diabetic may not be as good for another. Be sure to test your blood sugar reaction after introducing a new food or supplement into your diet.

FEET

Every piece of literature about managing diabetes stresses foot care. Follow simple precautions, such as:

- *Never* walk barefoot.
- After showering or bathing, wipe your feet thoroughly, particularly in between your toes.
- Inspect your feet daily (in the morning and/or at night). If you have a cut, bruise, or infection of any kind, get to a podiatrist immediately.
- Have diabetic podiatric examinations at least three times a year.
- Wear shoes that will help protect your feet. Make comfort and safety your priority, not fashion.
- Wear socks that don't create too much friction, and that allow moisture to ventilate properly. Researchers at the University of Missouri found that 100 percent cotton socks were the worst in terms of causing friction and trapping humidity. Socks made from nylon or a blend of materials were generally found to be best.

NOTEWORTHY: Crocs is becoming a leader in medical shoes. Check out Crocs Rx, a line of affordable shoes designed for specific medical and therapeutic podiatric considerations, the kinds of considerations associated with diabetes as well as other foot challenges.

There are three distinctive styles in the Crocs Rx line (probably more by the time you read this). All are made from Croslite material, which provides a super grip on wet surfaces and does not absorb moisture, so it stays odor-free and inhibits the growth of bacteria and fungi. All of the shoes have side air portals to keep feet cool and dry (just don't walk through puddles).

- *Cloud* is specifically designed with diabetic feet in mind. They feature a supersoft footbed and roomy toe box, which allows for wearing heavy socks without creating any tightness or pressure points on the foot. The protective front toe cap and elevated heel rim protect the foot from stubbing and bruising. The shoes also accommodate podiatrist-prescribed orthodics.
- *Silver Cloud* contains all of the benefits of the Cloud diabetic comfort shoe, plus an infusion of silver ions that's ideal for anyone susceptible to skin breakdown, ulcers, foot fungus, and infections.
- *Relief* is designed with an ultrasoft shock-absorbing sole and wide toe box. They provide therapeutic relief for plantar fasciitis, bunions, heel pain, and arthritis.

While you're at it, try Crocs' Ortho-cloud socks. They have a double cushion sole—extra padding that protects toes, heel, and the entire bottom of the foot. Also, there's no irritating toe seam.

continued

Their moisture-wicking fibers keep feet cool and dry. I'm wearing a pair of Crocs socks as I write this. They make my feet and legs feel embraced . . . in a good way.

The Crocs Rx shoes and socks are available through podiatrists, online at www.crocsrx.com, or by calling 877-238-4404.

NEUROPATHY

Diabetic neuropathy is nerve damage that affects approximately 50 to 70 percent of people with diabetes. This nasty condition usually impacts the limbs—hands and arms as well as feet and legs. The most common symptoms are tingling, loss of feeling or sensation, muscular weakness, discomfort, pain, immobility, and the unhappiness that accompanies any one of these symptoms.

Neuropathy Pain Reducer

Cayenne pepper has been used for its medicinal and nutritional properties for thousands of years.

In the form of capsaicin cream (available at health food stores), modest relief from diabetic nerve pain may be a shmear away. Do not apply the cream to broken skin.

Neuropathy Reversal

If your endocrinologist is like the typical diabetes doctor, his or her goal for treating diabetic neuropathy is to prevent progression by advising you to be sure to keep your blood-sugar numbers down. If you complain about pain, you may be given a prescription for a painkiller or told to buy an over-the-counter painkiller, both of which have long lists of possible side effects.

FYI: Pain medications work by suppressing the nerve signals and can actually make your neuropathy worse over time (not to mention what the possible side effects can do).

Yes, we're painting a bleak but realistic picture of most health care providers' approach to diabetic neuropathy. If you can identify with this, then it's time to take the lead to help your doctor take care of you.

NOTEWORTHY: There is a treatment that can relieve your pain and numbness, actually restore the feeling in your feet and hands, restore your balance and mobility, and reduce or eliminate the need for pain medication.

Internationally recognized electronic medical device inventor David B. Phillips, Ph.D. (inventor of the very first infrared ear thermometer), set out to create a device to help his father, who had peripheral neuropathy after heart surgery. Dr. Phillips discovered that nerves can be rebuilt and, in some cases, full function restored.

His invention, the ReBuilder Electronic Stimulator system, can be used in the comfort of your home, and provides a unique, nonsurgical treatment that is noninvasive, has no side effects, and (most important) can rebuild your nerves to stop numbness and pain while increasing blood flow to your legs and feet to support the nutritional needs of these newly awakened nerves. It can increase calf muscle strength to restore your mobility and help restore balance. Another important benefit is that it causes the brain to release endorphins, putting you in a much happier state of mind.

There's a lot more to say about the many benefits of the ReBuilder, but if you've read this far, you should know whether or not you're seriously interested in it. So if you are, we suggest you visit the ReBuilder Web site, www.rebuildermedical.com, to learn more, see Dr. Phillips' video interviews and demonstration, and to help you decide if you want to start rebuilding with a ReBuilder. The machine can also be used on the lower back, hands, and shoulders.

ReBuilder Medical Technologies has full-time, licensed medical professionals on staff to answer your questions and explain whatever you need to know. (We know from experience that they're very patient.) And the company offers a thirty-day money-back guarantee. Telephone 866-725-2202.

NUTRIENTS: GLUCOSE-LOWERING AGENTS

The goal of this category is to make you aware of supplements—herbs and minerals—known to help lower blood-sugar levels. Your mission, should you decide to accept it, is to talk to your diabetes team—doctor, diabetes educator, nutritionist, health food store manager (you should have at least two of the four)—for their feedback and dosage recommendations.

- *Gymnena sylvestre.* This plant from India has been credited with blocking the absorption of simple sugars, helping prevent elevated glucose levels, and regenerating the insulin-producing pancreatic tissues.

- *Banaba leaf.* This Asian plant contains corosolic acid, said to help fine-tune the damaged insulin receptor that is the cause of insulin-resistance diabetes. The corosolic acid in the banaba leaf activates glucose transport into the cells, which results in a lowering of blood sugar.

■ *Bitter melon.* Looking like a cucumber with warts, this tropical fruit has been used in traditional Asian medicine for a long time. Since bitter melon extract is being sold in capsules to help lower blood sugar levels, we would be remiss not to mention it here. We hope you take into consideration that while research and studies are being conducted, until there is conclusive scientific evidence of bitter melon's effectiveness, you should proceed with caution and the advice of a knowledgeable health care provider.

■ *Chromium.* This trace mineral, in the form of chromium picolinate or polynicolinate, makes insulin work more efficiently and facilitates the uptake of glucose into the cells. While supplements are available, you can also get chromium from broccoli, black pepper, dried beans, and whole grains.

■ *Magnesium.* The most common condition associated with low magnesium is diabetes. An adequate amount of magnesium (about 350 mg daily) can improve insulin resistance and blood sugar control. According to one study, magnesium citrate is well absorbed. Supplement your supplement by eating magnesium-rich foods such as green leafy vegetables, legumes, nuts, and whole grains.

■ *Alpha-lipoic acid.* This potent antioxidant helps with glucose utilization and supports peripheral nerves.

■ *Vanadium.* According to Julian Whitaker, M.D., founder of the Whitaker Wellness Institute (www.whitakerwellness.com), America's largest alternative medical clinic, "The single most effective and intriguing weapon for combating diabetes is vanadium. This unique trace mineral lowers blood sugar by mimicking insulin and improving the cells' sensitivity to insulin. Supplemention with vanadyl sulfate and other vanadium compounds markedly lowers fasting glucose and improves other measures of diabetes. Vanadium is quite safe. I and other physicians have utilized vanadyl sulfate with thousands of diabetic patients in doses of 100–150 mg per day with remarkable success and absolutely no adverse reactions, save slight GI distress in a few individuals."

CAUTION: Dr. Whitaker advises you to monitor your blood sugar levels carefully when you first start taking vanadyl sulfate, and let your doctor know what you're doing because blood sugar levels drop dramatically in some people.

■ *Milk thistle*. Generally linked to the treatment of liver problems, this flowering herb seems to be blossoming into a remedy for diabetics. The herb's active component, silymarin, may be helpful in lowering blood sugar levels and reducing the amount of sugar bound to the hemoglobin in a diabetic's blood.

■ *Sage*. Laboratory studies report that sage has been shown to help boost insulin activity in non-insulin-dependent type 2 diabetics. If you want to see if it works for you, keep taking your meds, and whenever you drink a cup of sage tea (up to 3 cups a day), check your blood sugar number. If your numbers seem to be going down consistently and significantly, work with your health care provider to reduce your medication dosage.

To prepare sage tea for the day, put 3 tablespoons of sage leaves in a pitcher and pour 3 cups of just-boiled water in it. Let it steep for 10 minutes. Strain and drink a cup during or after meals. If you use sage tea bags (instead of loose leaves bought in bulk), use two tea bags for each cup.

■ *Cinnamon*. This spice contains a bioactive component that scientists believe has the potential to help type 2 diabetics. As of this writing, the jury is still out as to whether or not cinnamon significantly decreases blood glucose levels. If you want to see if it works for you, take ¼ teaspoon of cinnamon two to three times a day, in tea, in food, or in capsules. It may take up to forty days to see results.

NOTEWORTHY: Not all cinnamon is created equal. If you appreciate the finer things in life, try Red Ape Cinnamon. It is harvested in Indonesia from cassia trees that are at least twenty years old. The older the tree, the higher the volatile oil content, resulting in a higher-quality cinnamon. This cinnamon is chemical-free and certified organic. After tasting it, you will understand why the country's top chefs use Red Ape Cinnamon. It's special, and so is Kestrel Growth Brands, the company responsible for it. Five percent of profits from sales of their cinnamon are donated to programs dedicated to the protection of orangutans (aka red apes). Visit www.redapecinnamon.com or call 888-343-0002.

■ *Vitamin D*. According to research in Italy, published in the journal *Diabetes Care*, approximately 61 percent of type 2 diabetics suffer from chronic vitamin D deficiency. The *New England Journal of Medicine* (July 2007) reported that studies showed 40 percent of children and nearly 100 percent of the elderly in the United States and Europe were deficient in vitamin D. The lack of vitamin D impairs a person's immunity and ability to produce insulin and respond to insulin.

NOTE: It is very important to have your doctor test your vitamin D level.

Ray D. Strand, M.D. (www.raystrand .com), refers to vitamin D as "the truly essential nutrient." Dr. Strand writes about the difference between DRI (Dietary Reference Intake) levels and what are considered to be optimal levels of nutrients. At the conclusion of Dr. Strand's newsletter about the importance of vitamin D, he says, "Clinical research of vitamin D has now reached a point that we can predictably state that several hundred thousand American lives could be saved each year if people supplemented their diets with 1,000 IU of vitamin D. Begin taking at least 1,000 IU of vitamin D today. Your body will love you for it."

We want to quote Dr. Strand's wonderful words in summing up this entire section: "This is what nutritional medicine is all about. It emphasizes the true health benefits of supplementing a healthy diet with these optimal or advanced levels of nutrients—not RDA levels."

Do not do it alone. Work with a savvy health care professional who can monitor you. If you need such a person, ask for recommendations at your local health food store, diabetes support group, or health insurance company. Keep looking until you find the right person for you.

NOTEWORTHY: Many companies have specialty supplements for diabetes that combine nutrients. One such company is Progressive Research Labs, at www .prlab.com, or call 800-877-0966 for the name of a store in your area that carries their products.

FOOD

Salba: The Just-About-Perfect Food

Dr. Vladimir Vuksan, professor of endocrinology and nutritional sciences, Faculty of Medicine, University of Toronto, has devoted over two decades searching for, finding, and testing dietary therapies. Salba (*Salvia hispanica L.*) is a registered variety of an ancient whole grain plant species belonging to the mint family. Dr. Vuksan has rediscovered the seed and has been studying it with amazing results for diabetics as well as for everyone else.

Total Health Magazine reports that Dr. Vuksan's studies were irrefutable evidence that consumption of Salba results in a simultaneous reduction of blood pressure, body inflammation, and blood clotting, while balancing after-meal blood sugar.

Salba is high in antioxidants, fiber, vegetable protein, and micronutrients (calcium, magnesium, and iron). As if that isn't enough, Salba is the richest whole food source of omega-3 fatty alpha-linolenic acid, which has been shown to be converted to EPA, the heart-protective omega-3 found in fish oil.

This translates into the following health benefits:

■ Promotes cardiovascular health

■ Supports joint function and mobility

■ Great source of fiber for digestive health

■ Assists bowel function and regularity in a gentle way

These are the results of the clinical studies conducted by Dr. Vuksan, using type 2 diabetics:

■ Reduced after-meal blood glucose and plasma insulin levels, improving the glycemic index of any food consumed with Salba

■ Significantly lowered C-reactive protein, a marker for low-grade body inflammation

■ Significantly lowered systolic blood pressure

■ Significantly decreased coagulation (blood thinning)

For those of you interested in reading the astounding results of the first-ever long-term study of Salba on type 2 diabetes patients (who were already taking medication and on dietary therapy for their diabetes), which appeared in the November 2007 issue of the American Diabetic Association's journal, *Diabetes Care*, visit http://care.diabetesjournals.org/cgi/content/full/30/11/2804, or you can order a copy of this study, Manuscript #1144, by calling 800-232-3472.

CAUTION: Continue taking your medication, monitor your blood sugar carefully, and work with your health care provider. Hopefully, your blood sugar numbers will improve and your medication dosage may need to be lowered.

Dosage: The recommended dosage for diabetics is 2 tablespoons of Salba daily.

That's 15 grams, supplying more than 100 percent of the recommended daily intake of omega-3 and omega-6 fatty acids in a perfectly balanced ratio.

NOTEWORTHY: Salba is available in many health food stores, and you can order it on the Internet. The two Salba companies that we wholeheartedly recommend for their integrity in terms of the quality of their ingredients, starting with the highest grade of Salba, are:

- Core Natural Products,
  www.salbausa.com,
  phone 888-895-3603
- Salba Smart Natural Products
  LLC, www.salbasmart.com,
  phone 303-298-3833

PLEASE KNOW: We are not working for either company, but after sampling their products and experiencing positive results, we want to sing the praises of Salba loud and clear . . . and are doing so throughout this book.

Salba comes in several forms: seeds (good tossed on salads, cereal, yogurt), ground (easy to use in food preparation—cooking and baking), oil, and gelcaps. There are also delicious products containing Salba—chips, salsa, tortillas, pretzels, bars—that make great snacks in addition to (not in place of) your daily recommended dose of Salba.

To learn more about incorporating Salba into your daily diet, see the "Food for Thought" chapter and be bedazzled by the rest of Salba's special qualities.

Shopping List Add-Ons

When it comes to food, we keep it simple. Fresh and raw is best. The foods we prepare are usually low in carbohydrates and high in fiber, and we use good fat—olive oil or coconut oil. We season food with garlic, curry, and pepper; on the rare occasions when we need to add salt to a dish, we use Himalayan Crystal Salt (see "High-Quality Energy and Balance and More . . . Much More" in the "Remedies in a Class by Themselves" chapter).

If you were to go food shopping with us, you'd have to have patience. We read every label, paying particular attention to the carb, fiber, fat, and sodium content, as well as the list of ingredients. You should, too. To know exactly what you're eating, you have to know exactly what you're buying.

Here are some foods that pass our label scrutiny:

A GOOD GO-WITH

GG Bran Crispbread is a high-fiber, low-carb, fat-free Scandinavian crispbread.

The official Recommended Dietary Allowance (RDA) of dietary fiber is from 20 to 35 grams daily, depending on age, sex, and reproductive state. Each slice of crispbread has 3 grams of fiber, 3 grams of carbohydrates, and 16 calories. It's wonderful for a snack—dip it in hummus, pair it with a salad, spread soy cheese on it, or dunk it—and a few slices take care of half the recommended fiber for the day. Salad and fruit should easily take care of the other recommended 12 grams of fiber.

Some people think it's a little like cardboard, but when you consider that the fiber count cancels out the carb count, we've learned to love cardboard.

If you can't find GG Bran Crispbread at your local health food store, go to the store locator at www.brancrispbread.com, or call the company directly at 843-522-0833, option 5, and you can buy it by the case.

BEFORE-BED OR DURING-THE-DAY SNACK

Francine Kaufman, M.D., an endocrinologist and past president of the American Diabetes Association, discovered that a mixture containing *uncooked* cornstarch would deliver the gradual conversion to glucose that diabetics need. Clinical studies proved her right. The doctor's formula for a guilt-free, gluten-free snack, with slow-burning carbs, high protein, and low fat, is the first snack bar to help stabilize blood glucose levels for up to 9 hours. The bars come in several delicious flavors.

Dr. Kaufman's ExtendBars may be appropriate for you as an answer to one or more of the following concerns:

■ An ExtendBar before bed can help reduce the chance of nighttime blood sugar dipping too low.

■ If you go to sleep with a normal blood sugar level yet wake up with it much higher, use ExtendBar at bedtime to stabilize your blood sugar through the night and reduce morning highs by 28 percent.

■ Grab an ExtendBar between meals as a snack to control your appetite and reduce calorie consumption at your next meal by 21 percent.

■ ExtendBar provides you with a sustained supply of energy and helps guard against low blood sugar for up to nine hours.

Read more about this sweet treat at www.extendbar.com, or call 800-887-2919.

PASTA POSSIBILITIES

Typically, pasta is a no-no for carb counters. There are four low-carb pastas that may satisfy a craving for pasta without sending blood-sugar numbers soaring . . . if eaten in moderation, of course. (See more about low-carb pastas in the "Weight Control" chapter.)

■ *FiberGourmet Light Pasta.* A 2-ounce (dry) portion has 20 grams of fiber. The pasta is delicious; the portion size is satisfying. If it's not on your local health food store shelf, ask the manager to order it, or order it directly from the company: www.fibergourmet.com, phone 786-348-0081.

■ *Dreamfields.* This line of pasta has twice the fiber, fewer digestible carbohydrates, and a 65 percent lower glycemic index than regular pasta. Its good taste and nutritional benefits make it a healthful option for people with diabetes and for the entire family. Dreamfields is available nationwide in supermarkets and online. For more information and recipe ideas, visit www.DreamfieldsFoods.com or call 800-250-1917.

■ *Miracle Noodle Shirataki Pasta.* This shirataki pasta, made from a healthy soluble plant fiber called glucomannan, has 0 calories and less than 1 gram of carbs per serving size, and is soy free and gluten free. It expands slightly in the stomach, which helps you feel full. The water the shirataki noodles are packed in has a slightly fishy smell that completely disappears when you rinse the noodles for a minute or two in warm water. The noo-

dles have no real flavor but will absorb the flavors of other ingredients or sauce. These products are worth a try, especially since the company has a refund-return policy. Also a portion of their profits goes to the Juvenile Diabetes Research Foundation. Learn about their selection of pasta products at www.miraclenoodle.com or phone 800-948-4205.

NOTEWORTHY: There's no reason to eat low-carb pasta and then kill all the benefits with high-carb ketchup when there's Wholemato Organic Agave Ketchup. The Glycemic Research Institute tested this ketchup and determined that it is low glycemic for diabetics. We determined that this ketchup is delicious, and a little goes a long way. Their Wholemato Organic Agave Spicy Ketchup is addictive! Love it! Find out for yourself: www.wholemato.com or phone 212-220-0039.

■ *House Foods Tofu Shirataki.* This soy version of shirataki says "guilt-free" on the package. One serving has 20 calories, 3 grams of carbs, and 2 grams of fiber. Don't get too excited—the serving is small. Remember, shirataki noodles do not have much taste, but they can satisfy the craving for pasta in soup, or can be seasoned in a stir-fry or served with sauce. Some health food stores, specialty food stores, and even some supermarkets carry shirataki, usually near tofu products or bagged salad greens (always in a refrigerated case). To see the stores in your area that may have this product, click on "Contact Us" at www.house-foods.com or phone 877-333-7077.

EDAMAME

Grown in clusters on bushy branches, edamame are green soybeans. Unlike fully mature soybeans, which can be like little rocks, edamame are easy to eat, and they're delicious. They come frozen or in snack bags, raw or dry roasted. They are high in protein and fiber, low in carbs and fat; what fat they do have is heart-healthy. They make a great snack or side dish. They're available at health food stores and most supermarkets.

As a bonus, soy protein may help reduce insulin resistance, kidney damage, and fatty liver in diabetics.

SUGAR-FREE CHOCOLATE

The entire line of YC Chocolate (www .ycchocolate.com, 800-433-2462) is sugar-free. The cofounder of the company, Diane K. S. Yamate, was inspired by her dad, who is a diabetic and loves chocolate.

The dark chocolate (70 percent cocoa) is also gluten-free, lactose-free, and peanut-free. To help eliminate a laxative effect, a minimal amount of maltitol sweetener is used. Diane stresses the importance of eating the chocolates in small quantities on a full stomach to test your tolerance of the level of their sweetener, maltitol.

The fats are from cocoa butter, a non-cholesterol-raising fat. It contains inulin (helpful in the management of diabetes) and additional probiotic healthful properties.

After interviewing Diane and learning about the integrity of the ingredients in her products, we're thinking YC Chocolate can almost be classified as delicious medication. But seriously . . . As with any new food introduced into your diet, it's a good idea to test your blood sugar a couple of hours after eating it.

SWEET AS SUGAR

Stevia is a nutritional supplement that is made from an intensely sweet extract of natural stevia leaves, said to be thirty times sweeter than sugar. It has no chemicals, zero calories, zero carbohydrates, and a zero glycemic index. Ya gotta love it!

It may take time to wean yourself off your favorite artificial sweetener and get used to stevia, but it seems worth it, even if it's just for the zero glycemic index (GI). The GI ranks foods on how they affect blood sugar levels, measuring how much the blood sugar increases in the two or three hours after eating. A GI value tells you how rapidly a particular carbohydrate turns into sugar; the lower the GI number the better. Stevia's GI is zero as compared to sugar at 70.

Stevia can be used in almost anything, including tea, coffee, whipped cream, yogurt, and smoothies. It's also good for cooking and baking.

We found two companies whose stevia is 100 percent natural—no chemicals, no preservatives: SweetLeaf Stevia, available in single-serving packets as well as liquid, powder, tabs, and concentrate (www.sweet leaf.com, phone 800-899-9908), and Stevita Simply Stevia, available in packets and jars (Stevita offers a free sample at www .stevitastevia.com, phone 800-337-5561).

Look for a selection of stevia products at your local health food store and some supermarkets.

DR. MAO'S HOME REMEDIES

Doctor of Chinese medicine, Taoist antiaging expert (www.taoofwellness.com), and cofounder of Yo San University in Los Angeles, Dr. Maoshing Ni (known as Dr. Mao—www.askdrmao.com) graciously agreed to share the home remedies from his book *Secrets of Self-Healing* (Avery):

▪ Eat a slice of baked pumpkin topped with olive oil and rosemary every day.

▪ Chop ½ medium head of cabbage. Cook the cabbage, 1 diced sweet potato, and ⅓ cup lentils in 8 cups of water for 30 to 45 minutes. Season lightly with herbs and spices and eat as a soup for dinner. Have this dish two to three times a week for a month.

▪ Juice 1 daikon radish, 3 stalks of celery, 1 cucumber, and 1 bunch of spinach. Drink 2 glasses a day.

GEM THERAPY

In *Gifts of the Gemstone Guardians* (Natural Healing Press), author and leading authority on therapeutic gemstones Michael Katz reports on a new field of energy medicine—one that uses the energy emanated by gemstone spheres to heal, nourish, and illuminate all aspects of our lives.

According to Michael Katz, the gems for diabetes support are:

- ▪ Carnelian
- ▪ Citrine
- ▪ Dark green aventurine
- ▪ Light green aventurine
- ▪ Emerald

There is a lot more to it than carrying around a chunk of the appropriate stone. Gemisphere, founded in 1988 by Michael Katz, is regarded as a world-class pharmacy of therapeutic-quality gemstones, offering a wide range of resources for learning how to choose and use these extraordinary healing tools. Visit www .gemisphere.com for a lot of helpful information, including the care and cleansing of the gemstones, or call 800-727-8877 for a free gemstone advisor consultation. Get answers about any aspect of gemstone energy medicine.

WORTHWHILE WEB SITES

Diabetes Health, a magazine whose motto is: "Investigate. Inform. Inspire." www.diabeteshealth.com

Diabetes Action, a research and education foundation. Innovation for prevention, healing and the cure. Have a question? Ask the Diabetes Educator. www.diabetesaction.org

dLife for Your Diabetes Life is the Web site part of the *dLife* TV show. Find lots of good information, recipes, resources and more. www.dlife.com

The American Diabetes Association provides a variety of information to educate the diabetic and the parents of diabetic children. In keeping with the mission of the association (to prevent and cure diabetes and to improve the lives of all people affected by diabetes), they offer free information packets for recently diagnosed diabetics, and free boxes of educational materials for newly diagnosed children. To request a packet, call 800-DIABETES (342-2383). www.diabetes.org

BOOK LIST

Check out the books listed here to get an idea of the range of information and programs available.

■ *Diabetes Survival Guide: Understanding the Facts About Diagnosis, Treatment, and Prevention* by Stanley Mirsky, M.D., and Joan Rattner Heilman (Ballantine). This book can answer many of your questions and give you sensible, easy-to-follow suggestions about what, when, and how much to eat; included are delicious choices.

■ *Beat Diabetes Naturally: The Best Foods, Herbs, Supplements, and Lifestyle Strategies to Optimize Your Diabetes Care* by Michael Murray, N.D., and Michael Lyon, M.D. (Rodale). The goal of this book is to help you balance your blood sugar, drop extra pounds, enhance the effectiveness of medications, and reduce your risk of complications.

■ *Transitions Lifestyle System: Easy-to-Use Glycemic Index Food Guide* by Dr. Shari Lieberman (Square One). The book explains how using the glycemic index can help manage a range of disorders, including diabetes. It answers the most commonly asked questions about carbohydrates, blood glucose, and the glycemic index.

■ *Diabetes for Dummies* by Alan L. Rubin, M.D. (Wiley). Although the third word of the title doesn't apply to you, dear reader, the book clearly states on the cover, "A Reference for the Rest of Us!" And it is a good and comprehensive guide to just about every aspect of diabetes for diabetics and their families.

If you plan on preparing diabetic meals, check out *Diabetes Cookbook for Dummies* by Alan L. Rubin, M.D., with Alison G. Acerra, M.S., R.D., and kitchen assistance from Chef Denise Sharf. The recipes are extremely user-friendly, and each has a nutrition breakdown of calories, carbs, fat, sodium, fiber, protein, cholesterol, and the diabetic exchanges. The book is also chock-full of all kinds of helpful food information, for eating in or out.

■ *The 30-Day Diabetes Miracle* by Franklin House, M.D., Stuart A. Seale, M.D., and Ian Blake Newman (Perigee). The book is based on the Lifestyle Center of America's complete program to stop diabetes, restore health, and build natural vitality. The authors believe that there is no better treatment for diabetes than lifestyle modification. (This program may be more extreme than most, and it has been proven very effective.) To know what to expect, here is an abridged version of the three pillars upon which this book is based:

* Reject the standard American diet (SAD) and adopt a plant-based diet. This means limit or eliminate animal products such as meat, dairy, and eggs. The idea here is to avoid animal fat and animal protein, as well as concentrated calories, all of which are associated with most of our chronic diseases, including diabetes.
* Reject exercise prescriptions based on the myth of "No pain, no gain," and adopt a sensible program of intermittent training. This means you make your body work a little, then you let it rest a little, then you make it work again, and so on. Remember that exercise is medicine.
* Reject the idea that it's too late to change your behaviors, eliminate your "stinkin' victim thinkin'," and adopt the right attitude. This means training your brain to make some big changes and make them stick. You can do this in a few key ways, including getting in touch with answers to the vital question "Good health—for what?" Realize why you want to get better. It's good

to be clear about your goals, set specific target behaviors to reach those goals, and make time and devote resources to reach the goals.

DIARRHEA AND DYSENTERY

DIARRHEA

Diarrhea is a common condition usually caused by overeating, a minor bacterial infection, or mild food poisoning, and sometimes by emotional anxiety or extreme fatigue.

Even a quick and simple bout of diarrhea depletes the system of potassium, magnesium, and sometimes sodium, too, often leaving the sufferer tired, dehydrated, and depressed. It's important to keep drinking during and after a siege in order to avoid depletion and dehydration.

NOTE: If diarrhea persists, it may be a symptom of a more serious ailment. Seek professional medical attention.

Drinks

A West Indian remedy for diarrhea is 1 pinch of allspice in a cup of warm water or milk. A Pennsylvania Dutch remedy is 2 pinches of cinnamon in a cup of warm milk. A Brazilian remedy calls for 2 pinches of cinnamon and 1 pinch of powdered cloves in a cup of warm milk.

The combination of cinnamon and cayenne pepper is known to be very effective in tightening the bowels very quickly. In fact, it probably takes longer to prepare the tea than for it to work.

Bring 2 cups of water to a boil and take it off the heat. Add ½ teaspoon of cinnamon and ¼ teaspoon of cayenne pepper. Let the mixture simmer for 20 minutes. As soon as it's cool enough to drink, have ¼ cup every half hour.

Drink black tea. That's it . . . just black tea. Okay, you can sweeten it with some honey, but don't drink or eat anything else until you're able to stay out of the bathroom for two hours. Then eat a little yogurt, and continue sipping a couple of cups of the black tea for a few more hours.

Add 1 teaspoon of powdered ginger to 1 cup of just-boiled water. Let it cool, then drink it. Do this throughout the day with 3 cups of this ginger tea.

Grate an onion and squeeze it through cheesecloth until you get 2 tablespoons (1 ounce) of onion juice. Take the onion juice every hour, along with 1 cup of peppermint tea.

◗ Since biblical times, the common blackberry plant has been used to cure diarrhea and dysentery. The berry remedy, in one form or another, has been passed down through the generations. Don't be surprised if your neighborhood bartender recommends some blackberry brandy.

Dose: 1 shot glass (1½ tablespoons) of blackberry brandy every 4 hours. Or 6 ounces of blackberry juice every 4 hours. Or 2 ounces (4 tablespoons) blackberry wine every 4 hours.

◗ Lactic acid drinks are effective in treating diarrhea and important in that they replenish the system's supply of friendly intestinal bacteria. Have 1 to 2 glasses of buttermilk, sauerkraut juice, or kefir (found in health food stores). Or eat a portion or two of yogurt with active cultures.

◗ Drink barley water. See the "Preparation Guide" for instructions.

Foods

Scrape a peeled apple with a spoon (preferably nonmetal) and eat the scrapings. In fact, eat no other food but scraped apple until the condition greatly subsides.

◗ Bananas may help promote the growth of beneficial bacteria in the intestine and replace some of the lost potassium. Three times a day, eat a banana that has been soaked in milk.

Supplement

An adsorbent (that's right, *adsorbent*) substance attaches things to its surface instead of absorbing them into itself. Activated charcoal is the most powerful adsorbent known. Charcoal capsules or tablets (available at health food stores) can help stop diarrhea quickly by adsorbing the bacteria or toxins that may have caused the problem. Follow the instructions on the label.

NOTE: Be sure to heed the warning and drug interaction precautions. Activated charcoal is not for everyday use because it adsorbs the vitamins and minerals you need to be healthy.

In place of charcoal, you might eat a slice or two of burned toast.

Acupressure

The navel is an acupressure point for treating diarrhea. Using your thumb or the heel of your hand, press in and massage the area in a circular motion for about 2 minutes.

CHRONIC DIARRHEA

This remedy goes to prove that you can't argue with success. A woman wrote to tell us that Archway Coconut Macaroons—two a day—put an end to her twelve-year bout with diarrhea. She has Crohn's disease, a chronic inflammation of the intestinal wall. Chronic diarrhea is one of the most common and debilitating symptoms of this condition. The woman asked that we include her remedy in our book, hoping it will help others with this problem.

Upon further investigation, we found that Joe Graedon, the People's Pharmacist, also reported on these Archway cookies (found at most supermarkets) and the success many people had with them.

One woman couldn't find the Archway cookies, so she made her own coconut macaroons and they, too, worked like magic. While they don't work for everyone, they may be worth a try.

> **CAUTION:** Take into consideration your dietary needs. The cookies are high in fat and contain sugar, so don't overdo it.

DYSENTERY

All of the above diarrhea remedies may help treat *bacterial* dysentery. However, *amoebic* dysentery (caused by amoebas living in raw green vegetables, usually in foreign countries) and *viral* dysentery are more severe forms and should be diagnosed and treated by a health professional.

Dysentery Prevention

To help prevent bacterial dysentery, two weeks before you travel to a foreign country, eat a finely chopped raw onion in a cup of yogurt every day. Before you dismiss this preventive measure, try it. You may be surprised at how good it tastes. Use plain yogurt that says it contains live or active cultures.

DRINKING TOO MUCH

Drinking alcohol in excess can make you look wrinkled and haggard, destroy vital organs, and in general ruin your life.

For the problem drinker, we strongly recommend the leading self-help organization for combating alcoholism: Alcoholics Anonymous. For more information go to www.aa.org, or check the white pages of the telephone book for your local chapter.

This section offers help for the social

drinker who occasionally has one too many.

SOBERING UP

The following remedies can help sober people up—that is, make them more alert and communicative. However, do not trust or depend on those drinkers' reflexes, especially behind the wheel of a car.

FACT: For every ounce of alcohol you drink, it takes an hour to regain full driving faculties. In other words, if you have 4 ounces of alcohol by 8:00 P.M., you should not drive until at least midnight. Actually, we don't think it's a good idea to drive at all on the same night you've done any drinking. Statistics can bear that out.

If a drunk person imagines that the room is spinning, have him or her lie down on a bed and put one foot on the floor to stop that awful feeling.

Honey contains fructose, which promotes the chemical breakdown of alcohol. If you know that the drunk person is not allergic to honey and is not a diabetic, give him 1 or 2 teaspoons of honey. Follow that up with 1 teaspoon of the sweet treat

every half hour for the next couple of hours.

Try sobering up someone who's tipsy by massaging the tip of his nose.

CAUTION: Stimulation of the tip of the nose can cause vomiting, so don't stand right in front of the person you're sobering up.

HANGOVERS

According to the Chinese:

■ A cup of ginger tea (see "Preparation Guide") will help settle an unsettled stomach caused by a hangover.

■ To relieve eye, ear, mouth, nose, and brain pain from the hangover, knead the fleshy part of the hand between the thumb and the index finger on both hands.

■ For the pounding hangover headache, massage each thumb just below the knuckle.

■ Eating a raw persimmon can also help relieve a hangover headache. If it works for you, and you insist on drinking, make sure it's persimmon season.

To ease the symptoms of a hangover, rub a wedge of lemon on each armpit. (An

M.D. who checked the safety of our reme-dies made a note next to this one in the margin of our manuscript. He wrote, "Great remedy! Helped get me through medical school.")

◗ If the hangover makes you feel like pulling your hair out, good. According to a noted reflexologist, hair pulling is stimu-lating to the entire body and can help lessen the symptoms of a hangover. Just pull your hair, clump by clump, until it hurts a little.

◗ According to Linda Van Horn, Ph.D., R.D., a nutritionist and professor of pre-ventive medicine at Northwestern Univer-sity, when you're throwing up because of a major hangover, it's likely you're low on potassium, calcium, and sodium. The body's depletion of that combination is what leaves you feeling sick and ex-hausted. To restore the potassium, cal-cium, and sodium, drink tomato juice. It's rich in those nutrients. Also, drink water to replace the fluids you've lost.

◗ Hangover sufferers are often advised to "sleep it off." That's smart advice, since a contributing factor to hangovers is the lack of REM (rapid eye movement) sleep, which alcohol seems to suppress. So yes, sleep it off!

◗ If you're anticipating waking up in the morning with a hangover, take a vitamin B complex with two or three glasses of water before you go to bed. If you pass out before remembering to take the B com-plex, when you awaken with a hangover take the vitamin as soon as possible.

Some of the B-complex vitamins—B_1 (thiamine), B_2 (riboflavin), B_3 (niaci-namide), and B_6 (pyridoxine)—are help-ful in aiding carbohydrate metabolizing, nerve functioning, the cellular oxidation process, and the dilation of blood vessels, which can help make your hangover a thing of the past.

MORNING-AFTER BREAKFAST

Banana and milk is the breakfast of choice for many hangover sufferers. It may be ef-fective due to the fact that alcohol depletes the magnesium in one's body, and bananas and milk help replenish the supply.

You may want to add to that tomato, car-rot, celery and/or beet juice to replenish the B and C vitamins along with some trace minerals that alcohol may also deplete.

◗ We were on a radio show in Boston when a caller shared his hangover break-fast that works for him every time: bagel, cream cheese, and lox (smoked salmon). He explained that he's an Irishman who discovered this sure cure after marrying a Jewish woman who served him the sandwich one morning-after-the-night-before, as a typical Sunday brunch.

HANGOVER PREVENTION ADVICE

According to a research team in England, drinkers are advised to guzzle clear alcohols—gin, vodka, or white rum—to lessen the chances of that "morning-after" feeling. Red wine and whiskey seem to have more hangover-promoting elements.

A SURE CURE

If you really need to recover rapidly from a hangover, go to your local doctor, dentist, or hospital, and, under medical supervision, take 10 snorts of oxygen.

INTOXICATION PREVENTION

We're reporting the remedies that supposedly prevent you from getting drunk, but we ask that you please take full responsibility for your drinking. No matter how sober you seem to feel, or which preventive remedies you take, *do not drink and drive*!

▶ Native Americans recommend eating a handful of raw (not roasted) almonds before drinking.

▶ This remedy comes from healers in West Africa. They suggest eating peanut butter before imbibing.

▶ Gem therapists tell of the power of amethysts. In Greek, amethyst is *amethystos,* which translates to "remedy against drunkenness." Please don't take this to mean that if you carry an amethyst and you drink, you won't get drunk. It's that carrying an amethyst should give one the strength to refuse a drink and, therefore, prevent intoxication.

▶ Before you have a drink, sprinkle nutmeg into a glass of milk and sip it slowly. It may help absorb and neutralize the effects of alcoholic beverages.

▶ While cabbage is said to be good for a hangover, according to Aristotle, eating a big chunk of cabbage before imbibing is an effective intoxication preventive.

Eating cole slaw—the combination of cabbage and vinegar—may be even more effective than cabbage alone.

WOMEN, LISTEN UP . . .

As if PMS was not bad enough, women who drink right before menstruating, when their estrogen level is low, get drunk more easily and usually become more nauseated, with rougher hangovers, than during the rest of their cycle. How does that song go? "I enjoy being a girl!"

GREAT ADVICE

The best way to hold your liquor is in the bottle it comes in! What may help you to do that is, when sober, look at a man or woman who is drunk.

EAR CONDITIONS

n the 1700s, satirist and physicist Georg Lichtenberg said, "What a blessing it would be if we could open and shut our ears as easily as we do our eyes."

If your ears are troubling you, keep your eyes open long enough to read the suggestions that follow.

EARACHES

An earache is generally an infection of the middle ear, usually as a result of a cold or the flu. The pain can be out of proportion to the seriousness of the problem . . . or not.

NOTE: If an earache persists, don't turn a deaf ear! Check it out with a health professional.

CAUTION: If your ear is draining—discharging thick or thin liquid material from the canal—it may be that the eardrum has ruptured and there is a potentially serious infection. Do not put anything in your ear. Get medical attention immediately.

There are times when you have an earache and can determine that medical care is not required at that moment. It is only at such times that you should consider the remedies below.

Eardrops

Fill the ear with 3 warm (not too hot) drops of olive oil and plug the ear with a puff of cotton. Do this three or four times a day until the earache is gone.

If you believe in the healing power of garlic and you don't mind the smell, puncture a garlic oil softgel and let the contents ooze into the ear. Gently plug the ear with a puff of cotton. The earache may ease considerably within a half hour.

This remedy is known for its fast relief. Grate fresh ginger and squeeze it through cheesecloth until you have a teaspoon of juice. Mix the juice with an equal amount of sesame oil. Drop 3 drops of the mixture into your ear and plug it with a puff of cotton. Keep it there for a few hours while your ear heals.

On the Ear

Put castor oil on a piece of cotton. Sprinkle the oiled cotton with black pepper and apply it to the aching ear—not *in* the ear canal, *on* the ear. Let it stay there until you get relief.

Mix ½ cup of unprocessed bran (available at health food stores) with ½ cup of coarse (kosher) salt and envelop it in a generous piece of folded-over cheesecloth. In other words, bundle it up so that the contents don't spill all over the place. Then heat it in a low oven until it's warm but bearable to the touch. Place it on the painful ear and keep it there for an hour.

Even though most earache remedies say to put something warm on the ear, herbalist Angela Harris feels that the infection-causing bacteria thrive on warmth, and so her approach is with cold on the ear.

Put an ice pack on the infected ear and, at the same time, put your feet in hot water—as hot as you can stand it without burning yourself. As if that weren't enough, slowly drink a mild laxative herb tea (available at health food stores). Do this cold-on-ear, feet-in-hot, drinking-tea remedy for about 15 minutes, long enough for the pain to be relieved.

Cut a large onion in half. Take out the inside of the onion so that the remaining part will fit over your ear. Warm the onion "earmuff" in the oven, then put it over your ear. Be sure it's not too hot. It should help draw out the pain.

Acupressure

This acupressure remedy requires something sterile you can bite down on. The ideal thing is one of those cotton cylinders the dentist uses. What we do is wad up a piece of cheesecloth and it works fine.

Place the wad of whatever in back of the last tooth on the side of the aching ear, and bite down on it for five minutes. This stimulates the pressure point that goes directly to the ear. Repeat this procedure every 2 hours until the earache is gone. This acupressure process relieves the pain of an earache and has been known to improve hearing as well.

INFLAMED EAR

Mix 1 tablespoon of milk with 1 tablespoon of olive oil or castor oil, then heat the combination in a nonaluminum pan.

Once the mixture has cooled off, put 4 drops into the inflamed ear every hour and gently plug it up with a puff of cotton. Be sure the drops are not too hot.

GETTING THE WAX OUT

Wax buildup? Warm 1 teaspoon of sesame oil and put ½ teaspoon in each ear. Be sure the oil is not too hot. Gently plug the ear with a puff of cotton and allow the oil to float around for a while. Once the sesame oil softens the wax, you can wash out the ears completely in the shower. No more oil; no more wax.

◗ Sprinkle black pepper into 1 tablespoon of warm corn oil, then dip a puff of cotton into it and gently put the cotton into your ear. Leave it there for 5 minutes, then remove the cotton. With luck, the wax will be removed, too.

GETTING THE BUGS OUT

It happens! Not often, but once in a blue moon, an insect will get inside a person's ear. Since insects are attracted to light, if it's daytime when an insect gets in your ear, turn your ear toward the sun. Chances are the insect will fly out and away. If it happens at night, shut off the lights in the room and shine a flashlight in your ear.

◗ If the insect in your ear doesn't respond to the light, pour 1 teaspoon of warm olive oil into your ear and hold it there for a minute. Then tilt your head so that the oil and the bug come floating out. If that doesn't work, gently fill your ear with warm water and let the insect and the oil glide out. If none of the above debugs you, get professional medical help to remove the insect.

RINGING (TINNITUS)

Ringing in the ears may be the result of a mild overdose of salicylate, which is found in aspirin and other drugs. The ringing should stop when the drug is discontinued.

◗ If your ringing or buzzing is not caused by medication you're taking and if your doctor doesn't know what it's from or what to do for it, you might want to try castor oil—3 or 4 drops a day in each ear. To get full benefit from the castor oil, plug the ear with cotton once you've put in the drops, and keep it there overnight.

We heard about a woman who had constant ringing in her ears for years. None of the specialists could help her. As a last resort, she started using castor oil. After a month, the ringing subsided considerably. Within three months, it was completely gone.

A massage therapist deals with ringing in the ears for herself as well as for her clients by applying gentle pressure to neck muscles and stretching the sternocleido-mastoid (the muscle that extends from behind your ear to the base of your neck).

To help yourself, stand or sit erect and do this stretching exercise.

1. Keep your head straight as you slowly tilt it over to the side with your ear toward your shoulder. Do not lift your shoulder to touch your ear.

2. Hold that posture for 10 seconds, then return your head to the center position.

3. Slowly tilt your head to the other side and hold for 10 seconds. Return your head to the center position.

4. Tilt your head back, hold for 10 seconds, and return your head to the center position.

5. Bend your head forward, chin toward your chest, hold for 10 seconds, and return to the center position.

6. Repeat the entire four stretches a second time.

Don't be surprised if you hear or feel a pop in your neck. For some, the ringing subsides or completely stops after the first set of stretches; for others, it may take a few days of stretching before there's a difference.

Believe it or not, a heating pad on your feet and one on your hands may ease the ringing in your ears. It all has to do with blood being redistributed, improving circulation, and lessening pressure in congested areas.

EARLOBE INFECTION

Men as well as women have been troubled with earlobe infections from ear piercing. Put castor oil on your lobes a few times a day—the more the better. The infection should clear up in two or three days at most. If it gets worse, seek professional help.

EAR PAIN IN AIRPLANE

The key to relieving the pressure caused by airplane takeoffs and landings is chewing and swallowing.

The American Academy of Otolaryngology advises that you chew gum or suck on mints—whatever causes you to swallow more than usual. Stay awake as the plane ascends and descends so that you can consciously increase the amount of times you swallow. If you're sleepy, that's good. The idea is to start yawning, which is even better than swallowing because it activates the muscle that opens your eustachian tube so that air can be forced in and out of the eustachian canal, and that's what relieves the pressure in your ears.

SWIMMER'S EAR

Soon after swimming, if you notice that it hurts when you touch or move your ear, you may have an ear canal infection known as "swimmer's ear."

Combine 1 drop of grapefruit seed extract, 1 drop of tea tree oil (both available at health food stores), and 2 drops of olive oil, and put it in your ear. Gently plug your ear with a cotton puff. After an hour, remove the cotton. The mixture should help clear up the infection.

Swimmer's Ear Prevention

Lots of people are plagued by recurrent, painful ear canal infections soon after swimming. Here's a solution that may prevent the problem. Add 1 teaspoon of distilled white vinegar to ¼ cup of just-boiled water. Once the liquid is cool, store it in a bottle that comes with a dropper, and take it with you to the beach or pool. Right

after swimming, put 2 drops of the vinegar mixture in each ear. Plug the ears with cotton puffs and leave them there for about ten minutes—long enough to destroy the infection-causing bacteria.

PREVENTING HEARING DETERIORATION

Aerobic exercise, including brisk walking or bicycling, can help prevent some age-related deterioration in the ears, as well as damage caused by exposure to loud noises. Exercise also increases the ability to hear faint sounds. This good news comes from results of studies conducted at Miami University of Ohio—you heard right, Miami U. of Ohio—which concluded that aerobic exercise improves hearing by circulating blood to inner ear cells and bringing them more oxygen and an increased supply of chemicals that help prevent damage to them.

RESTORE AND/OR IMPROVE HEARING

Pinch the tips of your middle fingers four times a day, 5 minutes each time. It may restore or even improve your hearing.

It's easy if you organize it this way: When you get up in the morning, and before every meal, pinch the right middle finger. After every meal, and when you go to bed, pinch the left middle finger. You may want to make it easy on yourself by clipping a clothespin on the tips of your fingers instead of doing all of that pinching.

▶ It's been said that nothing improves a person's hearing like overhearing.

EMPHYSEMA

If you've been diagnosed as having the lung condition known as emphysema and you're still smoking cigarettes, don't bother reading this. Turn to the "Smoking" chapter immediately and come back here once you've kicked the habit.

▶ Now then, combine ½ teaspoon of raw honey with 5 drops of anise oil (available at health food stores) and take this a half hour before each meal.

We've heard positive reports about this remedy. Anything that can help is worth a try.

▶ When you're having a hard time breathing, sit down, lean forward, and put your elbows on your knees. This position can make breathing easier because it elevates the diaphragm, the most important muscle used for breathing.

▶ Increase your lung power and breath control by taking up a musical instrument—the harmonica (mouth organ). It's fun! A Marine Band by Hohner is a good beginner's harmonica and is inexpensive. It comes with a little sheet of instructions. It's easy. Who knows—it may start you on a whole new career.

When we contacted the Hohner Harmonica Company, they sent us a big batch of unsolicited testimonials from people who had all kinds of lung conditions, including emphysema. Most of the letters said that playing the harmonica every day increased their lung power, made breathing easier, and made them happier.

We expect to be invited to your first concert!

EYE PROBLEMS

How very precious our eyes and sight are to us. Agreed? Agreed! Then what have you done for your eyes lately? Do you know there's eye food, eye-strengthening exercises, an acupressure eyestrain reliever, eyewashes to brighten those baby blues, browns, grays, or greens, and natural healing alternatives instead of chemical symptom cover-ups?

There is an optometrist with a sign in his office window: "If you don't see what you want, you're in the right place."

We're hoping you're in the right place to get the help you need. Read on . . . or get someone to read it to you.

NOTE ABOUT EYEDROPS: To get the most benefit from eyedrops, gently pull out your lower lid and let the liquid drop into the eye pocket. Then gently close your eye once the drop is in and keep your eye closed for at least a minute. That will prevent the fluttering and blinking process from releasing the drop from the eye.

EYE FOOD

"People with concerns over vision problems might wish to add more lutein-containing foods to their diets," advises certified nutrition specialist Shereen Jegtvig (whose last name, coincidentally, looks like the letters of an eye chart).

Jegtvig explains, "Lutein is found in the retinas of your eyes. It is necessary for good vision, and getting lutein from the foods you eat will lower the risk of cataracts and macular degeneration."

The richest sources of lutein are fruit,

particularly berries, and vegetables with red, orange, and yellow pigments—tomatoes, carrots, squash. Spinach and other green leafy vegetables also contain high amounts of lutein. Also, egg yolks.

Studies suggest that eating lutein-rich foods may be a more effective means of boosting lutein concentration in the eye than taking supplements. But if you eat fewer than five servings of fruit and vegetables a day, then consider taking a daily lutein supplement—20 mg (available at health food stores).

During World War II, British pilots ate bilberry jam before a flight and claimed that it improved night vision, sometimes dramatically. Modern research now supports those claims.

A relative of American blueberries, cranberries, and huckleberries, the European bilberry contains anthocyanosides (powerful antioxidants), shown to improve night vision, slow macular degeneration, and prevent cataracts and diabetic retinopathy.

Bilberry jam is not that readily available, but bilberry supplements can be found at health food stores. Follow the recommended dosage on the label.

BLOODSHOT EYES

Use any of the eyewashes listed at the end of this chapter. You might also want to try the grated potato remedy under "Black Eye" in the "Bruises, Cuts, Black Eyes, and More" chapter.

CATARACTS

There are amazing new surgical procedures now for removing cataracts. Know your options. While you're investigating them, you may want to try one of the following.

❱ Honey! No, we're not getting overly friendly here, we're just relaying a remedy to help clear away a cataract.

Every day for two weeks, put a drop of raw honey in the eye that has the cataract. It will sting like crazy until the tears wash away the pain. At the end of the two weeks, if you see an improvement, continue the daily regimen for another two weeks. Then have your eye doctor confirm the improvement. Or schedule an appointment for a cataract-removal procedure.

❱ Dr. Gladys McGarey of the Association for Research and Enlightenment Clinic of Phoenix, Arizona, recommends 2 drops of castor oil in each eye at bedtime. If there is no improvement after a month, chances are it's never going to help.

❱ English physician Nicholas Culpeper was a great believer in the healing effects of chamomile eyewashes to improve a cataract condition. (See "Eyewashes" at the end of this chapter.)

CHEMICALS

When chemicals such as hair dye get in your eyes, immediately wash the eyes thoroughly with lots of clean, tepid water. In most cases, the eyes should be checked by a doctor right after you've washed the damaging liquids out.

FOREIGN BODY IN THE EYE

When something gets in your eye, try not to rub the eye. You'll irritate it, and then it's hard to tell whether or not the foreign particle is out.

Get a tissue ready. With one hand pull your lashes so that the upper lid is away from your eye. With the other hand, appropriately position the tissue in the center of your face and blow your nose three times.

❱ Combine 1 drop of fresh lemon juice (1 drop only!) in 1 ounce of tepid water and wash your eye with it, using an eye cup (available at pharmacies) or an eyedropper. It should remove the particle, and it is surprisingly soothing.

If you have something in your eye besides a contact lens, do what our mother had us do: grasp the lashes of your upper lid firmly between your thumb and index finger. Gently pull the lashes toward the cheek as far as you can without pulling them out. Hold it, count to ten, spit three times, and let go of the lashes. Is it out? If not, repeat the procedure one more time. If it still didn't work, get an onion and read the next remedy.

Mince an onion, encouraging the onion's fumes to reach your eyes. Once your eyes tear, the tears should wash away the foreign body in your eye.

CONJUNCTIVITIS (PINKEYE)

NOTE: Conjunctivitis can be a severe and contagious infection. If the condition doesn't show signs of improvement within a couple of days, a health professional should have a look-see.

The plant eyebright is particularly effective in the treatment of conjunctivitis. Add 3 drops of tincture of eyebright (available at health food stores) to 1 tablespoon of just-boiled water. When the water is cool enough to use, bathe the eye in the mixture. Since this condition is a contagious one, wash the eye cup thoroughly after you've washed one eye, then mix a new batch of eyebright with water and wash the other eye. Do this three or four times a day for a day or two. If there is no improvement, make an appointment with an eye doctor.

Goat's-milk yogurt can help clear up this uncomfortable condition. Apply a yogurt poultice (see "Preparation Guide") to your closed infected eye(s) daily and leave it on for half an hour. Do it twice a day. Also, eat 1 or 2 portions of the yogurt each day. The active culture in yogurt can help destroy the infection-causing bacteria in your system.

If goat's-milk yogurt is not for you, make a poultice of grated apple or grated raw red potato and place it on your closed infected eye(s). Let it stay on for a half hour. Do it twice a day. Within two days, three at most, the condition should completely clear up.

DRY EYES

Tear ducts that do not produce enough fluid to keep the eyes moist can result in an uncomfortable dry eye condition that is characterized by irritation, burning, and a gravelly feeling.

You may be able to eliminate the need for artificial tears by adding omega-3 fatty acids to your diet, which may increase the viscosity of oils made by the body, mostly in the skin and eyes. Omega-3 is found abundantly in cold-water fish, flaxseed oil, and Salba. This means eating several servings a week of fish—all varieties of salmon (except smoked) and canned white tuna—and/or taking flaxseed oil or Salba. (See the "Diabetes" chapter for Salba information and recipes.)

> **CAUTION:** If you're on blood-thinning medication, have uncontrolled high blood pressure or bleeding disorders, or are going in for surgery, be sure to check with your doctor before taking flaxseed oil or Salba.

Help your eyes self-lubricate by opening the clogged oil glands in the eyelids. Take a warm, wet white washcloth and place it on your closed eyelids. Leave it on until it turns cool, 5 to 10 minutes. Do this a few times a day—the more the better.

Dry-Eye Don'ts

Don't use a blow dryer on your hair unless you absolutely have to, or can wear goggles while doing it.

■ Don't go outdoors without sunglasses. The wraparound kind are excellent for keeping the wind and the UV rays out.

■ Don't dry out your eyes with heating or cooling systems in your home, office, car, and even on an airplane. Keep the heat or air-conditioning to a minimum or turn it off completely unless it's really necessary, and then be sure the vents are not pointing in your direction.

■ Don't go for any length of time without blinking. According to Dr. Robert-Michael Kaplan, author of *Seeing Without Glasses,* you should blink every three seconds. That especially applies to people sitting at computers. Every time you click the mouse, blink. Every time you save a document, blink. Every time you swallow, blink. Do whatever it takes to make yourself conscious of blinking often, especially when you're sitting in front of the computer.

■ Don't wear contact lenses all the time. Give your eyes a rest from them on a regular basis.

■ Don't smoke! One more reason to quit is that smoke adds to the burning and other dry eye symptoms.

■ Don't cry about it. It makes the problem worse. Tears brought on by emotion wash away the oils that help prevent dry eyes.

EYE AND VISION STRENGTHENERS

Apply cold water on a washcloth to the eyelids, eyebrows, and temples morning, noon, and night, 5 to 10 minutes each time.

Eat a handful of shelled, raw, and unsalted sunflower seeds every day.

You know all the talk about carrots being good for your eyes? They are! Drink 5 to 6 ounces of fresh carrot juice twice a day for at least two weeks. Obviously, you'll need a juicer or a nearby juice bar. After two weeks, ease off to 1 glass of carrot juice a day or every other day . . . forever.

NOTE: If you are diabetic or have a candida/yeast problem, do not drink carrot juice because of its high sugar content.

We've thoroughly researched "palming" and no two resources agree on the procedure. We'll give you a couple of variations. Test them and see what works best for you.

Sit. (They all agree on that.) Rub your hands together until you feel heat. With your elbows on the table, place the heels of your hands over your eyes, blocking out all light. Some feel it's better to keep one's eyes open in the dark; others advocate closed eyes. The length of time to sit this way also varies—from 2 minutes to 10 minutes.

Eyes open or closed, any length of time, palming is beneficial for improving vision, for nearsightedness, tired eyes, astigmatisms, inflammations, and may even help squinters stop squinting. Do this energizing exercise twice a day or more.

EYESTRAIN (TIRED EYES)

If your eyes are strained and tired, chances are the rest of your body is also dragging. Lie down with your feet raised higher than your head. Relax that way for about 15 minutes. This gravity-reversing process should make you and your eyes feel refreshed and rarin' to go.

Cut two thin slices of raw red potato and keep them on your closed eyelids for at least 20 minutes. While red potatoes are said to have strong healing energy, any other kind of potato should work, too. (No, not potato chips.)

Steep 1 heaping teaspoon of rosemary in a cup of just-boiled hot water for 10 minutes. Or make a cup of tea with a rosemary teabag. Saturate cotton pads with the tea and keep them on your eyes for 15 minutes. Rosemary should help draw out that tired-eye feeling.

🔸 Looking at red ink on white paper for long periods of time can cause eyestrain and headaches. Stay out of the red!

Acupressure

Pinch the ends of your index and middle (second and third) fingers of each hand for 30 seconds at a time on each finger. If your eyestrain isn't relieved after 2 minutes, do another round of pinching.

Eyestrain Prevention at the Computer

When you're typing something from a book or sheet of paper, or answering a letter, chances are you rest the book or paper flat on the desk and take turns referring to the paper, then to the computer screen. By doing that, you cause your eyes to have to refocus from the paper to the screen and back to the paper. All of that refocusing puts a strain on your eyes.

If you use a standing document holder (available at office supply and stationery stores) and place it alongside the screen with your paper standing in it, both the paper and the screen will be the same distance from your eyes. No refocusing. No eyestrain. But do remember to keep blinking.

🔸 Also see the "Palming" exercise above under "Eye and Vision Strengtheners."

NIGHT BLINDNESS

Eat blueberries—lots of them—when they're in season, or buy frozen blueberries the rest of the year. Also consider taking blueberry extract (sold at health food and vitamin stores) as a supplement. Follow the dosage on the label.

INFLAMMATION AND IRRITATION

A poultice (see "Preparation Guide") of grated raw potato, fresh mashed papaya pulp, or mashed cooked beets is soothing and promotes healing. Leave the poultice on for 15 minutes twice a day.

🔸 If your eyes are irritated from a foreign particle, cooking fumes, cigarette smoke, dust, et cetera, put 2 drops of castor oil or 2 drops of milk in each eye to wash out and soothe your eyes.

🔸 Use any of the eyewashes listed at the end of this chapter.

STIES

When you feel and see the start of a sty—a small red bump on the edge of your upper or lower eyelid, caused by an infected gland—rub the sty several times with a gold wedding ring or any smooth gold ring. We were not going to use any ridiculous remedies that seemed more like superstitions than medically based cures, but this is one of the exceptions. As crazy as it sounds, it has worked for us many times.

❧ If a gold ring isn't your thing, moisten a black or green tea bag, put it on the closed eye with the sty, bandage it in place, and leave the bandage on overnight. By morning it may be bye-bye sty.

❧ Thyme is a soothing herb that can be used for its drawing-out qualities. Wet a thyme tea bag with boiled water, and as soon as it's cool enough to place on the eye with the sty, close that eye and put the tea bag on it. Let it stay there for about 10 minutes. Repeat the process an hour later, then an hour after that. By then, you should feel relief.

❧ Place a handful of fresh parsley in a soup bowl. Pour a cup of just-boiled water over the parsley and let it steep for 10 minutes. Soak a clean washcloth in the hot parsley water, lie down, and while the cloth is still warm but not burning hot, put it on your closed lid and relax for 15 minutes. Repeat the procedure before bedtime.

Parsley water is also good for eliminating puffiness around the eyes.

❧ Dab on castor oil several times throughout the day until the sty disappears.

EYEWASHES

Eyewash Directions
See "Preparation Guide."

> **REMINDER:** Always remove contact lenses before doing an eyewash.

You'll need an eye cup (available at drugstores). Carefully pour just-boiled water over the cup to clean it. Without contaminating the rim or inside surfaces of the cup, fill it half full with whichever eyewash you've selected. Apply the cup tightly to the eye to prevent spillage, then tilt your head backward. Open your eyelid wide and rotate your eyeball to thoroughly wash the eye. Use the same procedure with the other eye.

❧ Place a handful of scrubbed (preferably organic) carrot tops (just the green leaves) in a jar of distilled hot water. Let it stand. When it's cool, use the carrot water as an eyewash. Drink the remaining liquid. It should help your eyes be bright and clear, and also help strengthen your kidneys and bladder.

Mix 1 drop of lemon juice in 1 ounce of distilled warm water and use it as an eyewash. It's particularly effective when your eyes have been exposed to dust, cigarette smoke, harsh lights, and chemical compounds in the air.

For an eyebright eyewash, add 1 ounce of the whole dried herb eyebright to 1 pint of just-boiled water and let it steep for 10 minutes. Strain thoroughly through a superfine strainer or through unbleached muslin. Wait until the liquid is cool enough to use.

Or add 3 drops of tincture of eyebright to a tablespoon of just-boiled water, and again, wait until it's cool enough to use. (Health food and herb stores should have both forms of eyebright.)

EYEGLASS CLEANERS

To avoid streaks on your eyeglass lenses, clean them with a touch of distilled white vinegar or vodka.

BLACK EYE

See "Bruises, Cuts, Black Eyes, and More."

SUNBURNED EYES AND EYELIDS

See "Sunburn."

FAINTING

TREATING A FAINTER

In India, instead of smelling salts, people take a couple of strong whiffs of half an onion to bring them around.

CAUTION: If you faint and don't know why, consult a doctor. Fainting may be a symptom of an ailment that requires proper diagnosis and treatment.

PREVENTION

When you feel as though you're going to faint, sit down and put your head between your knees. If you're in an appropriate place, lie down with your feet and torso elevated so that your head is lower than your heart. That's the secret of preventing a faint—getting your head lower than your heart so the blood can rush to your brain.

If it's a scorcher of a day and you're feeling every degree of it, or if you're in a very warm room that's making you feel faint, just run cold tap water over the insides of your wrists. If there are ice cubes around, rub them on your wrists. Relief is almost immediate.

A friend of ours is a paramedic. When one of her patients is about to faint, she pinches the patient's philtrum—the fleshy part between the upper lip and nose. That prevents the faint from happening.

If you're prone to fainting—a case of the vapors, perhaps—keep pepper handy. Sniff just a few grains, enough to make you sneeze. The sneeze stimulates the brain's blood vessels and may help prevent fainting. It's good to remember, since not many households have smelling salts, but most have black pepper.

A drop in blood sugar can make you feel faint. Prevent that from happening by eating wholesome food regularly at mealtimes, snacking on fruit and nuts in between meals, and staying away from an excess of sweets and refined foods.

FATIGUE

f you're tired the second you awaken in the morning, try this Vermont tonic. In a blender, put 1 cup of warm water, 2 tablespoons of apple cider vinegar, and 1 teaspoon of honey. Blend thoroughly, then sip it slowly till it's all gone. Have this tonic every morning before breakfast, and

within days, you may feel a difference in your energy level.

Here's another way to wake up your metabolism in the morning. Squeeze the juice of half a grapefruit. Fill the rest of the glass with warm water. Drink it down slowly, then eat the fruit of the squeezed-out half grapefruit. Now that your thyroid is activated, have a productive day!

CAUTION: If you're taking medication, check with your doctor or pharmacist about negative grapefruit-drug interaction.

If, after a full night's sleep, you get up feeling sluggish, it may be due to a tired liver. Stand up. Place your right hand above your waist, on the bottom of your ribs on your right side, with your fingers apart, pointing toward your left side. Place your left hand the same way on your left side. Ready? You press your right hand in, then back in place. You press your left hand in, then back in place. You do the Hokey-Pokey and you— Just checking to see if you're paying attention. Now then, press your right hand in, then back in place. Press your left hand in, then back in place. Do it a dozen times on each side when you get up each morning. In a couple of weeks, this liver massage may make a difference in your daily energy level.

Cutting out heavy starches and sweets from your daily diet can also go a long way in adding to your get-up-and-go.

QUICK PICK-ME-UPS

Food and Drink

Mix ⅛ teaspoon (more if you can take it) of cayenne pepper into a cup of water. Drink it down and get a second wind.

If you're taking a long drive or have a night of cramming ahead, prepare a quart of juice—any kind of juice as long as it has no sugar or preservatives added—and mix in 1 teaspoon of cayenne pepper. As soon as you feel sleep overcoming you, take a cup of the cayenne-laced juice to keep awake and alert.

Tough day at the office? Want a lift? Ready for a drink? Tired of all these questions? Add 1 tablespoon of blackstrap molasses to a glass of milk—regular, skim, soy, coconut, almond, or rice milk—and bottoms up.

A bunch of grapes can give you a bunch of energy. Hey, maybe that's why you always see pictures of people eating grapes at those bacchanalian orgies.

Grapes may be too perishable for you to carry around, but dried figs aren't. And they sure can pack an energy punch. They're delicious and satisfying, plus they have more potassium than bananas, more calcium than milk, a very high dietary fiber content, and no cholesterol, fat, or sodium. Most important, figs have easily digestible, natural, slow-burning sugars that will get you going and keep you going, unlike the quick-fix, fast-crash processed sugar in junk food.

Herbalist Lalitha Thomas, who lists figs as one of the ten essential foods (in her book of the same name), says to make a serious effort to get unsulfured figs. (Health food stores have them.) Eat a few at a time, but don't overdo it . . . figs are known to help prevent or relieve constipation.

Physical Solutions

If possible, walk barefoot in dewy grass. The next best thing is to carefully walk up and back in six inches of cold bathwater. Do it for about 5 minutes in the morning and late afternoon.

A Chinese theory is that "tiredness" collects on the insides of one's elbows and the backs of one's knees. Wake up your body by slap-slap-slapping both those areas.

Call on your imagination for this visualization exercise. Sit up with your arms over your head and your palms facing the ceiling. With your right hand, pluck a fistful of vitality out of the air. Next, let your left hand grab its share. Open both hands, allowing all that energy to flow down your arms to your neck, shoulders, and chest. Start over again. This time, when you open your hands, let the energy flow straight down to your waist, hips, thighs, legs, feet, and toes. There! You've revitalized your body. Now stand up feeling refreshed.

When you just can't keep your eyes open or your head up and you don't know how you'll make it to the end of the day at your office, run away from it all. Go to the bathroom or a secluded spot and run in place. Run for 2 minutes and it should help you keep going the rest of the day.

MENTAL FATIGUE

Try this Austrian recipe: Thoroughly wash an apple, cut it into small pieces, leaving the peel on, and place the pieces in a bowl. Pour 2 cups of just-boiled water over the apple and let it steep for an hour. Then add 1 tablespoon of honey. Drink the apple-honey water and eat the pieces of apple.

We've read case histories in which, within weeks, the intake of bee pollen not only increased a person's physical energy but also restored mental alertness and eliminated lapses of memory and confusion. The suggested dosage is 1 teaspoon of granular bee pollen or two 500 mg bee pollen pills after breakfast.

FOOT AND LEG PROBLEMS

Our feet carry a lot of weight and are probably the most abused and neglected part of our anatomy. We put our poor, tired tootsies under all kinds of stress and strain. They get cold, frostbitten, and wet; they burn, blister, and itch; and they sweat as we walk, jog, run, dance, climb, skate, ski, hop, skip, and jump. And at some time or other, we're all guilty of the Cinderella's stepsister syndrome—pushing our feet into ill-fitting shoes. Then we wonder why our feet are just killing us. Well, we killed them first.

According to podiatrist Dr. Steven Baff, 40 percent of American children develop foot ailments by age six, and by adulthood, 80 percent of Americans suffer from foot problems.

Let's get to the bottom of our problems with some remedies for the feet.

> **CAUTION:** If you have circulation problems or diabetes, do not use any of these remedies without the approval and supervision of your health care provider.

ACHING FEET

This remedy requires two basins or four plastic shoe boxes. Fill one basin or two shoe boxes with ½ cup Epsom salts and about 1 gallon of hot (not scalding) water; fill the other basin or the other two shoe boxes with ice cubes.

Sit down with a watch or timer. Put your feet in the hot water for 1 minute and then in the ice cubes for 30 seconds. Alternate back and forth for about 10 minutes. Your feet will feel better. This procedure may also help regulate high blood pressure and may help prevent varicose veins, improve circulation, and, if done on a regular basis, relieve chronic "cold feet."

A modified version of the above is to stand in the bathtub and first let hot water run on your feet, then let ice cold water run on your feet, timing it the same as above.

Do not exceed 1 minute of hot or cold water on your feet!

▸ Add 1 cup of apple cider vinegar to a basin or two plastic shoe boxes filled halfway with lukewarm water. Then soak your feet in it for at least 15 minutes. The heat and hurt should be gone by then.

▸ Cut a large turnip into small pieces and boil it until the pieces are soft. Or roast it in a 450-degree oven for about half an hour, until it's soft. Then mash it and spread half of it on a white cotton handkerchief; spread the other half on another handkerchief. Apply the turnip mush to the bottoms of your bare feet, bandage them in place, and sit with your feet elevated for about a half hour. This "sole food" should draw out the pain and tiredness.

> **NOTEWORTHY:** After a tough day on your feet, you may not feel like giving yourself a foot massage. The Foot Choice Foot Massager may be the answer. This reasonably priced machine combines massage therapy and infrared heat with the ancient pain-relieving principle of reflexology.
>
> For more information, visit www.bio techresearch.com or call 800-895-0008.

▸ After a long day, when your feet hurt and you're actually feeling too tired to go to sleep, unwind as you soak your feet in a basin or two plastic shoe boxes filled with hot water for 10 to 15 minutes.

Then massage your feet with lemon juice. After you've done a thorough job of massaging, rinse your feet with cool water. Dry your feet completely and take five deep breaths. You and your pain-free feet should be ready and able to settle down for a good night's sleep.

ATHLETE'S FOOT

The fungus that causes athlete's foot dies in natural sunlight. So if you can spend the next couple of weeks barefoot in the Bahamas . . . If that's a bit impractical, then for 20 minutes a day expose your feet to sunlight—that may eliminate a mild case of athlete's foot. Be sure to cover all other exposed areas of your face and body with sunscreen.

> **NOTE:** To avoid reinfecting yourself with athlete's foot, soak your socks and hose in vinegar. Also, after taking off your shoes, wipe them out with vinegar. The smell of vinegar will vanish (say that three times fast) after being exposed to the air for about 15 minutes. If possible, don't wear the same pair of shoes two days in a row.

In between sunbaths, wear loose-fitting socks. The more air that gets to them, the better. At night, apply alcohol (ow!—it stings for a few seconds), and when your feet are completely dry, sprinkle on talcum powder (the unscented kind is preferable).

Apply 1 clove of crushed garlic to the affected area. Leave it on for half an hour, then wash with water. If you do this once a day, within a week you'll be smelling like a salami, but you may not have athlete's foot.

> **CAUTION:** When you first apply the garlic, there will be a sensation of warmth for a few minutes. If after a few minutes that warm feeling intensifies, the garlic may be burning the skin. Take off the garlic and wash the area with cool water. Wait a day, then try another remedy.

Grate an onion and squeeze it through cheesecloth to get onion juice. Massage the juice into the fungus-infected areas of your foot. Leave it on for 10 minutes, then rinse your foot in lukewarm water and dry it thoroughly. Repeat this procedure three times a day until the condition clears up.

Every evening apply cotton or cheesecloth that has been dipped in honey to the infected area. Tape it in place. To avoid a gooey mess (a possibility even with the tape in place) wear socks to bed. In the morning, wash with water, dry thoroughly, and sprinkle on talcum powder (preferably unscented). In a week's time, you may have every bear in the neighborhood at your feet, but they probably won't be athlete's-foot feet.

BURNING FEET

Wrap tomato slices on the soles of the feet and keep the feet elevated for about a half hour.

We heard from a woman whose husband was in the hospital. Among his many health challenges was the terrible discomfort of burning feet. Nothing that the doctors and nurses did could relieve the burning sensation. The patient's wife was told about this remedy. As ridiculous as it seemed, she bought big beefsteak tomatoes, brought them to the hospital, and got permission to slice them and bind them on her husband's feet. It worked like a fire extinguisher. The burning sensation disappeared and, for the first time in weeks, the man was comfortable. Throughout the following few years, whenever that burning feeling recurred, all the man had to say was, "Get some tomatoes!"

This 100 percent true—no exaggeration—story is one of many that have led us to include remedies that seem absurd but may make a major difference in someone's life.

Soak your feet in warm potato water (see "Preparation Guide") for 15 minutes. Dry your feet thoroughly. If you're going right to bed, massage the feet with a small amount of sesame or almond oil. You might want to put on loose-fitting socks to avoid messing up the sheets.

Bavarian mountain climbers, after soaking their feet in potato water, sprinkle hot roasted salt on a cloth and wrap it around their feet. It not only soothes burning and tired feet but relieves itchy ones as well.

CALLUSES

Soften your calluses by applying any of the following oils: wheat germ oil, castor oil, sesame seed oil, or olive oil. Apply the oil as often as possible day after day, throughout the day and night. It's a good idea to wear white socks after each application.

Cut two thick slices of onion (wide enough to cover the callused area of each foot). Let the onion slices soak in wine vinegar for 4 hours. Then place a slice of onion on top of each callus. Bind them in place with plastic wrap, put on white socks, and let it stay that way overnight. Next morning, you should be able to carefully scrape away the callus. Don't forget to rinse your feet to get rid of the smell of onion and wine vinegar.

CALLUS PREVENTION

Walking barefoot in the sand, particularly wet sand, is wonderful for your feet. It acts as an abrasive and sloughs off dead skin that could lead to calluses . . . corns, too.

If you're not near the beach for the remedy above, add 1 tablespoon of baking soda to a basin or two plastic shoe boxes filled halfway with lukewarm water, and soak your feet in it for 10 to 15 minutes. Then take a pumice stone (available at health food stores and drugstores) and carefully and gently file away the tough skin.

COLD FEET

Stand on your toes for a couple of minutes, then quickly come back down on your heels. Repeat toes/heels several times until your blood tingles through your feet and warms them up.

Before going to bed, carefully walk in cold water in the bathtub for 2 minutes. Then briskly rub the feet dry with a coarse towel. To give the feet a warm glow, hold each end of the towel and run it back and forth through the hollow or arch of the bottom of your feet.

If the thought of putting already cold feet into cold water is not appealing to you, then add 1 cup of table salt to a bathtub filled ankle-high with hot water, and soak your feet for 10 minutes. Dry your feet and massage them with damp salt. This will remove dead skin and stimulate circulation. After you've rubbed each foot for 3 to 5 minutes, rinse them both in lukewarm water and dry them thoroughly.

Warm your feet by sprinkling a little bit of black or cayenne pepper into your socks before putting them on. It's an old skier's trick, but you don't have to be an old skier to do it. If you use cayenne, your socks and your feet will turn red. Your feet will be fine, but your white socks may never be the same again.

CORNS

Hell hath no fury like a woman's corn!

The difference between an oak tree and a tight shoe is that one makes acorns, the other makes corns ache.

Okay, so we're a little corny. If not here, where? Here's also where you'll find help for those aching corns.

Rub castor oil on the corn twice a day and it will gradually peel off, leaving soft, smooth skin.

Every night, put a piece of fresh lemon peel on the corn, the inside of the peel touching the corn. Put a Band-Aid around it to keep it in place. In a few days, the corn should be gone.

Soak a piece of bread in distilled white vinegar for a half hour. Then apply it to the corn and tape it in place. Put a white sock over it and let it stay that way overnight. By morning, the corn should peel off. If it's a particularly stubborn corn, you may have to reapply the vinegar-soaked bread a few nights in a row.

Daily, wrap a strip of fresh pineapple peel around the corn (the inside of the peel should be touching the corn). Within a week, the corn should disappear, thanks to the enzymes and acid content of the fresh pineapple.

A Hawaiian medicine man recommends pure papaya juice on a cotton pad, or a piece of papaya pulp directly on the corn. Bind it in place and leave it on overnight. Change daily until the corn is gone.

Save your used tea bags. Tape a moist one on the corn for a half hour a day, and the corn should be gone in a week or so.

CRACKED HEELS

Before bedtime, wash your feet with warm water and dry them. Liberally apply petroleum jelly on your feet, massaging it into the rough and cracked areas. Wrap each foot with plastic wrap. Put socks on and sleep that way. Repeat the process nightly until your feet are fine. It shouldn't take more than a week . . . probably a lot less.

Then to keep them from cracking again, put olive oil on your feet at bedtime. It's surprisingly nonoily and doesn't seem to mess up the linens.

PLANTAR FASCIITIS (HEEL SPUR SYNDROME)

Plantar fasciitis is irritation and swelling of the thick tissue on the bottom of the foot. It's often referred to as a heel spur, probably because that term is easier to pronounce. Many people with plantar fasciitis have heel spurs, but it's not the spurs that cause the pain. The painful plantar fasciitis condition can be caused by inadequate flexibility in the calf muscles, lack of arch support, being overweight, a sudden increase in activity, and standing on one's feet for long periods of time.

There is a nonsurgical treatment—a

stretching exercise—that can relieve the pain and speed the healing of the condition.

Developed by Benedict DiGiovanni, M.D., associate professor of orthopedic surgery at the University of Rochester, and Deborah Nawoczenski, P.T., Ph.D., professor of physical therapy at Ithaca College, this exercise can help and potentially cure plantar fasciitis, according to the positive results of their two-year study.

The stretch requires patients to sit with one leg crossed over the other and stretch the arch of the foot by taking one hand and pulling the toes back toward the shin for a count of ten. The exercise must be repeated ten times and performed at least three times a day, including before taking the first step in the morning and before standing after a prolonged period of sitting.

Dr. DiGiovanni feels that "walking without stretching those foot tissues is just reinjuring yourself." Follow the doctor's directions and you'll be glad you did.

LEG CRAMPS

Frequent Leg Cramps

Leg cramps can be caused by a variety of nutritional deficiencies, for instance, magnesium, potassium, vitamin E, calcium, or protein. Are you eating lots of green? (We don't mean two olives in your martini.)

Cut down on fatty meats, sugar, and white flour. In a week, see if there's a difference in the frequency of leg cramps.

If you take a diuretic, you may be losing too much potassium from your system, which may be causing leg cramps. If that's the case, eat a banana or two every day. You may also want to ask your doctor to take you off the chemical diuretic and find a natural one, such as cucumber, celery, or lettuce.

Occasional Leg Cramps

This simple acupressure procedure helps relieve the pain and cramping almost instantly. The second you get a cramp, use your thumb and index finger and pinch your philtrum—the skin between your upper lip and your nose. Keep pinching for about 20 seconds, unless the cramp stops sooner.

This remedy is especially good to know if you get a cramp while swimming.

If you get leg cramps while you sleep, keep a piece of silverware—a spoon is the safest—on your night table. When the cramp wakes you up, place the spoon on the painful area and the muscle should uncramp. Incidentally, the spoon doesn't have to be silver; stainless steel will work as well.

Leg Cramp Prevention

Before you get out of bed in the morning, turn yourself around so that you can put your feet against the wall, higher than your body. Stay that way for 10 minutes. Do the same thing at night, right before you go to sleep. It will improve blood circulation and may prevent muscle cramps. It's also an excellent stretch that in itself may prevent cramps.

✺ Vermont's noted doctor D. C. Jarvis suggested taking 2 teaspoons of honey combined with 2 teaspoons of apple cider vinegar in a glass of water before each meal as a way to prevent muscle cramps.

✺ Take advantage of the therapeutic value of a rocking chair. Rock whenever you watch television and for at least 1 hour before bedtime. For those of you who sit most of the time, a rocking chair may help prevent varicose veins and blood clots, and improve circulation as well as relieve you of leg cramps.

✺ *Lancet,* the British medical journal, reports that vitamin E is helpful in relieving and preventing cramps in the legs. Take 100 IU of vitamin E before each meal. Within a week or two, the attacks of cramping should be ebbing off or stopping completely.

✺ Drink 1 cup of red raspberry leaf tea (available at health food stores) in the morning and 1 cup at night. Do this daily and you may no longer be troubled with leg cramps.

Leg Cramp Prevention for Joggers

After your run, find a cool stream of moving water in which to soak your feet for 15 to 20 minutes. For those of you who can only dream of that, every night, right before going to bed, walk in about 6 inches of cold water in your bathtub for about 3 minutes. The feedback from runners who do this has been very convincing that the cold-water walks do help prevent leg cramps.

Be sure to have those nonslip stick-ons on the floor of the tub.

RESTLESS LEG SYNDROME

A big bruiser of a guy said that drinking a 16-ounce bottle of tonic water (with quinine) daily has made his restless leg syndrome (RLS) disappear. He claims he had RLS both during the day and at night in his legs, as well as restlessness in both of his arms.

If you're not a big guy but want to try tonic water with quinine, start with a few ounces a day and slowly increase the dose up to whatever works for you.

If you don't want the high-fructose corn

syrup that's in tonic water, there is a homeopathic formula (available at health food and vitamin shops) that you may want to check out. It's Hyland's Leg Cramps with Quinine.

Every day, drink 1 tablespoon of apple cider vinegar mixed into a glass of water.

For those of you who absolutely cannot get used to the taste of apple cider vinegar, instead of drinking it, rub it on your legs.

We've heard several reports that blackstrap molasses does away with RLS symptoms—as little as 2 teaspoons and as much as 1 tablespoon daily. Someone said they mix it into a cup of warm soy milk. Don't say "Yuck!" if you haven't tried it. It happens to taste good.

Ever try jumping on a rebounder (minitrampoline)? It is said that a rebounder workout, for even short periods of time, benefits all the systems of the body—lymphatic, digestive, glandular, respiratory, cardiovascular, skeletal, muscular, and nervous. It may also do away with RLS symptoms.

If you're interested in buying a rebounder after trying one at a health club, sporting goods store, or fitness specialty shop, look for a sturdy style—one with six

legs, rather than four. You may also want one with a stabilizing bar to make you feel safer on it.

NEUROPATHY

See "Neuropathy" in the "Diabetes" chapter.

TOES: TINGLING AND NUMBNESS

Daily doses of a B complex plus extra vitamin B_6 have been known to eliminate tingling and numbness in toes. Take 100 to 200 mg B_6. Check the amount of B_6 in the B complex and make sure you are taking *less* than 300 mg of B_6 daily in total. Too much B_6 can be toxic.

INGROWN TOENAILS

We were surprised to learn that a tendency toward ingrown toenails is inherited.

If you have an ingrown toenail, relieve the pain with a footbath. In a plastic shoe box, add ½ ounce of comfrey root (available at herb and health food stores) to 2 quarts of warm water. Soak your foot in it for 20 minutes.

Once the nail is softened from soaking, take a piece of absorbent cotton and twist it so that it's like a thick strand of thread. Or you can twist together a few strands of unwaxed dental floss. Gently wedge the "thread" under the corner of the nail. That should prevent the nail from cutting into the skin. Replace the strands a couple of times a day, every day, until the nail grows out.

The nail should be cut straight across, not down into the corners, and not shorter than the toe. You may want to consider having a podiatrist trim the toenail properly. If you do have a podiatrist trim your toenails, pay careful attention so you'll be able to take care of your toes yourself, and avoid another ingrown nail (and another podiatrist bill).

TOENAIL FUNGUS

While fungal infections affect fingernails, this condition is much more common on toenails. There are several effective medications on the market, but the potential side effects—toxicity leading to liver damage—should make the following safe remedies your first and only course of action. And chances are it will not clear up overnight. It may take a month or two. Be patient and diligent.

Soak the infected toenail in 2 parts water to 1 part distilled white vinegar twice a day for 10 to 15 minutes, or apply the vinegar full strength on the nail at least twice a day.

Oil of oregano is strong, powerful, and a bit expensive, but worth it. Rub the oil on the nail several times throughout the day and night. (You will get used to the smell.) Drink 2 or 3 drops in a glass of water twice a day. Also take oregano softgels three to four times a day.

Tea tree oil is another strong, powerful, and pricey herb that can help heal toenail fungus. Rub it on your nail a few times a day. (You will get used to the smell.) Be consistent and don't stop the oil treatment until the thick, yellowish nail grows out completely.

NOTE: Do not polish your nails. The polish will seal in the fungus and prevent the healing process.

SWEATY FEET

The average pair of feet gives off about half a pint of perspiration daily. It's amazing we don't all seem to slosh around. Well, for those of you who feel like you do . . .

Put some bran or uncooked oat flakes into your socks. It should absorb the sweat and make you feel more comfortable. Start conservatively, with about 1 tablespoon per foot. Add more if needed.

WEAK ANKLES

This exercise will promote toe flexibility and strengthen the arches as well as the ankles.

Get a dozen marbles and a plastic cup. Put them all on the floor. Pick up each marble with the toes of your right foot and, one by one, drop them into the cup. Then do the same with the toes of your left foot. You may want to add to the fun by timing yourself and seeing if you can keep breaking your previous record. Whatever happens, try not to lose your marbles.

NOTEWORTHY: Z-CoiL Pain Relief Footwear is engineered to help relieve foot, leg, and back pain by reducing impact to the body. The shoes are unusual-looking. Someone described them as something Dr. Seuss would have created. Ya gotta see 'em to believe 'em! You also have to try them on to experience moving with a **spring** in your walk. They are on the pricey side, but may be worth it if you have or want to prevent foot problems such as tendonitis, bunions, Morton's neuroma, flat feet, hammertoes, and other foot and ankle pains. Visit www.zcoil.com to see the styles, read the testimonials, and find a store in your area that carries them.

GOUT

Simply put, gout is a form of acute arthritis (we know, there's nothing *cute* about it) that comes on suddenly, goes away after a week or two, and can keep recurring. (To keep it from recurring, see "Gout Prevention," below.)

Inadequate processing of purines, a component in certain foods, produces uric acid. Gout occurs when there are high levels of uric acid circulating in the blood.

If you have gout, you're one of an estimated million Americans—mostly men forty or older—hobbling along with pain and swelling in the joints, most commonly the big toe, although it may also affect the heel, ankle, hand, wrist, and elbow.

Gout is caused by food, and may be treated with food. Here are some suggestions.

The classic gout folk remedy: cherries. They seem to help prevent crystallization of uric acid and to reduce the uric acid levels in the blood. Eat cherries, any kind—sweet or sour, fresh, canned or frozen, black, Royal Anne, or Bing. Drink cherry juice, available without preservatives or sugar added and also in a concentrated form at health food stores.

The average portion of fresh cherries is a dozen a day. Let your size and diet help you determine the amount of cherries you eat.

Eating strawberries and very little else for a few days is said to be a possible cure for gout. Strawberries are a powerful alkalizer and contain calcium, iron, and an ingredient known as salacin, which soothes inflammatory conditions. It worked so well for botanist Linnaeus that he referred to strawberries as "a blessing of the gods."

A Russian remedy is raw garlic, 2 cloves a day. The best way to take raw garlic cloves is to mince them, put them in water (better yet, in unsweetened cherry juice), and drink it down. No chewing necessary. It doesn't linger on your breath, but it may repeat on you. Then again, so does a salami sandwich, and this is a helluva lot healthier.

PAIN RELIEF

Alternate 3-minute hot compresses with 30-second cold compresses to help dissolve the urate crystals in the tissues of the joints that are causing the pain.

GOUT PREVENTION

Lose weight! Avoid, or at least limit, your intake of purine-rich foods: organ meats, sardines, anchovies, shellfish, fried foods, rich desserts (anything with sugar and white flour is a no-no), mushrooms, broth, red meat, gravies, beans, spinach, peas, asparagus, and all alcoholic beverages including beer and wine.

Drink lots of water. And don't forget to eat lots of garlic.

HAIR PROBLEMS

In an average lifetime, the hair on the head grows about 25 feet. Each of us loses about one hundred hairs a day from our scalp. Mostly, the hairs grow back. When they don't, the hairstyle changes from parted or unparted to departed.

Hair is a secondary sex characteristic and seems to play a part in sexual attractiveness.

The biggest hair worries: too much or too little. Too much hair, especially in the wrong places, can be permanently removed by electrolysis. It's expensive and can be painful, but worth every penny and pain in exchange for better self-image.

Too little hair, especially in men, is usually hereditary baldness (alopecia). If the available hair-restoring treatments, including cosmetic surgery (implants and transplants), and the drugs currently on the market are not for you, you may want to try one of the folk remedies that people claim have stopped the loss of hair as well as restored the hair already lost. While neither of us has seen it happen to anyone we know, any one or more of these remedies may be worth a try. After all, what do you have to lose that you aren't already losing?

SLOWING DOWN HAIR LOSS

Experts agree that men prone to male pattern baldness may be able to delay or slow down hair loss by eating healthy—especially by limiting the amount of animal fat, animal protein, and salt in their diet.

STOPPING LOSS AND PROMOTING GROWTH

An hour before bedtime, slice open a clove of garlic and rub it on the hairless area, or puncture a couple of garlic softgels, squish out the oil, and massage it into your scalp.

It's been reported to us that raw onion massaged on the scalp is also an effective stimulant.

An hour after using either garlic or onion, put on a slumber cap and go to bed. Next morning, shampoo and rinse. Repeat the procedure night and morning

for a few weeks and, hopefully, hair will have stopped falling out and there will be regrowth showing.

An Asian remedy to stop excessive amounts of hair from falling out is sesame oil. Rub it on your scalp every night. Cover your head with a sleep cap, or wrap a hand towel around your head. In the morning, wash with an herbal shampoo. Your final rinse should be with 1 tablespoon of apple cider vinegar in 1 quart of warm water.

Another version of the above nightly/daily treatments calls for equal amounts of olive oil and oil of rosemary (available at health food stores). Combine the two in a bottle and shake vigorously. Then massage it into the scalp, cover the head, sleep, awaken, shampoo, and rinse.

A man who emigrated to the United States from Russia told us that many barbers in the former Soviet Union recommended this to their balding customers: Combine 1 tablespoon of honey with 1 jigger (about 1½ ounces) of vodka and the juice from a medium-size onion. Rub the mixture into the scalp every night, cover, sleep, awaken, shampoo, and rinse.

Three times a day, 5 minutes each time, buff your fingernails with your fingernails. Huh? In other words, rub the fingernails of your right hand across the fingernails of your left hand. Not only is it supposed to stop hair loss, it's also supposed to encourage hair growth and prevent hair from graying. It sounds ridiculous, but the price is right and it's not hard to do while watching TV, on an exercycle, or on the commuter train. Give it a few weeks and see if you notice a positive difference in your head of hair.

Prepare your own hair-growing elixir by combining ¼ cup of onion juice with 1 tablespoon of honey. Massage the scalp with the mixture every day. We heard about a man who had a bottle of this hair tonic. One day he took the cork out of the bottle with his teeth. The next day he had a mustache that needed to be trimmed. But seriously . . .

Stand on your head. If you can't, then get down on all fours, with your hands about 2 feet from your knees. Then carefully lift your rear end in the air so that your legs are straight and your head is between your outstretched arms. Stay in that position for 1 minute each day, and after a week, gradually work your way up to 5 minutes each day. The theory behind this is that you will bring oxygen to the hair follicles, which will rejuvenate the scalp and encourage hair to grow.

> **CAUTION:** Do not do this exercise if you have high or low blood pressure! Do not do this exercise without your doctor's approval if you are significantly beyond young adulthood!

We heard that the late comedian Rodney Dangerfield came up with a formula: alum and persimmon juice. It doesn't grow hair. It just shrinks your head to fit whatever hair you've got.

TEST YOUR HAIR'S HEALTHINESS

Human hair is almost impossible to destroy. Other than its vulnerability to fire, it cannot be destroyed by changes of climate, water, or other natural forces. When you think of the ways some of us abuse our hair with bleaches, dyes, rubber bands, permanents, mousses, sprays, and that greasy kid stuff, you can see how resistant it is to all kinds of corrosive chemicals. No wonder it's always clogging up sinks and drainpipes.

While hair may not be destroyed by the abuse mentioned above, it may look lifeless and become unmanageable and unhealthy.

One way to tell whether or not hair is

healthy is by its stretchability. A strand of adult hair should be able to stretch an additional 25 percent of its length without breaking. If it's less elastic than that, it's less than healthy, and there's room for improvement. The remedies on these pages may help.

BAD HAIR DAYS

If your self-esteem is in the cellar and you're feeling less than confident, it may be because you're having a bad hair day. The findings of a Yale University study confirmed the negative effect of a crummy coif on the psyche. The fascinating aspect of the study was that men were more likely to feel less smart and less capable than women when their hair stuck out, was badly cut, or was otherwise mussed up.

Here are remedies to help you have healthy hair, be the best-tressed person around, and boost your self-esteem.

Shampoo That Adds Body, Bounce, and Shine

Reduce 1 cup of beer (fresh or flat) to ¼ cup by heating it in a saucepan over medium heat. Let it cool, then mix the reduced beer into a cup of inexpensive commercial shampoo. Pour the mixture into a clean, empty shampoo bottle or squeeze bottle. No refrigeration is necessary. Use it as you would your regular shampoo. Rinse well. After seeing the results, you may never want to use any other shampoo.

Shampoo/Treatment for Correcting and Preventing Problems

This treatment is said to clean, condition, and give a shine to the hair. It should also help get rid of dandruff and nourish the scalp and hair. If it does only half of what it promises, it's worth doing. All you need is:

- 1 egg yolk and ½ cup warm water for thin and short hair
- 2 egg yolks and 1 cup warm water for average shoulder-length hair
- 3 egg yolks and 1½ cups warm water for thick and long hair

Combine and beat the egg yolk(s) and water thoroughly. Massage the mixture into your scalp and on every strand of hair. To make sure the entire head of hair is saturated and fed this protein potion, massage for 5 minutes, then put a plastic bag over your scalp and hair for another 5 minutes. Next, rinse with tepid water (hot water will cook the egg, making it difficult to remove). When you're sure that all of the egg is out of your hair, rinse one more time.

Use this as a maintenance shampoo

once or twice a month to help prevent problems from returning.

Dry Hair

Shampoo and towel-dry your hair. Then evenly distribute 1 tablespoon of mayonnaise throughout your hair. (Use more mayo if your hair is long.) After the mayonnaise has been on for an hour, wash your hair with a mild shampoo and rinse. The theory is that the flow of oil from the sebaceous glands is encouraged as the natural fatty acids of the mayonnaise help nourish the hair.

Mix together ½ cup water, ¼ cup olive oil, and 1 cup mild shampoo or liquid soap. Pour the mixture into a clean, empty shampoo bottle or squeeze bottle. Use it as you would any shampoo, but right before you use it, shake it to make sure the ingredients are completely blended. After shampooing, rinse well with cool water.

Frizzy Dry Hair

After shampooing, rinse with 1 tablespoon of wheat germ oil (available at health food stores), followed by a mixture of ½ cup of apple cider vinegar and 2 cups of water. It should tame the frizzies and add moisture.

Conditioner for Wispy Hair

This conditioning treatment comes highly recommended for taming flyaway hair. (If you don't know what we mean, you don't have it.) Beat an egg into 3 ounces (6 tablespoons) of plain yogurt. After shampooing your hair, vigorously rub this mixture into the scalp and hair for 3 minutes. Wrap a towel around your hair and leave it that way for 10 minutes. Rinse with tepid water. If this treatment works for your hair, repeat the procedure after every shampooing.

After-Shampoo Conditioning Rinse

Prepare any one of these herbal infusions and use it as an after-shampoo conditioning rinse for smooth, lustrous, bouncy tresses.

Boil 5 tablespoons of fresh parsley or fresh mint leaves, or a handful of fresh celery leaves, in a quart of water. Once the water boils, reduce the heat and let it simmer for about 15 minutes. Remove from the heat, cover it, and let it stand for 4 hours. Strain out the herbs, pour, and store the liquid in a bottle.

Right before you wash your hair, put 2 teaspoons of the herbal infusion in a plastic bottle with 8 ounces of water. If you've used the celery leaves to make the infusion, add a teaspoon of lemon juice—only for the celery leaves.

After you've shampooed and rinsed your hair, pour the herbal water on your hair as the final rinse. Good-bye to dull, limp hair; hello shiny, lovely locks.

Thin, Bodiless Hair

Add 2 egg whites and the juice of half a lemon to your shampoo. This should give your hair more body and volume.

DRY SHAMPOO

If your building is having plumbing problems, your city is having a water shortage, or you just don't feel like washing your hair, you can dry-shampoo it with cornmeal or cornstarch. Sprinkle some on your hair. Put a piece of cheesecloth or already-run pantyhose on the bristles of a hairbrush and brush your hair with it. The cornmeal/cornstarch will pull out the dust from your hair; the cloth will absorb the grease.

Complete the job with a silk scarf. Shine your hair with it, using it as you would a buffing cloth on shoes. After a few minutes of this, if your hair doesn't look clean and shiny, tie the scarf around your head and no one will know the difference.

Coarse or kosher salt is known to be an effective dry shampoo. Put 1 tablespoon of the salt in aluminum foil and set it in the oven to warm for 5 minutes. Using your fingers, work the warm salt into the scalp and throughout the hair. As soon as you feel that the salt has had a chance to absorb the grease and dislodge the dust, patiently brush it out of your hair. Wash the brush thoroughly, or use an already-clean brush and brush again to make sure all the salt has been removed.

NOTE: Do not use table salt. Not only will you still have dirty hair, but it will look as though you have dandruff, too.

Dull Hair with or without a Perm

After shampooing, rinse with a combination of 1 cup of apple cider vinegar and 2 cups of water. Your hair will come alive and shine. This treatment is especially effective on permed hair but can be used on any lifeless-looking hair.

Hair Revitalizer

This was our mom's favorite hair treatment. (Actually, it was the only hair treatment she ever used.) Slightly warm ½ cup of olive oil. You may want to add a few drops of an extract such as vanilla to make it more fragrant. Mom put it in a large eyedropper bottle and let it stand in very hot water for a few minutes. Then, using the eyedropper, she'd put the warm oil on the hair and massage it into the scalp. Once the entire head is oiled, shampoo the oil out.

Dandruff

Squeeze the juice of 1 large lemon and apply half of it to your hair. Mix the other half with 2 cups of water. Wash your hair with a mild shampoo, then rinse with water. Rinse again with the lemon and water mixture. Repeat every other day until dandruff disappears.

Massage 4 tablespoons of warm corn oil into your scalp. Wrap a warm, wet towel around your head and leave it there on the corn oil for a half hour. Then shampoo and rinse. Repeat this treatment once a week.

Prepare chive tea by adding 1 tablespoon of fresh chives to 1 cup of just-boiled water. Cover and let it steep for 20 minutes. Strain and, making sure it's cool, rinse your hair with it right after you shampoo.

Grate a piece of ginger and squeeze it through cheesecloth, collecting the juice. Then mix the ginger juice with an equal amount of sesame oil. Rub the ginger-sesame lotion on the entire scalp, cover the head with a sleep cap or wrap a dish towel around the head, and sleep with it on. In the morning, wash with an herbal shampoo. The final rinse should be with 1 tablespoon of apple cider vinegar in 1 quart of warm water. Repeat this treatment three or four times a week until there's no more dandruff.

We've gotten feedback from people with different kinds of scalp problems that have cleared up when using this remedy.

In a glass bowl, combine ½ cup apple cider vinegar, ½ cup fresh mint leaves or 1 tablespoon dried mint leaves, and 1 cup of just-boiled water. When the mixture is completely cool, strain out the mint leaves. Shampoo as usual, and as a final rinse, pour the mixture all over your scalp, then rinse with cool water.

This solution should be the solution for your scalp's dry flakes and dead skin cells.

ENERGIZING HAIR ROOTS

According to reflexology expert Mildred Carter, "To energize the hair roots, grab handsful of hair and yank gently. Do this over the whole head. This is also said to help a hangover, indigestion, and other complaints. To further stimulate these reflexes in the head, lightly close your hands into loose fists. With a loose wrist action, lightly pound the whole head. This will not only stimulate the hair, but also the brain, bladder, liver, and other organs."

HELPFUL HAIR HINTS

No-No Number 1: Rubber Bands

We've always been told not to wear rubber bands in our hair. We just found an explanation for it: The rubber insulates the hair and stops the normal flow of static electricity, so hair elasticity is reduced and the hair breaks more easily.

No-No Number 2: Combing Wet Hair

Combing wet hair stretches it out, causing it to be less elastic and break more easily.

Hair Spray Remover

In the middle of shampooing, massage 1 tablespoon of baking soda into your soaped-up hair. Rinse thoroughly. The baking soda should remove all the hair spray buildup.

Chewing Gum Remover

To remove gum from hair without doing a Delilah, take a glob of peanut butter, put it on the gummed area, then rub the gum and peanut butter between your fingers until the gum is on its way out. Use a comb to finish the job. Then get that kid under the faucet for a good shampooing.

Ground Your Fly-Away Hair

Rub a fabric-softening dryer sheet on your hair as well as on your brush or comb.

For a chronic wispy hair condition, see "Conditioner for Wispy Hair," above.

Odor Remover for Permed Hair

The distinctive and unpleasant smell of a hair permanent has a habit of lingering. Tomato juice to the rescue! Saturate your dry, permed, stinky hair with tomato juice. Cover your hair and scalp with a plastic bag and stay that way for 10 minutes. Rinse hair thoroughly, then shampoo and rinse again.

SETTING

Setting Lotions

Don't throw away beer that's gone flat. Instead, dip your comb in it and comb it through your hair for a wonderful setting lotion. Incidentally, the smell of beer seems to disappear quickly.

A friend of ours is a professional model and knows many tricks of her trade. Her favorite hair-setting lotion is fresh lemon juice. The hair takes longer to dry once the juice is dabbed on it, but the setting stays in a lot longer. If she runs out of lemons, she uses bottled lemon juice from the fridge, and that works well, too.

If beer or lemon isn't your cup of tea, try milk. Dissolve 4 tablespoons of skim milk powder in 1 cup of tepid water. Use it as you would any commercial hair-setting lotion. Unlike most commercial products, the milk helps nourish the scalp and hair.

Improvised Setting Rollers

If you have long hair and want to experiment setting it with big rollers, try used frozen juice cans that have been opened at both ends and washed clean. Roll your hair on them and use long hair clips or bobby pins to hold the rollers in place.

HAIR COLOR

According to a French proverb, "A fool's hair never turns white." The Russians say, "There was never a saint with red hair." "Pull out a gray hair," according to the German Pennsylvanians, "and seven will come to its funeral."

For those of you who want to use herbal or vegetable dyes, beware that they take time to cover gray or whatever color you currently have, because the color must accumulate. If you've got the patience, we've got the suggestions.

Brunettes

We have two hair-darkening formulas, both with dried sage, which adds life to hair and prevents dandruff.

Prepare dark sage tea by adding 4 tablespoons of dried sage to 2 cups of just-boiled water and letting it steep for 2 hours. Strain. This dark tea alone will darken gray hair, but for a stronger hair color, add 2 cups of rum and 2 tablespoons of glycerin (available in pharmacies). Bottle this mixture and be sure to label it. Every night, apply the potion to your hair, starting at the roots and working your way down. Stop the applications when your hair is as dark as you want it to be.

Or, if you're a teetotaler and don't want to use the rum, combine 2 tablespoons of dried sage with 2 tablespoons of black tea and simmer in 1 quart of water for 20 minutes. Let it steep for 4 hours, then strain and bottle. Massage it into your hair daily until your hair is the color of your choice. When you need a touch-up, mix a fresh batch of tea.

Drinking sesame-seed tea has been known to darken one's hair. Crush 2 teaspoons of sesame seeds and bring to a boil in 1 cup of water. Then let it simmer for 20 minutes. As soon as it's cool enough to drink, drink it, seeds and all. Have 2 to 3 cups daily and keep checking the mirror for darkening hair.

If you brunettes want to add a little life to your hair, pour a cool cup of espresso through your hair. Let it remain there for 5 minutes and then rinse.

Blondes

Dried chamomile (available at health food stores) can help add golden highlights to wishy-washy blond hair. Add 4 tablespoons of dried chamomile to 2 cups of just-boiled water and let it steep for 2 hours. Strain and use it as a rinse. Be sure to have a basin set up so you can catch the chamomile and use it over again for the next two or three shampoos.

As with most herbal rinses, you mustn't expect dramatic results overnight . . . if ever. Chamomile tea, no matter how strong you make it, will not cover really dark roots.

Squeeze the juice out of 2 big lemons, strain, and dilute with 1 cup of warm water. Put sunscreen on your face, neck, and other exposed body parts. Comb the lemon juice through your hair. Be very careful not to get any of it on your skin, even though you're wearing sunscreen. Why? Because you should sit in the sun for fifteen minutes in order to give your hair the glowy highlight of a summer day. If your skin has lemon juice on it, it can cause a burn and give your skin mottled stains. Be very careful!

Redheads

Add radiance to your red hair right after you shampoo by pouring a cup of strong Red Zinger tea (available at health food stores and many supermarkets) through your hair. Let it remain there for 5 minutes and rinse.

Juice a raw beet in a juice extractor and add 3 times the amount of water as there is juice. Use this as a rinse after shampooing.

NOTE: Since there are many shades of red, we urge you to do a test patch with the beet juice to see how it reacts on your specific color.

Gray, Gray, Go Away!

Many vitamin therapists have seen proof positive that taking PABA (para-aminobenzoic acid)—not more than 300 mg a day—plus a good B-complex vitamin, also daily, can help change hair back to its original color if the hair turned gray due to trauma, stress, or a nutritional deficiency.

We got this suggestion from a nutritionist who doesn't have one gray hair on his head. (Of course, he's only twelve years old. Just kidding.)

In a glass of water, mix 2 tablespoons of

each of the following: apple cider vinegar, raw unheated honey (available at health food stores), and blackstrap molasses. Drink this mixture first thing in the morning. Not only should it help you get rid of gray hair, but it should also give you a lot more energy than people who haven't gotten gray yet.

> **CAUTION:** Clearly, you should not try this if you have diabetes or any other health challenge that requires you to limit your sugar and carbohydrate intake.

Prevent Gray Hair from Yellowing

By adding a couple of teaspoons of laundry bluing to a quart of warm water and using it as your final rinse after shampooing, you can prevent gray hair from turning that yucky yellow.

Make Green Hair Disappear

Don't you just hate it when you get out of the pool and your blond hair has a greenish tinge? Next time, take a clean sponge, dip it in red wine, and dab it on your 'do. The chemicals in a chlorinated pool will be neutralized by the tannic acid in the wine.

Dissolve 6 aspirins in a pint of warm water and massage it into your wet hair.

Rinse thoroughly with clear water, and the green will never be seen.

Keep a bottle of lemon juice and a box of baking soda in your locker. After your swim and before you hit the shower, mix ½ cup of the baking soda into a cup of lemon juice. Wet your hair, then rinse it with this bubbly mixture to get the green out. (Maybe blondes *don't* have more fun.)

HAIR SPRAY

If you don't want to inhale the chemicals in commercial hair spray, all you have to do is dissolve 1 tablespoon of sugar into 1 cup of hot water. Once the mixture cools, pour it into a clean spritzer bottle. Hair spray!

Spritz before setting, or to hold your hairdo in place.

> **CAUTION:** Do not use this hair spray if you are going to be outdoors when there are mosquitoes, bees, or yellowjackets around.

HAND AND NAIL PROBLEMS

Each hand contains 29 major and minor bones, 29 major joints, at least 123 named ligaments, 34 muscles that move the fingers and thumb, 48 nerves, and 30 named arteries. About a quarter of the motor cortex in the human brain (that part of the brain that controls all movement in the body) is devoted to the muscles of the hands. So use the rest of your brain to learn to take care of your hands. Here's how.

PROTECT YOUR HANDS

Wear gloves when you go out in cold weather. Duh!

ROUGH AND CHAPPED HANDS

The ideal remedy for people with rough and chapped hands is their own sheep as a pet. Sheep's wool contains lanolin. By rubbing your hands across the animal's back every so often, you'll keep them in great shape.

If you aren't getting a sheep anytime soon, try any of the remedies that follow.

◗ For chapped hands, try some honey. Wet your hands and shake off the water without actually drying them. Then rub some honey all over your hands. When they're completely honey-coated, let them stay that way for 5 minutes. Next, rub your hands as you rinse them under tepid water. Then pat your hands dry. Do this daily until you want to clap hands for your unchapped hands.

◗ Red, rough hands should be relieved with a coating of lemon juice. After you rinse off the lemon juice, massage the hands with olive oil, coconut oil, or wheat germ oil and leave it on overnight.

NOTE: To maximize the moisturizer's effectiveness, and to protect your bed linens, wear white cotton gloves to bed after applying the oil. If you don't have white cotton gloves (and who does these days?), you can probably find them at a drugstore, or go to a photographic supply store and pick up the inexpensive gloves that photographers and film editors wear when handling film.

ROUGH, CHAPPED, AND DIRTY HANDS

Tired of being called "lobster claw"? Take 1 teaspoon of granulated sugar in the palm of your hand and add a few drops of castor oil and enough fresh lemon juice to thoroughly moisten the sugar. Vigorously massage your hands together for a few minutes. Rinse in tepid water and pat dry. This hand scrub should leave hands smooth, and will remove stains.

⯈ This folk remedy for rough, chapped, and soiled hands is a favorite among farmers. In a bowl combine about ¼ cup of cornmeal, 1 tablespoon of water, and enough apple cider vinegar to make the mixture the consistency of a loose paste. Rub this mildly abrasive mixture all over your hands for 5 to 10 minutes. Rinse with tepid water and pat dry. This treatment not only removes dirt, it will also soften, soothe, and heal the hands.

⯈ Take a palmful of oatmeal or baking soda and moisten with a little milk. Rub and rinse. It will clean your hands as well as make them feel smooth.

CLAMMY HANDS

In a basin, combine ½ gallon of water with ½ cup of rubbing alcohol and bathe your hands in the mixture. After a few minutes, rinse your hands with cool water and pat dry. This is especially useful for clammy-handed hand shakers, such as politicians on the campaign trail.

ELIMINATE GARLIC AND ONION SMELLS

This helpful hint works like magic. Take a piece of silverware (any metal spoon, knife, or fork will do), pretend it's a cake of soap, and wash your hands with it under cold water. The garlic or onion smell will vanish in seconds.

Those pungent garlic and onion odors can also be removed by rubbing your hands with a slice of fresh tomato.

NAILS

It takes six months for your fingernails to grow all the way from the root to the tip. Your toenails take two to three times as long. While they're growing, here's how to care for them.

Strengthening Nails

If you're having problems with breaking, splitting, and thin nails, you may need to supplement your diet with vitamin B complex and zinc sulfate, along with garlic—raw and/or supplements. Follow the suggested dosage on the bottle.

⯈ In addition to a well-balanced diet and the supplements mentioned above, soak your fingers daily for 10 minutes in any one of these oils:

- Warm olive oil
- Warm sesame oil
- Warm wheat germ oil

As you wipe off the oil, give your nails a mini-massage from top to bottom.

Faster-Growing Nails

While tapping your nails on a table can be very annoying to people around you, it is very good for your nails. The more you tap, the faster they will grow. You may need long fingernails to defend yourself against those annoyed people around you.

Fingernail Fungus

See "Toenail Fungus" in the "Foot and Leg Problems" chapter.

Nicotine Nails

If your nails are cigarette-stained, we'll tell you how to bleach them back to normal if you promise to stop smoking, okay? Now then, rub half a lemon over your nails. Then remove the lemon's pulp and, with the remaining rind, concentrate on one nail at a time, rubbing each one until it looks nice and pink.

NOTE: If you have citrus juice on your skin and you go in the sun, your skin may become permanently mottled. Be sure to wash the lemon juice off before you go outdoors.

Stained Nails

Want natural, healthy-looking, pinkish nails? Stop staining them with colored nail polish. From now on, first wear a protein-based coat under nail polish to protect your nails from the polish's color pigments, which cause staining and oxidation.

To get rid of the stains, toss 2 denture-cleansing tablets into ¼ cup of water. Soak your fingertips in the solution for about 15 minutes. If your nails are not as stain-free as you had hoped, gently brush them with a nailbrush. Rinse and dry.

Put tooth-whitening paste on a toothbrush and gently distribute the paste on your nails. Leave it on for about 15 minutes. Brush the nails as you rinse off the paste, and then dry your nails.

NOTE: It may take several tries, day after day, before the stains are completely gone. We think you'll find it's worth it.

Nail Grooming Tips

POLISH PRIMER

Wipe your unpolished fingernails with distilled white vinegar to clean and prime the surfaces of your nails before polishing. This treatment will help the polish stay on longer.

MANICURE PROTECTION

Use a toothbrush and toothpaste to clean office-type stains (ink, toner, etc.) off your fingertips without damaging your manicure.

NAIL FILE SUBSTITUTE

When you need an emery board and nobody has one, chances are somebody will have a matchbook you can borrow. File down a jagged-edged fingernail with the rough, striking part of the matchbook.

HEADACHES

Take a holistic approach to yourself and your headache. Step back and look at the past twenty-four hours of your life. Have you eaten sensibly? Did you get a decent night's sleep? Have you moved your bowels since awakening this morning? Are there deadlines you need to meet? Do you have added pressures at home or at work? Is there something you're dreading?

Now that you probably realize the reason for your headache, what should you take for it? Don't refuse any offer.

Since studies show that more than 90 percent of headaches are brought on by nervous tension, we're starting with remedies for the common tension headache, and we follow those with remedies for migraines.

In the case of regularly recurring headaches, they can be caused by eyestrain, an allergy, or something more serious, and should be properly diagnosed by a health professional.

Headaches are a headache! Use your instincts, common sense, and patience to pinpoint the cause. Meanwhile, get rid of the headache you have with one or more of these remedies.

TENSION HEADACHES

External Applications

Peel the rind off a lemon. Make the piece(s) as long and as wide as possible. Rub the pith (the white spongy part of the rind) on your forehead and temples. Then place the rind on the forehead and temples with the pith on the inside, securing it with a scarf or Ace bandage. Keep it there until the headache goes away, usually within a half hour.

When our grandmother had a headache, she would dip a large white handkerchief in distilled white vinegar, wring it out, and tie it tightly around her forehead until the headache disappeared.

A variation of the handkerchief soaked in vinegar is to soak a piece of brown grocery-bag paper in vinegar. Shake off the excess liquid and place it on your forehead. Keep it in place with a handkerchief or Ace bandage and let it stay there for a half hour. By then the headache should be gone.

Get a little bottle of rosemary essential oil (available at health food stores) and rub a small amount of the oil on your forehead and temples, and also behind your ears. Then inhale the fumes from the open bottle four times. If your headache doesn't disappear within a half hour, repeat the rubbing and inhaling once more.

This seems to be a favorite of some Indian gurus: In a small pot combine 1 teaspoon of dried basil with 1 cup of hot water, and bring it to a boil. Take it off the stove, then add 2 tablespoons of witch hazel. Strain and let it cool, then saturate a washcloth with the mixture, wring it out, and apply it to the forehead. Keep it in place with an Ace bandage and let it stay there until the washcloth dries or your headache disappears . . . whichever comes first.

The fact that you have this book leads us to believe that you're a person who's interested in and open to all kinds of alternatives, variety, and new adventures. Usually, when people are adventurous, it extends to their eating habits. And so we would like to introduce you to daikon, a Japanese radish, available at most green-grocers. (It wouldn't surprise us if you are already familiar with it. Well, yes, it would.) It's delicious eaten raw in salads, and wonderful for digestion, especially when eating oily foods.

Meanwhile, back to the headache remedy. Make a poultice (see "Preparation Guide") using a grated piece of daikon. Apply the poultice to your forehead. It should help draw out the pain by the time the daikon dries out.

In Jamaica, a popular headache remedy requires the leaf of an aloe vera plant. Carefully cut the leaf in half the long way and place the cut side on your forehead and temples. Keep it in place with a handkerchief or Ace bandage and let it stay there until your headache is history.

Grate a potato (a red one if possible) or an apple and make a poultice out of it. (See "Preparation Guide.") Apply the poultice to your forehead and keep it in place with a handkerchief or Ace bandage.

Within an hour, the headache should be gone and you can remove the poultice.

Food

In one of our books we reported that almonds contain salicylates, which is the pain-relieving ingredient in aspirin. Eat 15 raw almonds to do the work of 1 aspirin. While it may take a little longer for the headache to vanish, you don't run the risk of side effects as you may from aspirin. (What scientists need to work on now are fast-acting almonds.)

Recently, we received an impactful e-mail from a man who read the remedy. He wrote and asked us to share his story with our readers, hoping that others may benefit from his incredible experience. And so, with permission from Joel F., we quote his e-mail.

"I am a seventy-three-year-old male in good health. I have been a headache sufferer for over fifty years (three or four headaches a week). Six weeks ago I started eating 1.5 ounces of almonds (about 30 to 35 almonds) a day. From day one, my headaches vanished, and as of now, I am in my forty-third day headache-free. My neurologist and internist are totally amazed. This is positively a miracle for me."

It may not work as dramatically as it did for Joel, but it sure is worth a try. If you don't have almonds on hand but you do have some strawberries, eat them. They also contain salicylates.

A very old American remedy says to swallow 1 teaspoon of honey mixed with ½ teaspoon of finely minced garlic. This healthful combination will make a headache disappear within 20 minutes.

Gomasio—that's Japanese sesame salt—is something you may want to know about even if you don't have a headache. The interesting thing about this seasoning (available at health food stores and Asian markets) is that the oil from the crushed sesame seeds coats the sea salt so that it doesn't cause an excessive attraction for water. In other words, you can season food with it and it won't make you thirsty the way regular salt does.

To get relief from a headache, eat 1 teaspoon of gomasio. Chew it thoroughly before swallowing.

CAUTION: If you are on a salt-restricted diet, gomasio is not for you.

If you grow or can buy fresh mint, take a large mint leaf, bruise it, then roll it up and stick it in your nostril. It may not be a pretty picture, but if it helps you get rid of a headache . . .

Water Therapy

This will either work for you or it won't. You'll find out quickly and easily. Dunk your hands into water that's as hot as you can stand without scalding yourself. Keep them there for 1 minute. If you don't start feeling relief within 5 minutes, go on to another remedy.

◗ Let ice-cold water accumulate ankle-high in the bathtub. Dress warmly except for your bare feet. Carefully, very carefully, take a leisurely stroll in the tub for 1 to 3 minutes—as long as it takes for your feet to start feeling warm in the ice-cold water. When that happens, get out of the tub, dry your feet, and go directly to bed. Cover up, relax, and within no time, your headache should be a pain of the past.

◗ If the tension headache seems to stem from the tightness in your neck, wet a cloth or towel with hot water and put it around your neck. An electric heating pad may be used instead of the wet cloth. The heat should relax you and improve circulation.

Vaporizing

In a medium-size pot, combine 1 cup of water with 1 cup of apple cider vinegar and bring it to a slow boil. When the fumes begin to rise, reduce the heat as low as it can go. Put a towel over your head, bend over the pot (be careful—steam can burn if you get too close), and inhale and exhale deeply through your nose about eighty times, or for about 10 minutes. Be sure the towel is far enough away from the burner so that it doesn't catch fire but does catch the vapor for you to inhale.

Mental Exercise

At a self-help seminar, we were told that whatever you fully experience disappears . . . headaches included.

Sit down. Close your eyes. Have someone walk you through this process by asking you the following questions:

■ Do you *really* want to get rid of the headache? (Don't laugh. A lot of people want to hang on to their headaches. It's a great excuse and cop-out from all kinds of things.)

■ What kind of headache is it? Be specific. Is it a pounding over one eye? Does it throb each time you bend down? Do you have a dull ache at the base of your neck?

■ What size is your headache? Describe the exact dimensions of it. Start with the length from the front of your face to the back of your head, the width from ear to ear, and the thickness of it from the top of your head down toward your neck.

■ What color is your headache?

■ How much water will it hold? Visualize yourself filling a cup with the amount of water needed to fill the area of the headache. Then pour the water from the cup into the space of your headache. When you've completed that, open your eyes.

You should have experienced away your headache.

The first time I (Lydia) used this process, my results were quite dramatic. I went from having an all-day bangeroo to no headache whatsoever. If I hadn't experienced it myself, I'd probably think it's as crazy as you're probably thinking I am right now.

Acupressure

Stick out your tongue about ½ inch and bite down on it as hard as you can without hurting yourself. Stay that way for *exactly 10 minutes,* not a minute more! (Some people would rather have a headache than do this.)

This is another acupressure remedy that should be done in private. Press your right or left thumb against the roof of your mouth for 4 to 5 minutes. Every so often, move your thumb to another section of the roof of your mouth. This should greatly relieve the nerve pressure in your head.

Vigorously rub the second joint of each thumb for 2 minutes on the right hand and 2 minutes on the left hand, until you've done it 5 times each, for a total of 20 minutes. Use hand lotion on the thumbs to eliminate friction.

Enlist the help of someone who will slowly move his or her thumb down the right side of your back, alongside your shoulder blade and toward your waist. Let that person know when (s)he hits a sore or tender spot. Have your helper exert steady pressure on that spot for a minute. By then you should have relief from the headache.

Supplements

Some people rid themselves of headache pain by taking vitamin C—500 mg every hour—to dilate the constricted blood vessels that are thought to cause the pain. If, after two hours, you still have a headache, this isn't working for you. Stop taking vitamin C and try another remedy.

Niacin has helped many headache sufferers when all else has failed. See "Migraine Headaches," below, for more information.

MIGRAINE HEADACHES

A migraine is a legitimate, biological disease affecting 28 million Americans—

that's about 13 percent of the U.S. population. Women experience migraines more often than men by a ratio of 3 to 1, and the peak prevalence for migraines is between the ages of twenty and forty-five, according to the National Headache Foundation (NHF, www.headaches.org).

The NHF says that practically anything may trigger a migraine, and triggers are not the same for everyone. In fact, what causes a migraine in one person may relieve it in another.

The most common triggers are in food. Sharon Herzfeld, M.D., an integrative neurologist with a holistic approach to practicing medicine, goes into detail about food triggers.

> **NOTE:** Following this advice takes more of a commitment than most of our remedies throughout this book. We're including the information because migraine sufferers are usually desperate to find the cause and, in so doing, find the solution. It very well may be on this page. And, when Dr. Herzfeld talks, we listen.

According to Dr. Herzfeld, the four main substances that have been found to trigger headaches are tyramine, nitrates, MSG (monosodium glutamate), and caffeine.

■ *Tyramine.* This substance, derived from the amino acid tyrosine, is found in aged cheese (avoid all cheese except ricotta, cottage cheese, and cream cheese), beans, miso soup, red wine, grapes, grape juice, and soy sauce.

The tyramine content of foods differs greatly due to processing, aging, fermentation, ripening, or contamination. Spoiled, aged, or fermented foods may develop greater amounts of tyramines. All overripe and spoiled foods should be avoided.

Limit the following foods to 4 ounces of only one per day: avocado, banana, raspberries, red plums, canned figs, citrus fruits/juices, and raisins. All other fruits are permitted.

■ *Nitrates.* They are naturally occurring in many foods and are added to some foods to retain freshness and the pink color. These foods include all smoked, aged, pickled, fermented, or marinated meats.

Avoid all nitrate-containing foods: salami, bologna, pepperoni, hot dogs, bacon, liverwurst, luncheon meats, ham, herring, and smoked food such as smoked salmon (lox).

■ *MSG.* This is a food additive found in many processed foods and widely used in Chinese food (especially soups). Check the labels on canned soup, barbecue sauce, potato chips, and spices such as adobo, Accent, and Sazón Goya.

■ *Caffeine.* Avoid this natural stimulant, found in coffee, some tea (check labels), chocolate, colas, some orange sodas, and Mountain Dew.

■ *Yeast.* While yeast is not one of the four main culprits, consider it a contender. Avoid sourdough and fresh, yeast-leavened breads. Yeast extracts are also found in canned and frozen foods. Check labels on everything!

■ *Dairy.* Limit your intake of buttermilk, yogurt, and sour cream to ½ cup per day maximum, or avoid them completely.

Dr. Herzfeld advises you to eliminate these foods and beverages for one month if possible. After the first month, reintroduce them—one at a time—into your diet. Pay attention to the frequency and severity of the migraines to help you determine the effect of each reintroduced substance and learn what agrees with you and what may be giving you a headache.

More Triggers

Dr. Sharon Herzfeld dealt with food (above), the most prevalent migraine trigger. There are other common triggers that you may want to look at:

■ Environment (bright lights, smoke)

■ Emotions (stress, anxiety)

■ Activity (irregular exercise, lack of sleep)

■ Hormones (menstrual cycle, oral contraceptives)

■ Medications (overuse of over-the-counter analgesics/pain relievers)

When you get a migraine, re-create (on paper) what you've eaten, where you've been, and what has gone on in your life for the last two days leading up to the headache. You may eventually notice a pattern and be able to pinpoint your migraine trigger. Until then, see if any of the following remedies can help you.

Supplement

Niacin, when taken at the first sign of a migraine, has been known to prevent a full-blown headache. To prevent or get rid of a headache, take anywhere from 50 to 100 mg at a time. The higher the dosage, the stronger the side effects. For most people, the side effects are felt when they take 100 mg or higher. Both of us get the "niacin flush" that makes us look like we've been in the sun too long. It's usually accompanied by itching and/or tingling. It lasts about 15 minutes and is not at all harmful.

Niacinamide is said to be as effective as niacin but without the side effects. Both are available at vitamin and health food stores.

NOTEWORTHY: Dr. Sharon Herzfeld recommends that you explore Petadolex Butterbur Gelcaps to help reduce the frequency and intensity of migraine attacks. We visited their Web site (www .petadolex.com) and found impressive results from controlled studies. We also discovered that not all medications said to be made with "butterbur" are the same. Not all of them are safe. The butterbur plant in its natural state contains pyrrolizidin alkaloids (PAs), which may cause liver cancer. However, Weber and Weber, responsible for Petadolex, has developed a patented method for extracting the beneficial ingredients of the butterbur plant without the PAs. It guarantees that its product is free of all detectable PAs.

Free samples are given to neurologists for their patients. Talk to your neurologist about it, or call this toll-free number to find a neurologist in your area who knows about this product: 888-301-1084.

Health food stores carry a variety of butterbur brands. Be sure the name "Petadolex" is somewhere on the label, to ensure you are getting the best-quality, safest herb.

Dr. Herzfeld stresses the importance of consulting with your health care provider to be sure that butterbur does not interfere with medication or supplements you are currently taking.

Foot Bath

Bathe your feet in a basin or two plastic shoe boxes filled with very strong, comfortably hot black coffee. Some medical professionals recommend drinking a cup or two of coffee as well.

If coffee isn't for you, put 1 teaspoon of mustard or ginger powder into each plastic shoe box, along with comfortably hot water. Then sit down, put your feet in the shoe boxes, place a towel over them to help keep the heat in, and soak your feet for about 15 minutes. You may want to turn on some soothing music, close your eyes, and relax. Your headache may be gone by the time the water cools.

Dry Heat

Sit under a hair dryer. The heat and high-pitched hum may relax the tension that brought on the headache. According to Dr. Robert B. Taylor, the dryer brings relief to 67 percent of the migraine sufferers who try it.

Your local beauty salon will probably be happy to accommodate you as long as you don't get a headache during their busy time.

NOTE: If you have chemical sensitivities, do not go to a hair salon.

Inhalant

Open a jar of strong mustard and slowly inhale the fumes several times. This has been known to help ease the pain for some people.

External Applications

Dip a few cabbage leaves in just-boiled water to make them soft. As soon as they're soft and cool enough, place one or two thicknesses on your forehead and on the back of your neck. Secure them in place with a scarf or Ace bandage, then relax as the cabbage draws out the pain.

▶ Boil 2 Spanish onions. Eat one and mash the other. Make a poultice (see "Preparation Guide") out of the mashed onion by rolling it in cheesecloth. Put the poultice on your forehead, lean back, and relax until the headache disappears.

Acupressure

Apply pressure to the palm of one hand with the thumb of the other hand. Then reverse the order. If you feel a tenderness in either palm, concentrate the massage on that area. Keep up the firm pressure and massage for 10 minutes—5 minutes on each hand. Better yet, get someone to do this acupressure remedy to you.

Food

For those of you who have migraines without having severe headaches but with impaired vision—auras, jagged edges, spots, seeing double—eating a handful of raisins may give you some relief. Be sure to chew the raisins thoroughly before swallowing.

▶ We heard about a woman who would take 1 tablespoon of honey the second she felt a migraine coming on. If the headache wasn't gone within a half hour, she would take another tablespoon of honey with 3 glasses of water and that would do it.

NOTE: Please remember that we're reporting on what works for others. Use common sense when deciding which remedy may be for you.

SINUS HEADACHES

Sniff a little horseradish juice—the stronger the horseradish, the better. (Horseradish in a jar is available at supermarkets.) Remember to sniff it slowly.

▶ Prepare three poultices (see "Preparation Guide") of grated onion and apply them to the nape of the neck and to the soles of the feet. Leave them on for an hour. Then take a shower in cool water. It will wash off the onion smell and may help clear your sinuses, too.

HEADACHE PREVENTION . . . SORT OF

A three-year study at the University of Michigan showed that students who ate 2 apples a day had far fewer headaches than those who didn't eat any apples. The apple eaters also had fewer skin problems, arthritic conditions, and colds.

You may want to have an apple for breakfast and one as a late-afternoon snack. Chances are, eating two apples a day will also prevent constipation, which is a leading cause of headaches.

HEART CONDITIONS

HEART ATTACK FIRST AID

If you feel as though you're having a heart attack, call 911 *immediately*, tell them you may be having a heart attack, and give them your exact location. Meanwhile, cough, and then take a deep breath. Again, cough, then take a deep breath. Keep doing this until the chest pain subsides and you can do more. Chew an adult aspirin and, if available, a magnesium capsule. If you have a cardiac history, take nitroglycerine.

▶ Put 1 teaspoon of cayenne pepper in a glass of warm water and force yourself to drink it all, advises Dr. John R. Christopher, master herbalist. Cayenne pepper is hotter than hot and hard to take, but so is having a heart attack.

▶ While you're waiting for help to arrive, squeeze the end of the pinky (the little finger) on the left hand. Squeeze it hard! Keep squeezing it. This acupressure procedure has been said to save lives.

NOW THEN . . . THE HEART

The heart is a four-chambered hollow muscle and double-acting pump located in the chest between the lungs. This hardworking, fist-size muscle pumps blood through the blood vessels in all parts of the body at the rate of about 4,000 gallons a day. (No wonder so many of us have "tired blood.")

The heart is so complex and heart trouble is so serious that the best preventive suggestions we can offer are:

■ Follow an eating plan that will promote a healthy heart.

■ Don't smoke! (See the "Smoking" chapter.)

■ Exercise. (See specifics below under "Heart Helpers.")

■ To help others who may have heart problems, take a cardiac pulmonary resuscitation (CPR) course through your local Red Cross chapter.

HEART HELPERS

According to the results of a study, orchestra conductors live an average of seven and a half years longer than the average person.

To strengthen your heart, tone up your circulatory system, and have some fun, go through the motions of conducting an orchestra. Do it for at least 10 minutes a day, or 20 minutes three times a week. Conduct to music that inspires you. If you don't have a baton, use a ruler or chopsticks. Pretend each day of exercise is a command performance. Throw your whole self into it physically and emotionally.

> **NOTE:** If you have a history of heart problems, be sure to check with your doctor before you begin conducting.

Two teaspoons of raw honey a day, either in a glass of water or straight off the spoon, is thought by many nutritionists to be the best tonic for strengthening the heart, as well as for general physical repair.

> **NOTE:** If you're on a sugar-restricted diet, this is not for you.

After researching the benefits of hawthorn berries, we now take it as part of our daily supplement regimen. Hawthorn berries are said to normalize blood pressure by regulating heart action, improve heart valve defects, help people who are stressed, strengthen weakened heart muscle, and help prevent arteriosclerosis (hardening of the arteries).

Check with your health professional for dosage, depending on your size and the state of your heart health.

For the best exercise and the perfect body stimulator, just take an old-fashioned walk—make it a brisk old-fashioned walk—daily. Brisk means walking a mile every 20 minutes (3 miles an hour). It's slower than running or race-walking, and faster than a stroll. A mile every 20 minutes is ideal, but less and slower is great, too.

The *New England Journal of Medicine* reported the findings of a long-term study of 72,000 women ages forty to sixty-five.

The heart attack risk was reduced 30 to 40 percent in the women who did at least 3 hours of brisk walking a week.

In addition to the walking, those who did vigorous exercise for 90 minutes a week cut their risk almost in half. Gardening and housework are considered vigorous exercise. You can have a clean house, a beautiful garden, and a healthy heart.

Incidentally, walking is believed to use the same amount of energy as running.

◗ Eat onions once a day. Eat lots of garlic. You may also want to take a garlic supplement. Both onions and garlic are great for . . . well, for just about everything except your breath.

◗ Omega-3 fatty acids impact many factors linked to cardiovascular challenges. Flaxseed oil, fish oils, and Salba (available at health food stores) are rich sources of omega-3 fatty acids. Add one or more to your daily diet. Prepare food with flaxseed meal or Salba. (See the "Food for Thought" chapter to learn more about Salba.)

HISTORY OF HEART PROBLEMS?

According to Dr. Richard Passwater (that's really his name), vitamin B_{15} (also sold as pangamic acid or DMG) quickens the healing of scar tissue around the heart and also limits the side effects of some heart medications. The suggested dosage is 150 mg a day, along with a B-complex vitamin. (Of course, check with your doctor first.) Food rich in B_{15} are sunflower seeds, nuts, brown rice, brewer's yeast, pumpkin seeds, and sesame seeds.

◗ Right before going to bed, take a 10-minute footbath. Get into calf-high water, as hot as you can take it without scalding yourself. As the minutes pass and the water cools, add more hot water. After 10 minutes, step out of the tub and dry your feet thoroughly, preferably with a rough towel. Once your feet are dry, give them a 1-minute massage, manipulating the toes as well as the entire foot. This footbath/massage may help circulation, remove congestion around the heart, and pave the way to a peaceful night's sleep.

Anticlotting Medication Alert

Broccoli and turnip greens are rich in vitamin K, the clot-promoting vitamin. If you take anticlotting medication, be aware that eating big portions of these vegetables can counteract the effects of the medicine.

HEART PALPITATIONS

CAUTION: If you have palpitations often, see a doctor for a diagnosis.

If you occasionally have palpitations (and who hasn't at one time or another?), take a holistic approach. Look at exactly what's going on in your life right now that may have caused the palpitations. Did you have MSG in the Chinese food you had for lunch? Or is it the caffeine in the chocolate mocha cappuccino? Or too much sugar? Is a deadline closing in on you at the office? Are you dreading a telephone call you have to make? Were you in the same room with a cigarette smoker? Work at figuring it out so that you can avoid setting up the same situation that caused palpitations.

Meanwhile, here's a natural sedative to subdue the thumping. Steep 2 chamomile tea bags in 2 cups of just-boiled water. Steam a few shredded leaves of cabbage. Then, in a soup bowl, combine the steamed leaves with the chamomile tea. This tea-soup may not taste great, but it can help overcome the *thump-thump-thump* of your heart.

Drink peppermint tea—a mugful a day. This caffeine-free herb seems to have a calming effect.

NOTE: Peppermint is a powerful herb that can undermine or negate the effectiveness of some medicines, including homeopathic formulas. Check with your doctor, nutritionist, or pharmacist before drinking it.

ATHEROSCLEROSIS (ARTERIOSCLEROSIS)

Whichever you call it, *atherosclerosis* or *arteriosclerosis,* it's hardening of the arteries, in which cholesterol and other fatty deposits build up on the inner walls of the arteries, limiting the flow of blood. This buildup is called plaque. It may develop over years of eating unhealthy foods, lack of exercise, and smoking.

Now is the time to take responsibility for your arteries. Improve your diet, start exercising, and stop smoking. It's doable. Read the "Cholesterol" and "Smoking" chapters . . . after you finish reading this one.

A couple of cloves of garlic a day has been known to unplug arteries. It seems to really do a job cleansing the system, and collecting and casting out toxic waste. Mince 2 cloves, put them in ½ glass of orange juice or water, and drink it down. There's no need to chew the pieces of garlic. When you just swallow them, the garlic smell doesn't stay on your breath.

In conjunction with a sensible diet, garlic can also help bring down cholesterol levels in the blood. No wonder this beautiful bulb has a fan club, appropriately called Lovers of the Stinking Rose.

Rutin is one of the elements of the bioflavonoids. Bioflavonoids are necessary for the proper absorption of vitamin C. Taking 500 mg of rutin daily, with at least the same amount of vitamin C, is said to increase the strength of capillaries, strengthen the artery walls, help prevent hemorrhaging, and help treat arteriosclerosis.

HARDENING OF THE ARTERIES PREVENTION

Red Wine

Yes, red wine, in moderation, helps reduce the risk of heart disease, as well of as stroke and other health problems that can lead to heart disease. But wait, not just any red wine.

Roger Corder, Ph.D., the William Harvey Research Institute's professor of experimental therapeutics and author of *The Red Wine Diet* (Avery), reveals the beneficial ingredients in wine, names some of the most healthful wines, and explains

how much to drink and when. Also, for abstainers, there are nonalcoholic options.

WHY RED WINE?

Polyphenols, found in dark red and purple grapes (also found in cocoa and pomegranates), can help stop atherosclerosis. The most potent polyphenols in red wines are procyanidins.

In connoisseur's terminology, wines described as having "firm" tannins are more likely to have high levels of procyanidins than wines with "soft" or "ripe" tannins.

Which Ones: The Wine List

William Harvey Research Institute's laboratory analyses of more than four hundred red wines discovered the richest sources of healthful procyanidins. Here is a round-the-world sampling of those wines:

- Cabernet sauvignons from Bodegas Catena Zapata, Argentina

- Cabernet sauvignons from Wynns, Australia

- Cabernet sauvignons from Robert Mondavi Napa Valley Reserve, as well as many other Napa Valley cabernets

- Cabernet sauvignons from Veramonte, Chile

■ France's many Bordeaux wines—from top-end to modestly priced—have high or better-than-average procyanidin levels

■ Tuscan wines made from Sangiovese grapes, including Il Colombaio di Cencios Chianti Classico Riserva

■ Rosso Superiore del Mandrolisai, Sardinia

When and How Much to Drink

Since food slows alcohol absorption, drink one or two small glasses at lunch and/or with dinner, and drink slowly. Drinking wine quickly or on an empty stomach speeds alcohol absorption, increasing the risk for high blood pressure.

Most research shows that women should not exceed 5 ounces of wine per day; men should limit their daily intake to 10 ounces daily.

NOTE: Consuming red wine in excess negates its benefits and increases the drinker's risk for many health challenges.

Nonalcoholic Procyanidin-Rich Options

■ *Dark chocolate.* Extra-dark with 70 percent to 85 percent cacao is best. One ounce of dark chocolate is equal to the amount of procyanidins in 4 ounces of red wine. Since it's high in calories and fat, limit your intake to 1 or 1½ ounces of dark chocolate daily.

NOTEWORTHY: Found in health food stores and some supermarkets, Chocolove (www.chocolove.com, phone: 888-CHOCOLOVE) has several dark chocolate bars with 70 percent to 76 percent cocoa content. Along with tasting notes on the back of each wrapper describing the distinct flavor profile of that particular bar, the package design resembles a love letter sent from a distant land, and inside each wrapper is a classic romantic poem. It does a heart good!

■ *Apples.* Red Delicious and Granny Smith are best. One medium-size apple is equivalent to 4 ounces of red wine.

■ *Cranberry juice.* An 8-ounce serving of juice containing 25 percent cranberry is equal to about a 4-ounce glass of red wine. (Be sure to look for low sugar and 25 percent cranberry content.)

■ *Foods.* Raspberries, blackberries, strawberries, pomegranates, walnuts, pinto beans, and cinnamon.

HEMORRHOIDS (PILES)

Hemorrhoids, or piles, are varicose veins in or around the rectum. It truly is a pain in the anus. Two out of every three adults have had, currently have, or will have hemorrhoids. Chances are, if you're reading this page, you are one of the two out of the three.

Along with treating your condition with natural, nonchemical remedies, here are ways of speeding up the healing process:

■ Keep the bowels as clear as possible. Eat a fiber-rich diet, and drink lots of vegetable juices. Stay away from hard-to-digest, overly processed foods and drinks, especially white flour, sugar, and alcoholic beverages.

■ Do not strain or hold your breath while you have a bowel movement. Make an effort to breathe evenly.

■ Take a brisk walk as often as you can, especially after meals.

Heed the suggestions above as well as the ones below, and we hope that in a few days you'll have this problem behind you.

▶ Take 100 mg of rutin (a bioflavonoid that's obtained from buckwheat leaves and available at health food stores) three times a day. This has helped hemorrhoid sufferers when all else has failed.

▶ Apply liquid lecithin (available at health food stores) directly on the hemorrhoids once a day until they completely disappear.

▶ Eat a large boiled leek every day as an afternoon snack or with dinner. Also, eat 3 raw almonds daily, chewing each one at least twenty times.

▶ Take advantage of the healing properties of the enzymes in papaya by putting papaya juice on a sanitary napkin and positioning it on the hemorrhoid area. The juice should help stop the bleeding and bring the irritation under control.

SUPPOSITORIES

Cut a peeled, raw (preferably red) potato in the shape of a suppository (like a bullet) and insert it in the rectum. This folk remedy has had dramatic, positive results.

▶ Insert a peeled clove of garlic in the rectum right after a bowel movement. Keep it in as long as possible. Then, before bedtime, remove it and insert another peeled clove, as high as you can push it with your finger. In order to keep it in overnight, you might have to put on a T-bandage. Garlic should help reduce the swelling quite quickly. Repeat the procedure daily until you're hemorrhoid-free.

Carefully carve or melt an ice cube down to the size and shape of a bullet. Use it as a suppository. The cold may give you a start, but it may also start reducing the swelling and help to heal the hemorrhoids.

Put ¼ cup of cranberries in a blender or food processor and chop finely. Place 1 tablespoon of the chopped cranberries in a piece of cheesecloth and insert it in the rectum, making sure a little piece of cheesecloth is hanging out. An hour later, remove the cheesecloth insert and replace it with another tablespoon of cranberries in cheesecloth for another hour. This is a great pain reliever. By the end of two hours, you should feel much better.

BATHS

A consulting doctor for the Denver Broncos and Denver Nuggets has had success in speeding up athletes' hemorrhoid healing processes with vitamin C baths. The doctor recommends 1 cup of ascorbic acid powder (available at health food stores) to every 5 quarts of cool bathwater.

Sit in the tub for 15 minutes at a time, two or three times a day. Ascorbic acid powder is expensive. If you can fit your tushy into a basin with ½ cup of the powder to 2½ quarts of cool water, or if you're really slim and can use ¼ cup of the powder in 1¼ quarts of water, you'll save a lot of money. Whatever you do, don't wedge yourself into a basin that you have to oil yourself out of or, worse yet, call the fire department to free you from.

If you have a basin that you can comfortably fit in, add ¼ cup of witch hazel and as much warm water as you can, then sit in it for about 15 minutes at least two times a day. Complete cures have been reported within three days.

> **NOTEWORTHY**: Dr. Leonard's health care catalog (www.drleonards.com or 800-785-0880) has a portable bidet that fits on any standard toilet bowl and is perfect for this kind of sitz bath.

EXERCISE

Psychic healer Edgar Cayce recommended this exercise:

1. Stand with your feet about 6 inches apart, hands at sides.

2. Raise your hands up to the ceiling.

3. Bend forward and bring your hands as close to the floor as you can.

4. Go back to the first position, hands at sides.

Repeat the entire procedure thirty-six times. It should take just a few minutes to do. Do it an hour after breakfast and an hour after dinner every day until the hemorrhoids are history.

HEMORRHOID PREVENTION

To help prevent a recurrence, increase the fiber and fluids in your diet.

⬤ Eat at least 3 raw almonds daily. According to psychic healer Edgar Cayce, the almonds will help prevent hemorrhoids.

⬤ Since hemorrhoids are a sitter's ailment, get up! Take a long walk daily at a fairly fast pace. Enroll in a yoga class once or twice a week, and do the yoga exercises daily.

HERPES AND SHINGLES

HERPES (GENITALIS, SIMPLEX, ETC.)

Twenty million Americans (one out of every five sexually active adults) have herpes. Each year 300,000 to 500,000 more get it.

We spoke with a man who did extensive research and came up with a remedy for overcoming the symptoms (fever blisters, cold sores, etc.). He tested it and had friends test it. The results were impressive. First, we'll give you the remedy, followed by the explanation, and then more about the results.

Remedy: Do not eat nuts, sesame seeds, chocolate, cocoa, or squash. At the first sign of a herpes flare-up, eat 1 pound of steamed flounder. That's it. That's the remedy.

Explanation in simple terms, as best we understand it: There's a certain balance in the body between two amino acids, arginine and lysine. To contract herpes and to have the symptoms recur, one's body has to have a high level of arginine compared with the level of lysine. The secret, then, is to reduce the amount of arginine (that's why you must eliminate nuts, chocolate, and chicken soup from your diet) and increase the amount of lysine (eat flounder). The pound of flounder has 11,000 mg of lysine. You can take lysine supplements, but you would have to take a huge number of them, and besides, they contain binders and other things you just don't need. Also, supplements are probably not nearly as digestible or as absorbable as the lysine in flounder. By steaming the fish, you help retain its nutrients. Also, you can add the sauce of your choice to the flounder after it's been steamed. Who would believe that your meal is medicine?

Results: The man and his friends have had their symptoms disappear, literally overnight, after eating flounder and never eating nuts, chocolate, or chicken soup.

Lemon balm is an herb that contains tannins, which are credited for giving it antiviral power. Lemon balm also contains eugenol, a bacteria killer.

To help prevent herpes outbreaks, drink a cup or two of lemon balm tea (available at health food stores) daily. If you have an outbreak, steep three or four tea bags in a cup of just-boiled water for about 15 minutes. By then the tea should be strong and cool. Using cotton balls, apply the tea to the sores throughout the day.

SHINGLES (HERPES ZOSTER)

Did you have the chicken pox when you were a kid? Herpes zoster virus is the chicken pox virus, which is also the shingles virus. After you get over the bout of chicken pox, the virus stays dormant until your immune system is compromised by something such as trauma, severe stress, a nutritional deficiency, or certain medications (e.g., cortisone). The resulting painful, blistery flare-up is shingles.

Oil of oregano (available in health food stores) should be applied to the affected areas. Repeat as often as needed to reduce pain and inflammation. To stop the growth of the virus, take 3 to 4 drops of the oil in water or juice twice a day.

CAUTION: Shingles that affect the face or forehead—anywhere near the eyes—can lead to cornea damage and/or temporary facial paralysis. If your face or forehead is affected, be sure to see your health care provider immediately.

For some relief, make a paste of baking soda and water, and apply to the affected area.

Aloe vera gel is a soothing, cooling antiseptic. You can buy a bottle of it at a health food store, or you can buy an aloe vera plant. They're inexpensive and easy to grow, and they look a lot prettier than a refrigerated bottle. Look for the aloes with the little spikes on the edge of the leaves. When using the plant, cut off the lowest leaf, then cut that leaf into 2-inch pieces. Slice one of the pieces in half and apply the gel directly on the affected area. Individually wrap the remaining pieces of the leaf in plastic wrap and keep them in the freezer. Every few hours, take a piece of leaf from the freezer and reapply the gel on the affected area.

▶ Prepare a paste of Epsom salts and water. Place the paste directly on the affected area, and when it starts to dry up and crumble off, gently wash it all off with cool water. Repeat the procedure as often as possible.

▶ St. John's wort is an antiviral, anti-inflammatory herb that can also strengthen the nervous system. Drink St. John's wort tea to help you de-stress, and gently massage the tincture directly on the affected area. (Both tea and tincture are available at health food stores.)

CAUTION: St. John's wort is a strong herb. Before taking it, check with your health professional.

▶ Apply any of the following to relieve the itching and speed the healing: witch hazel (an astringent), apple cider vinegar (an infection fighter), and red raspberry tea (particularly good for viral eruptive problems).

▶ Lysine may help stop the spread of the herpes zoster virus. Take lysine supplements (follow the recommended dosage on the label), or eat flounder. See "Herpes," above, for one man's success story. You may want to follow his lead.

HICCUPS

A hiccup is a spastic contraction of the diaphragm—the large circular muscle that separates the chest from the abdomen.

Hiccups are a great conversation starter. If you're in a room with thirty people, ask each one of them how they get rid of the hiccups and you will probably get close to thirty different remedies.

According to the *Guinness Book of World Records,* the longest recorded attack of hiccups is the one that afflicted Charles Osborne of Iowa. He was born in 1894 and got the hiccups in 1922, when he was slaughtering a hog.

The hiccups continued but didn't stop him from marrying twice and fathering eight children. (Who knows . . . maybe it helped.)

In 1983, Guinness reported that Mr. Osborne had hiccupped about 420 million times—and was still hiccupping. By the time he died in 1990, the hiccupping had slowed down from forty times a minute to twenty times a minute. Had he lived another ninety-six years . . . well, you do the math.

To cure a case of the hiccups, try one or more methods from this intriguing, makes-you-want-to-get-the-hiccups collection of remedies to find the one that works for you.

DRINK REMEDIES

Drink a glass of water that has a tablespoon in it—the bowl of the spoon being the part that's in the water. As you drink, be sure the metal stem of the spoon is pressed against your left temple.

Drink a glass of pineapple or orange juice or just plain sugar water.

This is one of the hiccup-cure classics: Drink a glass of water from the far side of the glass. You have to bend far forward to do this without dribbling all over yourself.

Another hiccup-cure classic: Fill a glass with water and take seven drinks of the water without taking a breath in between swallows. Also, while you're drinking the water, keep turning the glass to the left.

Put a handkerchief over a glass of water and drink the water as you suck it through the fabric.

Mix 1 teaspoon of apple cider vinegar in 1 cup of warm water and drink it down. For some people, just the thought of it scares away the hiccups.

Place a pencil between your teeth so that it sticks out on both sides of your mouth. Chomp down on it while drinking a glass of water.

PHYSICAL REMEDIES

Make believe your index finger is a mustache. Place it under your nose and press in hard for 30 seconds.

Locate the area about 2 to 3 inches above your navel and between the two sides of your rib cage. Press in with the fingers of both your hands and stay that way long enough to say to yourself: "One, two, three, four, I don't have the hiccups anymore." If you still have the hiccups, do it again while reciting the Declaration of Independence.

Close your eyes, hold your breath, and think of ten bald men. Let us start you off: Bruce Willis, Sean Connery, Montel Williams, Howie Mandel, Danny DeVito . . .

Pretend you're singing at the Metropolitan Opera House without a microphone and the foremost opera critic is in the last row of the uppermost tier. One aria and the hiccups should disappear. (So might everyone else in your home.)

Stick out your tongue as far as possible and keep it out for 3 minutes. Be careful—one big hiccup, and ouch!

Turn yourself into the letter *T* by spreading your arms. Then give a big yawn.

Pretend you're chewing gum while your fingers are in your ears, gently pressing inward. "What? I can't hear you. My fingers are in my ears."

Just visualizing a rabbit—its cute little face, quivering nose, white whiskers, big ears—has been known to make the hiccups disappear.

PHYSICAL REMEDIES WITH PROPS

Lay a broom on the floor and jump over it six times. If you want to update this remedy, try jumping over a vacuum cleaner. For all you rich people, jump over your housekeeper.

Place an ice cube right below the Adam's apple and count to 150.

Gently inhale a little pepper—enough to make you sneeze a couple of times. Sneezing usually makes the hiccups disappear.

FOOD REMEDIES

Our great-aunt Molly used to soak a cube of sugar in fresh lemon juice and then let it dissolve in her mouth. She did it to get rid of the hiccups. She also did it as a shortcut whenever she drank tea.

Pardon our name-dropping, but . . . Years ago, when we were on the *Today* show with Jane Pauley, she told us that her husband, cartoonist Garry Trudeau, gets painful hiccups. His remedy is to put a teaspoon of salt on half a lemon and then suck the juice and salt out of the lemon.

One of the most common remedies for hiccups is eating a teaspoon of granulated sugar. It supposedly irritates the throat, causing an interruption of the vagus nerve impulse pattern that is responsible for triggering the spasms of the diaphragm. (Just reading the previous sentence aloud may help you get rid of the hiccups.) In Arabia, people have been known to use sand in place of sugar. Stick with the sugar.

LAST-RESORT REMEDY

If nothing else works, take a hot bath. This has helped cure severe cases of hiccups.

WHEN SOMEONE ELSE HAS HICCUPS

Take something that's made of metal—a spoon is good. Tie a string around it and put it in the freezer for a minute. Take it out and, while it's still ice-cold, lower it down the hiccupper's back.

INDIGESTION

Mae West said, "Too much of a good thing is wonderful!" We say, "Too much of a good thing can cause indigestion!"

There are different types of indigestion: mild, severe, and persistent. Persistent indigestion may be a food allergy. Get professional medical help to check it out. Severe indigestion may be something a lot more serious than you think. It may not be indigestion, but rather some health challenge that needs tending to immediately. Seek professional help immediately.

CAUTION: *Never* take a laxative when you have severe stomach pain!

Mild indigestion usually produces one or a combination of the following symptoms: stomachache, heartburn, nausea and vomiting, and/or gas.

The first thing a person suffering from a mild case of indigestion usually does is promise never to overindulge again. That takes care of next time. As for now, relief is just a page or two away.

INDIGESTION (STOMACHACHE)

According to a Chinese massage therapist, if you are having stomach discomfort, there will be tender areas at the sides of your knees, just below the kneecaps. As you massage those spots and the tenderness decreases, so should the corresponding stomachache.

◈ This remedy from India is recommended for quick relief after a junk-food binge. Crush 1 teaspoon of fenugreek seeds and steep them in 1 cup of just-boiled water for 5 minutes. Strain and drink slowly. You should feel better in about 10 minutes.

◈ Mix 1 tablespoon of honey and 2 teaspoons of apple cider vinegar into a glass of hot water and drink the mixture.

◈ Put on a yellow slicker—not because it's raining, but because color therapists claim that the color yellow has rays that can help heal all digestive problems. Eat yellow foods such as bananas, lemons, pineapple, squash, and grapefruit. Lie down on a yellow sheet and get a massage with some yellow oil. What could be bad?

◈ Take some form of papaya after eating. Fresh papaya (the yellow ones are ripe), papaya juice, or papaya pills help combat indigestion, thanks to the potent digestive enzyme papain.

◈ Chamomile and/or peppermint teas (both available at supermarkets and health food stores) are very soothing. At the first sign of indigestion, drink a cup of either one.

ACID INDIGESTION

Thoroughly chew a teaspoon of dry rolled oats, then swallow them. The oats soothe the acid condition as well as neutralize it.

◈ Potato juice neutralizes acidity. Grate a raw potato and squeeze it through cheesecloth to get the juice. Dilute 1 tablespoon of potato juice with ½ cup of warm water. Drink it slowly.

STOMACH CRAMPS

We have come across some strange remedies for which there seem to be no logical explanations. We've included a few of them simply because they sometimes work. This is one of them: When you have a stomachache, tie a red string around your waist, under your clothing. If the pain disappears, great. If not, go on to another remedy.

◈ Steep 1 teaspoon of fresh or dried parsley in a cup of hot water. After 5 minutes, strain and slowly drink the parsley tea. Remember that parsley tea acts as a diuretic, so make sure you plan accordingly, because you may have to eat and run.

❧ Slice 1 medium onion and boil it in 1 cup of milk. Drink this concoction warm. It sounds awful and probably is, but it's a classic folk remedy that seems to work.

❧ Water has amazing healing power. Get in a hot shower and let the water beat down on your stomach for 10 to 15 minutes. By the time you dry off, you should be feeling a lot better.

❧ This is an old Native American stomachache remedy: Pour 1 cup of just-boiled water over 1 teaspoon of cornmeal. Let it sit for 5 minutes. Add salt to taste and drink slowly. .

SOUR STOMACH

Chew a few aniseeds, cardamom seeds, or caraway seeds. They'll sweeten your stomach and your breath as well.

NERVOUS STOMACH

Add ¼ teaspoon of oregano and ½ teaspoon of marjoram to 1 cup of hot water. Let it steep for 10 minutes. Strain and sip slowly. If you still have stomach uneasiness 2 hours after drinking the oregano-marjoram tea, drink another cup and that should do it.

AFTER-MEAL SLUGGISHNESS

Take a wire hairbrush or a metal comb and brush or comb the backs of your hands for 3 to 4 minutes. It's said to relieve that sluggish feeling you get from eating one of those old-fashioned, home-cooked, the-cholesterol-can-kill-ya meals.

INDIGESTION PREVENTION

Preventing indigestion may be as simple as not drinking any beverages during or after meals. Wait at least 1 hour and preferably 2 or 3 hours after eating before drinking any liquids. This no-beverage plan may help you digest your food a lot better. It's worth a try.

❧ Daikon, a Japanese radish, is white, crisp, and delicious, and it has a kick. It is available at greengrocers and Asian markets. It's an effective digestive aid, especially when eating heavy, deep-fried foods. It also helps detoxify animal protein and fats in your body. Either grate 1 to 2 tablespoons or have a couple of slices of raw daikon with your meal. It's great in salads.

❧ Cayenne pepper sprinkled sparingly (no more than ¼ teaspoon) on food or in soup will aid digestion.

Add basil to food while cooking. It will make the food more digestible and also help prevent constipation. If you really have a taste for basil, add ⅛ to ¼ teaspoon to a glass of white wine and drink after (not during) the meal.

Digesting Raw Vegetables

If you have trouble digesting raw vegetables, sprinkle the veggies with fresh lemon juice at least 3 hours before eating. Somehow the lemon, as wild as this sounds, partly digests the hard-to-digest parts of the greens.

Digesting Spicy Foods

A doctor we know practices preventive medicine on himself before eating Szechuan or Mexican food, or any other "hot" food that would ordinarily given him an upset stomach. He takes 1 tablespoon of extra-virgin olive oil about 15 minutes before the meal.

NAUSEA AND/OR VOMITING

When you have an upset stomach and you're feeling nauseous, take a carbonated drink. Ginger ale is best. Seltzer or club soda is good, too. If you don't have any of those and you're not on a sodium-restricted diet, mix 1 teaspoon of baking soda with 1 glass of cold water and drink it slowly. Within a few minutes, you should burp and feel a lot better.

If you have cola or even root beer, let it go flat by stirring it. Once the fizz is gone, drink 2 or 3 ounces to help ease the nausea.

This remedy is the pits . . . the armpits. Peel a large onion and cut it in half. Place a half under each armpit. As nauseating as it sounds, we've been told it stops vomiting and relieves nausea in no time.

Steep 2 cloves in 1 cup of just-boiled water for 5 minutes. Strain and drink it. If the taste of the cloves reminds you too much of the dentist, which makes you more nauseous, then steep a piece of cinnamon stick in just-boiled water, or 1 teaspoon of powdered ginger. Drinking any of those spices in water should stop nausea and vomiting.

Crack an ice cube and suck on the little pieces. It's worth a try, especially if you have none of the above ingredients in your home.

Needing to Throw Up?

When the food you ate seems to be lying on your chest, making you miserable, and you know you'd feel much better if you threw up, reach for the English mustard (available at specialty food shops). Mix 1 teaspoon into a glass of warm water and drink it. If you don't upchuck in 10 minutes, drink another glass of the mustard water. After another 10 minutes, if it still hasn't worked, the third time should be the charm. We're getting nauseous just thinking about all that watered-down mustard.

After Upchucking

To help ease a severe bout of vomiting, warm ½ cup of distilled white vinegar, saturate a washcloth in it, wring it out, and place the wet cloth on your bare stomach with a hot-water bottle on top of it.

BELCHING

This is a Taoist remedy that dates back to the sixth century B.C. Scrub a tangerine, then peel it and boil the pieces of peel in 2 cups of water for 5 minutes. Strain, let cool, and drink the tangerine tea. The tea should stop you from belching. You can also eat the tangerine peel as a digestive aid.

HEARTBURN

This painful condition—a burning sensation in the chest—most often is the result of stomach acid backing up (reflux) into the esophagus.

Our mother used to get heartburn. One of us asked her, "How do you know when you have it?" Our mother's answer was, "You'll know!" She was right.

▶ When you have heartburn, it's best not to lie down. The backflow of stomach acid into the esophagus increases when you lie on your right side. If you *have* to lie down, stay on your left side.

▶ Our surefire family remedy that stops the burning is almonds. We always have a jar of almond slivers in the kitchen. On the rare occasion that one of us gets heartburn, we take a handful of the almonds and chew them thoroughly, and by the time we finish the last mouthful, the heartburn is gone.

▶ Eat a slice of raw potato. Or grate a raw potato and put it in cheesecloth, squeeze out the juice in a glass, add twice the amount of warm water as potato juice, and drink it down slowly.

▶ Keep chewable papaya tablets with you, and at the first sign of heartburn or any kind of indigestion, pop papaya pills in your mouth, chew, and swallow.

▶ The flow of saliva can neutralize the stomach acids that slosh up and cause heartburn. According to Dr. Wylie Dodds at the Medical College of Wisconsin, chewing gum (we suggest sugarless) can increase the flow of saliva by eight or nine times and reduce the damage caused by stomach acids.

Heartburn Prevention

Turmeric (found on the supermarket spice shelf), a basic ingredient in curries, is also a digestive aid. It stimulates the flow of saliva (saliva neutralizes acid and helps push digestive juices back down where they belong). If you're about to eat food that gives you heartburn, spice up the food with turmeric. If it's not an appropriate ingredient for the food, take 2 or 3 turmeric capsules (available at health food stores) before the meal.

GAS (FLATULENCE)

Do you have a pain in your stomach area? Are you sure it's gas and not your appendix? To test for appendix problems, in a standing position, lift your right leg and then quickly jut it forward as though kicking something. If you have an excruciating, sharp pain anywhere in the abdominal area, it may be your appendix, in which case get medical attention immediately. If there is no sharp pain when you kick, it's probably just gas, but you may want to check with your doctor to be sure.

Gas is caused by swallowing air when you gulp down food. It can also be caused by drinking through a straw, drinking carbonated beverages (with or without a straw), chewing gum, sucking on candy, loose-fitting dentures, smoking, and constipation. Most cases of gas are caused by specific foods (such as beans), foods that contain certain sugar substitutes (such as maltitol), and bad food combinations (such as eating melon soon after a meal).

Once you figure out the cause, you can prevent it from happening again. Meanwhile, here are some remedies for when you're cooking with gas.

Drinks

A strong cup of peppermint tea will give you relief quickly, especially if you walk around as you drink it.

▶ Add 1 teaspoon of anisette liqueur to 1 cup of warm water. Stir and sip.

▶ Add ½ teaspoon of bay leaves to 1 cup of boiling water. Let it steep, then strain it and drink it down slowly.

▶ Each one of the following seeds is known to give fast relief from the pain of gas: aniseeds, caraway seeds, dill seeds, and fennel seeds (available at health food stores). To release the essential oils from any of these, gently crush 1 teaspoon of seeds and add it to a cup of just-boiled water. Let it steep for 10 minutes. Strain and drink. If the gas pains don't disappear right away, drink another cup of the seed tea before eating your next meal.

❧ Allspice is the unripe berries of a pimento evergreen tree. It was given its name because it tastes like a combination of spices: cloves, juniper berries, cinnamon, and pepper. Allspice is said to be effective in treating flatulent indigestion. Add 1 teaspoon of powdered allspice to 1 cup of just-boiled water and drink. If you have the dried fruit, chew ½ teaspoon, then swallow.

Physical Maneuvers

This gas-expelling yoga technique should be done in the privacy of your bedroom. Lie on the bed facedown with one leg tucked under you. Got the picture? Your knee is under your chest. Stay that way for 3 or 4 minutes, then stretch out that leg and bring the other leg up, with the knee under your chest. Every 3 or 4 minutes reverse the legs. Stop when you've expelled the gas.

If you feel you have a gas pocket, or trapped gas, lie down on the floor or on a bed and slowly bring your knees up to your chest to the count of ten, then back down. In between this exercise, massage

your stomach in a circular motion with the top half of your fingers, pressing hard to move that gas around and out.

Water

Take a shower and let warm water beat down on your stomach. It works for stomach cramps and it also helps move out gas.

❧ A hot-water compress or a heating pad or hot-water bottle placed directly on the stomach can relieve gas pains.

Gas Prevention

Drink ginger tea after a heavy, gassy meal. Steep ¼ teaspoon of powdered ginger in 1 cup of just-boiled water for 5 minutes, or let a few small pieces of fresh ginger steep. Drink the tea slowly.

❧ See "Preparation Guide" for instructions for reducing the gas effect when cooking beans.

ITCHING

SKIN ITCHING

It's difficult to pinpoint the cause of itching, which can be anything from seasonal allergies to psychological anxiety. Chances are, the itching will go away just as mysteriously as it came. Until it does, try not to scratch. (Easy for us to say.) If you really can't control yourself, consider wearing gloves (cotton or latex) to keep from scratching your skin bloody with your nails.

Meanwhile, here are remedies that may offer some relief. Apply any one of the following to your itchy areas, but only if the skin is not broken:

■ Fresh sliced carrots

■ 1 vitamin C tablet dissolved in 1 cup of warm water

■ Fresh lemon juice

■ Raw potato slices

■ A paste of uncooked oatmeal with a little water

■ A paste combining distilled white vinegar and cornstarch

■ A paste combining 1 teaspoon of water with 3 teaspoons of baking soda

■ An infusion of ½ ounce of dried basil leaves steeped for at least 10 minutes (until cool) in 1 pint of just-boiled water. (Basil is rich in eugenol, a topical anesthetic.)

■ An infusion of 1 ounce of dried mint leaves, steeped for at least 10 minutes (until cool) in 1 pint of just-boiled water

■ A cold compress using 2 percent milk on the itchy area for 10 to 15 minutes, then rinsed with cool water

■ The gel from a leaf of the aloe vera plant

■ A fine paste of equal amounts of honey and cinnamon powder

■ Equal amounts of coconut oil and lime juice

■ Almond oil, baby oil, or olive oil

■ A mixture of equal amounts of tomato juice and coconut water (available at the supermarket)

■ Neem oil (known for its antibacterial properties and its effectiveness in fighting epidermal dysfunctions), as oil, lotion, salve, or capsules from your health food store

Itch-Stopping Tea

Oolong tea (available at health food stores and most supermarkets) tastes good and may stop the itching. Drink 3 to 4 cups a day of oolong tea.

Anti-Itching Bath

Add 2 cups of apple cider vinegar, or 1 cup of baking soda, or 1 12-ounce can of evaporated milk to your warm bathwater and bathe in it for about a half hour. If possible, air-dry.

▶ Prepare a pint of thyme tea and add it to your bathwater, then bathe in it for about a half hour. Thyme has thymol, an antiseptic substance that may make your itch disappear.

RECTAL ITCHING

Rectal and genital itching may be due to an allergy, yeast overgrowth, poor hygiene, or parasites. Find the cause and you can eliminate the problem. Meanwhile, these suggestions may help:

■ Pumpkin seeds are used as a folk treatment to control and prevent intestinal parasites. Buy the shelled and unsalted seeds, and eat a handful daily.

■ Soak a cotton pad in apple cider vinegar and place it on the affected area. If it's raw from scratching, be prepared for a temporary burning sensation. Leave the cotton pad on overnight. (You can keep it in place with a sanitary napkin.) If itching starts again the next day, repeat the procedure instead of scratching.

■ Before bedtime, take a shower, then pat dry the itchy area and apply wheat germ oil. To avoid messy nightclothes and bed linens, put a sanitary napkin over the oily area.

GENITAL ITCHING

See above under "Rectal Itching."

■ Sprinkle cornstarch all over the area to stop the itching.

■ Dip a cotton pad in buttermilk and apply it to the problem spot to stop the itching and help heal it.

■ Dilute ¼ cup fresh lemon juice in ½ cup water and apply to the itchy area.

ITCHING UNDER A CAST

When the itching under a cast is driving you crazy, scratch the same place on the other limb—the arm or leg—*without* the cast. Your brain may be fooled into believing that you're scratching the real itch.

MEMORY AND BRAINPOWER

"I told my doctor that my memory has gotten terrible lately."

"What did the doctor do about it?"

"He made me pay in advance."

Sure, it's easy to make jokes, but we know how frustrating it is to feel your memory is slipping. Lately, we hear people of all ages saying things like, "I don't remember a thing anymore." "I feel as though I'm losing my mind." "The only thing my memory is good for is to make me wonder what I've forgotten."

Neither of us believes a not-so-good memory is a matter of age. We think we're all victims of data overload.

A remedy for remembering a familiar name, place, or fact is to simply relax and forget that you can't remember. When you're not thinking about it, it will pop into your mind. The less tense you are, the better your memory.

The great scientist Albert Einstein didn't believe in remembering anything he could look up. That's a tension-relieving thought. And now, with the Internet, there's a lot you can look up.

Meanwhile, we have some remedies that may help you re-create a wonderful memory.

MEMORY BOOSTERS

Remember to Eat and Drink the Following . . .

Take 1 teaspoon of apple cider vinegar in a glass of room-temperature water before each meal. Not only is it said to be an excellent tonic for the memory, but it also curbs the appetite.

Ah, the healing powers of almonds. Eat 6 raw almonds a day to improve your memory.

Two mustard seeds, taken as you would take pills, first thing every morning, are said to revive one's memory.

Eat a handful of sunflower seeds daily. These seeds are beneficial in many ways, one being memory improvement.

Yerba maté is a form of holly and is the national beverage of Paraguay, where it's grown. One of the many positive effects of this herb (available at health food stores), according to South American medical authorities, is that it strengthens one's memory. Drink 1 cup early in the day.

> **NOTE:** Be aware that yerba maté contains caffeine, although less than coffee or regular tea.

Combine half a glass of carrot juice with half a glass of milk for a memory-improving drink to have once a day.

Eating three prunes daily is said to improve the memory. It can also help prevent constipation, and constipation paralyzes the thinking process.

Our research led us to a Japanese doctor whose records show that he successfully treated more than five hundred patients who were having memory problems. How? Eyebright. It's the herb best known for treating eye disorders . . . until now. Add ½ ounce of eyebright (available at health food stores) and 1 tablespoon of clover honey to 1½ cups of just-boiled water. When it's cool, strain the mixture and put it in a bottle. Drink ¾ cup before lunch and ¾ cup before dinner. After doing this every day for a week or two, you should notice an improvement in your memory.

Ginger helps the memory. Use fresh ginger (available at greengrocers) in cooking, and drink ginger tea. Steep a few quarter-size pieces of ginger root in just-boiled water for 6 minutes. Strain and drink. It's also good for digestion, so you might want to have it after meals.

Add 4 cloves (the kind used for preparing a ham) to a cup of sage tea. Steep for 10 minutes, then strain and drink. Sage and cloves have been said to strengthen the memory. Remember to drink a cup every day.

Color Counts

What's the most prevalent color in legal pads? In Post-its? Notice a pattern forming here? According to color therapy research, yellow most stimulates the brain. Writing on yellow paper may help you better remember whatever it is you've written.

Physical Exercise

Walking increases oxygen flow to the brain—and it's never too late! In adults between the ages of sixty and seventy-five, the group that walked briskly three days a week, starting with 15 minutes a day and working their way up to walking 45 minutes a day, had a 15 percent boost in mental functioning. That 15 percent could mean an end to the frustration of *not* remembering things . . . at any age.

If you have seen this simple yoga exercise in a magazine, on TV, or on the Internet, chances are you are doing it and reaping the rewards. If not, it's time to start.

These are some of the reported benefits:

■ Pumps up cell and neuron activity in the brain

■ Helps counter the common mental effects of aging and memory loss, as well as Alzheimer's disease and other types of dementia

■ Provides the energy fuel that can keep brains fit and functional

- Makes thinking and focusing easier

- Stress reduction

- Helps develop a stronger, healthier, more coordinated body

- A study of children with ADD, ADHD, developmental and cognitive delays, Down syndrome, and specific learning disabilities showed significant increases in academic and behavioral performance, greater class participation, and improved social skills.

Here is the exercise that's said to stimulate neural pathways in the brain by activating acupressure points on the earlobes:

Step 1. Get into position.
- Stand with your feet about a foot apart.
- Grasp your right earlobe with your left thumb on the front of the earlobe and your left index finger on the back of the earlobe.
- Grasp your left earlobe with your right thumb on the front of the earlobe and your right index finger on the back of the earlobe.

Step 2. Now that your left arm is on your chest and your right arm is on top of your left arm, and you're holding your earlobes:
- Gently squeeze your earlobes.

- Inhale through your nose as you do a deep-knee bend (squat), keeping your back straight.
- Exhale through your mouth on your way up.

Step 3. Repeat steps 1 and 2 about ten to twelve times daily.

If you cannot do a deep-knee bend or are afraid of falling, put a chair underneath you until you build up strength in your thighs.

To learn more, visit www.superbrain yoga.org and read *Superbrain Yoga* by Master Choa Kok Sui.

Mental Exercise

Dr. David Bilkey, an associate professer in the Department of Psychology at the University of Otago in New Zealand, says, "Science has proven that *physical* exercise has been shown to promote neurogenesis, the growth of new neurons in the brain." According to Dr. Bilkey, *mental* exercise is just as important. He believes that people need to think of their brains as being a muscle. "If you use it, it will get larger and better, and if you don't, it will atrophy." It's the old adage: Use it or lose it!

Writer and scholar Sir Harold Acton said, "Some people take no mental exercise apart from jumping to conclusions." Don't be one of those people.

Give your brain a daily workout. Start by figuring out what will be your first mental challenge. Here are some suggestions:

■ Do a crossword puzzle. Start with an easy one, either in your local newspaper or in an inexpensive book of puzzles, and work your way up to more difficult levels. To get the most out of this exercise, fill in the answers by writing with the hand you never use for writing.

■ Use your nondominant hand to brush your teeth and to use the mouse on your computer. It makes for great mental gymnastics.

■ If you are on the Internet, go to Google and type in "mental exercises," "puzzles," "brainteasers," or "mind games." Click and play! Here are two free sites to start you off: www.puzz.com and www.pogo.com.

■ Go to your local library and find books of word puzzles and games. They're fun and they're free.

NOTEWORTHY: *Mind Aerobics,* a series of three CDs or cassettes, from the New You Enterprises, uses Holosync audio technology, which is precisely engineered tones to stimulate the mind, in turn creating different combinations of alpha, theta, and delta brain-wave patterns. The result should be a number of positive changes in the brain, including:

■ Greatly improved mental abilities
■ Heightened learning ability and creativity
■ Enhanced memory
■ Production of vital neurochemicals that help keep the body alive and fully functioning
■ Dramatic reduction in stress and anxiety
■ Improved health and emotional well-being
■ Better, more restful sleep

If only half of the changes take place, it's worth checking out. To get an idea of the Mind Aerobics soundtracks, take advantage of the eight-minute demo at www.mindaerobics.com/demo.html.

NOTE: In order to experience the effects of Holosync, you must have stereo headphones so that each ear can receive a discrete and different stimulus.

Learn more about how this mind science can improve the quality of your life by visiting www.mindaerobics.com, or phone 818-906-0860.

Also see "Mental Fatigue" in the "Fatigue" chapter.

SHORT-TERM MEMORY ENHANCER

The sleep cycle that assists the learning process has usually been credited to rapid eye movement (REM) sleep. New studies prove that performance-enhancing naps consist mostly of a non-REM sleep stage known as slow-wave sleep.

This means a nap can improve your ability to recall just-learned information. "That's a reason to take a nap during the day," says Dr. Robert Stickgold, neuroscientist and associate professor of psychiatry at Harvard Medical School. "It helps clear out the brain's 'inbox' and integrates that information into memory." Dr. Stickgold adds, "Napping may protect brain circuits from overuse until those neurons can consolidate what's been learned."

> **BONUS BENEFIT:** Dr. Dimitrios Trichopoulos, at the Harvard School of Public Health, reported that the results of a six-year U.S. study showed that those who took a midday 30-minute snooze at least three times a week had a 37 percent lower risk of a heart attack.

Take a 30-minute after-lunch nap, and add your name to the list of prestigious daily-napping achievers: Albert Einstein, Winston Churchill, Margaret Thatcher, Florence Nightingale, John F. Kennedy, Ronald Reagan, and Bill Clinton.

ALERTNESS BOOSTER

Ian MacDonald, professor of metabolic physiology at the University of Nottingham, England, designed a study using MRI (magnetic resonance imaging) to detect increased activity in specific areas of the brain after his test subjects drank specially prepared flavonoid-rich cocoa. The results showed a boost in blood flow to key areas of the brain for two to three hours.

When you need to be most mentally alert—taking a test, going for an interview, meeting new people—have a cup of cocoa right before the event. Stick with cocoa instead of dark chocolate—even if the chocolate has at least 70 percent cocoa content, it also is more processed and has way more sugar and fat.

Other flavonoid-rich drinks and foods are green and black tea (especially Ceylon tea), sweet cherries, apples, apricots, purple grapes, blackberries, blueberries, raspberries, and garlic.

MEN'S HEALTH CHALLENGES

To relax tension, stimulate circulation, and generally soothe the male organs, massage the area behind the leg in back of the ankle, about 1 or 2 inches higher than the shoe line of each foot.

Also, nearly everything works more smoothly when it's used regularly. Many men enjoy better urination by seeing to it that appropriate ejaculation occurs on a regular basis.

That said, here are remedies for more specific problems.

> **CAUTION #1:** If you have pain, burning, testicular or scrotal swelling, or any other prostate-related symptoms, have your condition diagnosed and evaluated by a health professional as soon as possible.

PROSTATE

The bad news is that it is estimated that one out of every three men over the age of sixty has some kind of prostate problem, such as inflammation (prostatitis), enlargement (benign prostatic hyperplasia),

or prostate cancer. The good news is that there are many effective new as well as old treatments for all of the above.

> **CAUTION #2:** If you have been diagnosed with prostate cancer, we strongly urge you to check with your doctor before trying any of these prostate remedies, to make sure that they are not counterproductive.

Corn silk tea has been a popular folk remedy for prostate problems. Take the silky strings that grow around an ear of corn and steep them in a cup of just-boiled water for 10 minutes. Strain, then drink the corn silk tea. Prepare and drink the tea a few times throughout the day.

If it's not fresh-corn season, buy corn silk extract in a health food store, add 10 to 15 drops to 1 cup of water, and drink it several times a day.

Prostate Pain

To help relieve prostate pain, massage the area above the heel and just below the inner ankle of each foot and/or the inside of the wrists, above the palm of each hand, using a circular motion. Keep massaging until the pain and soreness disappear.

Enlarged Prostate

> **CAUTION:** Do not rely on a self-diagnosis. Consult an appropriate health care provider. If you do have an enlarged prostate and want to use any of these remedies, first run it by the doctor.

Grate part of a yellow onion and squeeze it through cheesecloth. Take 1 tablespoon of onion juice twice a day.

In extremely painful cases, get slippery elm capsules at a health food, herb, or vitamin store. Take the capsules apart and empty the contents—enough for ½ teaspoon of slippery elm powder—into a cup. Mix the powder with water (preferably distilled). Drink the mixture before breakfast and a couple of hours after dinner. If it relieves the pain, take the drink for a few days.

Asparagine, a health-giving alkaloid found in fresh asparagus, is said to be a healing element for prostate conditions. Use a juicer and juice equal amounts of fresh asparagus, carrots, and cucumber—enough for an 8-ounce glass of juice.

Organic vegetables are preferable. If not available, wash the asparagus thoroughly (see "Pesticide Removal for Fruits and Vegetables" in "Preparation Guide," or check your supermarket for a natural product called Veggie Wash), scrub the carrots, and peel the cucumber. Drink a glass of the juice daily.

A teaspoon of unrefined sesame oil (available at health food stores) taken every day for 1 month has been known to reduce an enlarged prostate back to normal size.

A warm milk compress is soothing when applied to the prostate area. Warm (do not boil) 1 cup of milk. Saturate a white towel with the milk, and when you apply it to the appropriate area, put a hot-water bottle on top to keep the towel warm longer. Leave it on for at least 20 minutes.

Lecithin (available at health food stores) comes highly recommended from many sources. Take 1 lecithin capsule—1,200 mg each—or 1 to 2 tablespoons of lecithin granules three times a day, after each meal.

Prostate Inflammation

Inflammation is usually caused by an infection, for which you may need antibiotics. Yes, seek professional health care. While waiting for your appointment, you may want to try one of these inflammation reducers.

■ Apply a watercress poultice (see "Preparation Guide") to reduce the inflammation.

■ Bee pollen is said to be effective in reducing swelling of the prostate as well as treating other prostate disorders. Pollen contains the hormone testosterone and traces of other male hormones. It seems to give the prostate a boost so that it may heal itself. Take 5 pollen pills daily—2 in the morning, 2 in the afternoon, and 1 in the evening—or the equivalent in bee pollen granules (both available at health food stores).

Prostate Congestion

If your doctor hasn't already told you to do so, eliminate all coffee and alcoholic beverages from your diet.

And now for a self-help prostatic massage: Lie down on the floor on your back. Put the sole of one foot again the sole of the other foot so that you're at your bow-legged best. While keeping the soles of your feet together, extend your legs as far as possible and then bring them in as close as possible to your chest. Do this exercise ten times in the morning and ten times at night.

Dr. Ray C. Wunderlich Jr., of the Wunderlich Center for Nutritional Medicine in St. Petersburg, Florida, recommends that you empty the gland by having ejaculations at a frequency that you can tolerate. It will improve your urinary stream.

Prostate Tone-Up

Drink 2 to 4 ounces of coconut milk (available at health food stores) every day to tone up the prostate gland. The milk is pure, uncontaminated, and loaded with minerals. It's also a soothing digestive aid.

Prostate Cancer Prevention

Eat two Brazil nuts daily. That's it.

The reasoning behind this prevention precaution is that Brazil nuts are an extraordinarily rich dietary source of selenium—about 90 mcg per nut.

While we couldn't find any studies substantiating this health hint, we have read reports saying that selenium has been shown to reduce the risk of prostate cancer by as much as 60 percent.

So, do we think it's worth doing? It's easy to do, inexpensive, and tastes good! You decide.

BLOODY URINE AFTER JOGGING

Some men pass bloody urine after jogging. It's especially common in men who have scrotal varicocele (varicose veins of the testicles). It's usually due to repeated impact of the empty bladder against the prostate. Some doctors recommend that men *not* empty their bladders completely before running.

IMPOTENCE

See "For Men Only" in the "Sex" chapter.

PREMATURE EJACULATION

See "For Men Only" in the "Sex" chapter.

MOTION SICKNESS

The story is told about the captain of the ship who announced, "There is no hope. We are all doomed. The ship is sinking and we'll all be dead within an hour." One voice was heard after the announcement. It was the seasick passenger saying, "Thank heavens!"

If you have ever been seasick, you probably anticipated that punch line.

Most people think motion sickness starts in the stomach. Wrong! Guess again. Constant jarring of the semicircular canals in the inner part of the *ears* causes balance problems that produce those awful motion sickness symptoms. What to do? Here are some remedies that may help you get through that miserable feeling.

EXTERNAL TREATMENTS

At the first wave of motion sickness, take a metal comb or wire brush (available in pharmacies and beauty supply stores) and run the teeth over the backs of your hands, particularly the area from the thumb to the first finger, including the web of skin in between those two fingers. You may have relief in 5 to 10 minutes.

▶ Pull out and pinch the skin in the middle of your inner wrist, about an inch from your palm. Keep pulling and pinching, alternating wrists, until you feel better.

▶ Briskly massage the fourth and fifth fingers of each hand, with particular emphasis on the vicinity of the pinky's knuckle. You may feel relief within 15 minutes.

FOOD AND DRINK

Take a teaspoon of gomasio (sesame seeds and sea salt, available at health food stores) and keep chewing it as long as you can before swallowing it.

▶ A cup of peppermint or chamomile tea may calm down the stomach and alleviate nausea.

▶ Mix ⅛ teaspoon of cayenne pepper in a cup of warm water or a cup of soup and force yourself to finish it, even if you think it'll finish you. It won't. And it may stop the nausea.

As soon as you get that queasy feeling, suck a lemon, or drink some freshly squeezed lemon juice.

MOTION SICKNESS PREVENTION

On any form of transportation, sit near a window so you can look out. Focus on things that are far away, not nearby objects that move past you quickly.

To ensure yourself the smoothest flight possible on a plane, select a seat that's over the wheels, not in the tail. There's a lot more movement in the tail end of a plane.

Take 2 or 3 capsules of powdered ginger a half hour before the expected motion, whether by car, boat, plane, or train. Or stir ½ teaspoon of ginger powder into 1 cup of warm water and drink it about 20 minutes before you travel.

Marjoram tea is an aid to help prevent seasickness. Have a cup of the tea before hitting the deck.

Off-the-Wall Preventive Remedies

This is a we-don't-know-why-but-it-just-seems-to-work remedy: Tape an umeboshi (Japanese pickled plum—available at Asian markets) directly on your navel right before you board a bus, train, car, plane, or ship. It's said to prevent motion sickness. Incidentally, the plums (which are salty, not sweet) are very rich in calcium and iron. To reap those benefits, one must *eat* them rather than tape them on one's tummy.

A Mexican method of preventing motion sickness is to tape a copper penny over the navel. It is supposed to work especially well on crowded bus rides over bumpy roads.

This remedy came to us from Hawaii, Afghanistan, and Switzerland. Take a big brown paper bag and cut off and discard the bag's bottom. Then slit the bag from top to bottom so that it's no longer in the round but is instead a long piece of brown paper. Wrap the paper around your bare chest and secure it in place. Put your regular clothes on top of it and travel that way. It should prevent motion sickness. This is particularly good for children who get queasy when traveling.

JET LAG

Travel Considerations

Generally, it takes a day to recover for each time zone you pass through. New York to California: three time zones, three days of jet lag. Actually, going east to west and gaining a few hours is better, jet-lag-wise, than west to east, when you lose a few hours.

In terms of getting that first good night's sleep at your destination, it seems best to plan on arriving in the evening. England's Royal Air Force Institute of Aviation Medicine suggests that when you're flying east, fly early; when heading west, fly late.

Surely you've heard that alcohol is one of the most powerful dehydrators there is. And you must know that just being in an airplane is dehydrating. But do you know that dehydration makes jet lag worse? Conclusion: *Do not drink any alcoholic beverages while airborne. Do drink lots of water and juice.* If you have to keep going to the lavatory, good. Walking up and down the aisles will help refresh and prepare you for your new time zone.

Jet Lag Prevention

It's been reported that taking 0.5 to 1 mg of melatonin right before boarding the plane has prevented jet lag. If you know that you really suffer from jet lag, ask your doctor about taking melatonin before your upcoming flight.

This is the U.S. Department of Energy's Anti-Jet-Lag Diet to help travelers quickly adjust their bodies' internal clocks to new time zones.

Start three days before departure day.

- Day 1: Have a high-protein breakfast and lunch, and a high-carbohydrate (no meat) dinner. No coffee except between 3:00 P.M. and 5:00 P.M.

- Day 2: Have very light meals—salads, light soups, fruit, and juices. Coffee only between 3:00 P.M. and 5:00 P.M.

- Day 3: Same as Day 1.

- Day 4, departure (listen up, this gets complex): If you must have a caffeinated beverage, you can have a cup in the morning when traveling west, or between 6:00 P.M. and 11:00 P.M. when traveling east. Have fruit or juice until your first meal. To know when to have your first meal, figure out when breakfast time will be at your destination. If your flight is long enough, sleep until normal breakfast time at your destination, *but no later* (that's important). Wake up and eat a big, high-protein breakfast. Stay awake and active. Continue the day's meals according to mealtimes at your destination and you'll be in sync when you arrive. No alcohol on the plane!

This is a modified version of the remedy above that may help minimize jet lag.

As soon as you board the plane, pretend it's whatever time it actually is at your destination. In other words, if you board the plane at 7:00 P.M. in New York, and you're headed for London, where it's 1:00 A.M., pull down your window shade or wear dark glasses, and if possible, go to sleep. If you board a plane late that night and it's daylight at your destination, force yourself to stay awake during the flight. Making believe you're in the new time zone at the very start of your trip should help you acclimate quickly once your plane touches down.

William F. Buckley, author and commentator, got this remedy from a world traveler friend of a British doctor specializing in jet lag.

NOTE: This is definitely not for anyone who has to watch their sodium and/or caffeine intake.

The theory behind the remedy is that jet lag comes from internal perspiring, which causes a salt deficiency. According to Buckley, the doctor said to put a heaping teaspoon of salt in a cup of coffee and drink it the minute you get into the plane. Five hours later, drink another cup of coffee with salt and you will experience a miracle. The salted coffee will taste like ambrosia. That will be your body talking, telling you how grateful it is that you have given it the salt it so badly needed.

NOTEWORTHY: We hope you're familiar with Magellan's, billed as "the world's most trusted source of travel supplies." If not, visit their Web site at www.magellans.com. They have valuable travel information, and a great selection of products that can make your comings and goings safer, more efficient, healthier, and happier. A free catalog is available by calling 800-962-4943.

ALTITUDE SICKNESS PREVENTION

The symptoms of altitude sickness can be headache, sluggishness, and excessive thirst due to the decrease in available oxygen. It usually happens to recreational hikers traveling from a low elevation up to the mountains.

The best way to avoid those awful high-mountain symptoms is by gradual acclimatization to higher altitudes. But if you're planning a day trip and not allowing yourself the time to adjust to the progressing heights, prepare four-spice tea and drink it before you start your climb.

Stir ⅓ teaspoon each of powdered cinnamon, clove, ginger, and thyme into 1 cup of just-boiled water. Let it steep for 5 minutes, then strain it through a coffee filter and drink it.

The cinnamon may help control blood

sugar levels, the eugenol in clove may thin the blood, ginger is known for preventing motion sickness, and thyme has soothing, antispasmodic qualities.

You may also want to prepare a thermos of the tea to take with you.

NECK PROBLEMS

PAIN-IN-THE-NECK PREVENTION

It's quite common for those of us who are under pressure to have a pain in the neck. People tend to tense up in that area, which is the worst thing to do.

Your neck connects your brain and nervous system to your body. When you create tension in your neck, you impair the flow of energy throughout your system. To prevent tension buildup, do these simple, basic neck exercises very slowly:

■ Sit or stand relaxed. Bend your head forward, chin on chest, then back to the original position.

■ Bend your head to the right, then back to the original position.

■ Bend your head backward, then back to the original position.

■ Bend your head to the left, then back to the original position.

Do it from start to finish five times in a row, two or three times a day.

You may hear lots of crackling, crunching, and gravelly noises coming from your neck. As tension is released, the noises will quiet. See the next remedy to help rid yourself of gravel.

CAUTION: Many exercise gurus do not recommend neck rolls in which the neck is rotated around clockwise and then counterclockwise. Neck rolls may impact the side joints of the neck, which can cause inflammation.

NECK GRAVEL

If you turn from side to side and you hear and feel as though there's gravel in your neck, do the exercises described above, and eat 3 to 4 cloves of raw garlic a day. You may have to work your way up to that amount.

STIFF NECK

Medicine men from several Native American tribes prescribe daily neck rubs with fresh lemon juice, as well as drinking the juice of half a lemon first thing in the morning and last thing at night.

According to the ancient principles of reflexology, the base of the big toe affects the neck. Rub your hands together vigorously until you feel heat. Now you're ready to massage your big toes with circular motions. Spend a few minutes massaging the bottoms of your feet at the base of the toes and the area surrounding them. As a change of pace, you might want to massage the base of your thumbs, also for a few minutes at a time. Keep at it, at least two times a day every day, in addition to doing the neck exercises described at the beginning of this chapter.

When you have neck discomfort, wear a silk scarf. It has been known to help blood circulation and relieve muscle pain and tension in the neck.

NOSEBLEEDS

Most of us have had a nosebleed at one time or another. It's usually nothing serious, just a little scary and inconvenient. Whether it's brought on by allergies, cold weather, sinus infection, or another illness, you rub, pick, or blow your nose, breaking the tiny blood vessels that cause a bloody nose.

NOTE: Nasal hemorrhaging—blood flowing from both nostrils—requires immediate medical attention. Rush to the nearest doctor or hospital emergency room.

Also, recurrent nosebleeds may be a symptom of an underlying ailment. Be sure to seek appropriate medical attention.

WHAT TO DO, WHAT NOT TO DO

When you have a nosebleed, sit or stand. Do *not* lie down. Do *not* put your head back. It will cause you to swallow blood and make you feel worse.

Now that you're sitting or standing, gently blow your nose. It will help rid your nostrils of blood clots that may prevent a blood vessel from sealing. Then try any of the following remedies.

We know that cayenne pepper stops the bleeding of a cut or gash. We've been told that drinking ⅛ to ¼ teaspoon of cayenne in a glass of warm water will stop a nosebleed and help normalize your blood pressure, calming you down.

Take your thumb and forefinger and pinch your nose right below the hard, bony part, about halfway down the nose.

Stay that way for 7 minutes, and you should no longer have a nosebleed.

▶ Fold a small piece of brown grocery bag paper and place it between your upper lip and your gum. If you don't have a grocery bag, use a dime instead. If you're outdoors without a bag or a dime, pick a stiff green leaf from a tree, place a piece of it under your upper lip, and press down on it with your finger.

▶ The dime remedy reminds us of our father's remedy. When either of us had a nosebleed, he would take a half-dollar, put it on a frozen ice cube tray for a few seconds, then press it to the back of the bleeder's neck. We looked forward to getting nosebleeds, since we would get to keep the half-dollar.

Ice at the nape of the neck has also been known to work, as has raw onion, but neither is as profitable.

▶ Gem therapists say that a nosebleed can be stopped by placing a piece of amber on the nose.

▶ Immerse your hands in warm water to stop a nosebleed. If you have a sink filled with dishes, you can multitask, and do the dishes while getting rid of a bloody nose.

Nosebleed Prevention

Bioflavonoids help prevent nosebleeds. Eat at least one citrus fruit a day and be sure to include the pith, or white spongy skin under the peel, which is extremely rich in bioflavonoids. In addition, take a vitamin C supplement with bioflavonoids. Also, add green leafy vegetables—lots of 'em—to your diet. They're rich in vitamin K, needed for the production of prothrombin, which is necessary for blood clotting.

OSTEOPOROSIS

Osteoporosis is a condition of decreased bone mass. It can lead to fragile bones and an increased risk for fractures.

While researching this chapter, we were horrified by the statistics of how many are affected by this condition, and the possible down-the-road consequences. Since it's too depressing and scary to report any of that, we decided to deviate from our usual style of one remedy after another, hoping to raise your calcium consciousness and make you aware of ways to turn things around so that you can be responsible for helping yourself and for lowering those negative statistics.

Testing

Your doctor may recommend that you take a bone density test. DEXA is today's established standard for measuring bone mineral density. According to Mary Beth Augustine, R.D., director/owner of the Natural Nutritionist in Brewster, New York, "Many health care providers are cavalier about DEXA's 'low-level radiation exposure' and often order the test every two years, or even yearly—yikes!"

Mary Beth enlightened us about there being a totally safe bone resorption assessment that can be done once or twice annually, in between DEXA scans (which shouldn't be done more than once about every five years). This test involves a urine specimen that's sent to a lab. Many doctors aren't familiar with the bone resorption test. Check it out with your insurance company and then enlighten your doctor.

Here are the names of two labs that do bone resorption testing:

■ Genova Diagnostics, www.genova diagnostics.com, phone: 800-522-4762

■ Metametrix Bone Resorption Assay, www.metametrix.com, phone: 800-221-4640

CALCIUM AND VITAMIN D

Getting the daily recommended amount of calcium is necessary for maintaining bone strength and helping to prevent osteoporosis-related fractures.

Vitamin D_3 (cholecalciferol) is the form of vitamin D that best supports bone health, and it increases calcium absorption by as much as 30 to 80 percent.

Recommended Dosage

Based on extensive research findings along with the consensus of leading experts on this topic, the National Osteoporosis Foundation (www.nof.org) updated its recommendations for daily adequate calcium and vitamin D_3 intake to the following amounts:

■ Adults under age fifty need 1,000 mg of calcium daily, and 400–800 IU of vitamin D_3 daily

■ Adults age fifty and over need 1,200 mg of calcium daily, and 800–1,000 IU of vitamin D_3 daily

NOTE: The extensive research findings of Osteoporosis Canada, an organization dedicated to educating, empowering, and supporting people about the risk, reduction, and treatment of osteoporosis, recommends that adults age fifty and over get 1,500 mg of calcium daily. They also recommend 1,500 mg of calcium daily for adults age fifty and under who have osteoporosis.

Calcium-Rich Foods

To give you some means of calculating your daily calcium intake, here is a list of calcium-rich foods. You do the math.

	Amount	Calcium (mg)
Dairy Foods		
Whole milk	1 cup	290
Lowfat (1 percent) milk	1 cup	300
Evaporated milk	1 cup	658
Sour cream	2 tbsp.	28
Cottage cheese	½ cup	68
Yogurt, lowfat, plain	8 oz.	415
Swiss cheese	1 oz.	272
Cheddar cheese	1 oz.	204
Mozzarella, part skim	1 oz.	207
American cheese, processed	1 slice	129
Cream cheese	1 oz.	23
Ricotta cheese	¼ cup	169
Macaroni and cheese, box	1 cup	100
Macaroni and cheese, homemade	1 cup	362
Cheeseburger	average	141
Cheese pizza	1 slice	117
Taco, small	6 oz.	221
Nondairy Foods		
Calcium-fortified soy milk	1 cup	350
Calcium-fortified orange juice	1 cup	350
Oatmeal made with milk	1 cup	300
Ocean perch	3 oz.	116

continued

	Amount	Calcium (mg)
Nondairy Foods		
Sardines with bones (no salt)	3 oz.	325
Salmon with bones (canned)	3 oz.	180
Shrimp	3 oz.	45
Calcium-fortified dry cereal	1 oz.	200–300
Acorn squash	1 cup	90
Broccoli, cooked	1 cup	94
Collard greens, cooked	1 cup	300
Mustard greens, cooked	1 cup	104
Kale, cooked	½ cup	90
Spinach	1 cup	291
Turnip greens, cooked	½ cup	124
Blackstrap molasses	1 tbsp.	172
Figs, dried	5 medium	135
Kelp (seaweed)	1 cup	170
Tofu with calcium	3 oz.	30–100
Almonds	1 oz.	72
Almond butter	2 tbsp.	86
Sesame seeds	2 tbsp.	176
Great Northern beans	1 cup	140
Kidney beans	1 cup	105
Pinto beans	1 cup	90
Navy beans	1 cup	130

We culled the list from a half-dozen lists. Since none of them agreed on the amount of calcium in any food, we did the best we could by averaging the amount from the sources we used.

How Much Calcium Should You Take?

You and your health care provider (doctor and/or nutritionist) should determine the amount of calcium and vitamin D_3 to take daily, considering your age, size, physical condition (after having a bone density test), and whether you consume a daily diet that includes calcium-rich foods.

Calcium Thieves

Acid-forming foods rob calcium from your bones as your body neutralizes the acidity and tries to keep itself in balance.

Make a difference in your diet by staying away from or greatly limiting your intake of acid-forming foods, including (for starters) pastries made with white flour, artificial sweeteners, soft drinks, alcoholic beverages, sugar, table salt, and caffeinated beverages.

There is evidence that excess salt and caffeine may cause you to lose an increased amount of calcium through the urine.

The current tolerable upper limit (UL) is 2,300 mg of sodium a day. That's about 1 teaspoon of table salt per day. Pay attention to sodium counts on labels, think twice before reaching for the salt shaker on the table, and when ordering at a restaurant, ask them to go easy on the salt.

Maximizing the Absorption of Calcium Supplements

Osteoporosis Canada (www.osteoporosis.ca) offers this important advice about taking calcium supplements:

1. Take calcium carbonate with food or immediately after eating. It is absorbed more effectively when there is food in the stomach. Calcium citrate, calcium lactate, and calcium gluconate are well absorbed at any time.

2. Take calcium with plenty of water.

3. Take no more than 500 mg of calcium at one time.

4. Antacids are an acceptable source of calcium. The calcium in these products is calcium carbonate and should be taken at mealtime to facilitate absorption.

5. Take vitamin D along with calcium in order to better absorb it.

When Selecting a Calcium Supplement

■ Read the ingredients on the label. Do not buy supplements that contain unrefined oyster shell, dolomite, or bone meal. These products may also contain toxic substances, such as mercury, arsenic, and lead.

■ Calcium carbonate and calcium citrate have the lowest lead content.

■ Do not pay more for chelated calcium tablets. They are not more beneficial than other types of calcium.

BONE DENSITY BOOSTERS

Vitamin K

An adequate amount of dietary vitamin K is said to be necessary to help prevent excess bone loss. In other words, vitamin K is a good thing!

The George Mateljan Foundation (www.whfoods.org), dedicated to making the world a healthier place by providing cutting-edge information about the world's healthiest foods, reports that a study of more than 70,000 women who consumed larger amounts of vitamin K in their diets had a lower risk of hip fracture. Also, lower levels of vitamin K were associated with lower bone mineral density. (That's not a good thing.)

It's clear that by adding the following foods rich in vitamin K to your daily diet, you will be protecting and possibly improving your bone health.

■ Kale, boiled

■ Spinach, boiled

■ Collard greens, boiled

■ Swiss chard, boiled

■ Turnip greens, cooked

■ Mustard greens, boiled

■ Broccoli, steamed

■ Parsley, fresh

■ Romaine lettuce

■ Liver

■ Tomatoes

■ Green beans

■ Asparagus

■ Green peas

■ Carrots

CAUTION: If you are taking anticoagulant medications, such as Coumadin, you and your health care provider must monitor vitamin K intake. Eating a diet high in vitamin K can make anticoagulant medications less effective.

Boron

Boron is a mineral that improves calcium absorption and helps reduce the amount of calcium excreted in the urine. Foods rich in boron are:

■ Red apples

■ Avocado

■ Banana

■ Broccoli

■ Celery

■ Hazelnuts

■ Peanut butter

■ Raisins

■ Walnuts

■ Cabbage

■ Dandelion tea

■ Parsley

Exercise

Help strengthen bones with weight-bearing exercise. That simply means any activity done to support one's body weight—walking, dancing, climbing stairs, vacuuming, grocery shopping.

You don't have to do high-impact exercise, such as jogging, to strengthen your bones. Walking will do just as well. Be as active as possible. Don't take shortcuts, literally. Take the long way around, just so you get more walking into your day.

To help strengthen your muscles, lift weights. Start with small weights—a pound in each hand—and gradually work your way up.

AN ENCOURAGING THOUGHT

We've given you lots to think about and act on. You probably have to rethink your diet and implement changes that will make a difference. You may want to add daily supplements, and you surely need to increase your daily activity.

In the realistically hopeful words of chiropractor and acupuncturist Dr. Ben Kim (www.drbenkim.com), "Weakened bones can become healthy again if you consistently make the right choices in the days ahead."

SEX

Researchers tell us that about 90 percent of the cases of decreased sexual ability are psychologically caused. Since a psychological placebo has been known to evoke a prize-winning performance, we're including rituals, recipes, potions, lotions, charms, and all kinds of passion-promoting spells that can help spell success.

For history buffs and for history in the buff, we culled the ancient Greek, Egyptian, Indian, and Asian sex secrets that are still being used today.

So if you did but don't, should but won't, can't but want to, or do but don't enjoy it, please read on. Help and newfound fun may be waiting on the following pages.

FOR MEN ONLY

Erectile Dysfunction (Impotence)

Most men at some time during their lives experience the dreaded inability to have an erection. That's the bad news. The good news is that it is usually a temporary condition commonly caused nowadays by prescription drugs or by some kind of psychological trauma and emotional tension. If you're taking prescription drugs, check their side effects. If you suspect that a drug is causing the problem, talk to your doctor about using an alternative or lowering the dosage. If it's not drugs, check what's going on in your life that may be causing this emotional (and physical) upheaval. You may want to consider seeing a professional sex therapist or analyst to help you sort through your situation, figure it out, and deal with it.

While you're examining your psyche, there are things you can do that just may make the difference.

In the Mexican pharmacopoeia, damiana is classified as an aphrodisiac and a tonic for the nervous system. It's been known to be an effective remedy for "performance anxiety."

Add 1 teaspoon of damiana leaves (available at herb and health food stores) to 1 cup of just-boiled water. Let it steep for 10 minutes. Strain and drink before breakfast on a daily basis.

Eat a handful of raw, hulled pumpkin seeds every day. (The cooking process may destroy some of the special values of the seeds, so steer clear of the roasted ones.) Pumpkin seeds contain large amounts of zinc, magnesium, iron, phosphorus, calcium, vitamin A, and the B vitamins. According to a German medical researcher, there are one or more substances not yet isolated that have vitalizing and regenerative effects and actually cause additional sex hormones to be produced. Many health authorities agree that a handful of pumpkin seeds a day may help prevent impotence and prostate problems, too.

Premature Ejaculation

According to the teachings of Yogi Bhajan, the revered Sikh leader in the Western Hemisphere, a man should never have sexual intercourse within two and a half hours after eating a meal, the length of time it takes to digest food.

The sex act is strenuous and requires your mind, your entire nervous system, and all your muscles needed for the digestion process. Yogi Bhajan felt that lovemaking right after eating could ruin your stomach and, if done often, could eventually result in premature ejaculation.

While he said that four hours between eating and sex is adequate, he thought that for optimal sexual function, a man should have nothing but liquids and juices twenty-four hours before making love.

According to sex therapists, premature ejaculation seems to be one of the easiest conditions to cure, simply by behavior modification. This is Masters and Johnson's conditioning treatment.

Enlist the assistance of your mate, who should be very willing to comply. Lie on your back with your legs straddling your partner. Have her stimulate your penis until you feel that orgasm is just around the corner. At that second, give her a pre-arranged signal. In response to the signal, she should stop stimulating and start squeezing the penis just below the tip. She should squeeze it firmly enough to cause you to lose your erection, but not so hard as to cause you pain. When the feeling that you are about to ejaculate leaves you, have her stimulate you again. As before, signal her when orgasm is imminent and, once again, she should stop stimulating and start squeezing the penis. The erection should go down and you will not ejaculate. Keep this up (and down) for a while and soon you will be able to control ejaculation.

The next step is intercourse. As soon as you feel you are about to climax, signal your partner, withdraw from her, and have her squeeze your penis until you lose the erection. Practice makes perfect.

Masters and Johnson reported that in just two weeks of using this behavior modification program, 98 percent of men with premature ejaculation are cured.

Sexual Stamina

It is said that the higher a man's voice, the lower his masculine vitality. The theory is based on the fact that the vortex at the base of the neck and the vortex in the sex center are directly connected and affected by each other. Men, lower your voice and you'll increase the speed of vibration in these vortexes, which in turn may increase your sexual energy.

Hindi records, circa the tenth century, tell about men who went to view the famous Temple of Khajuraho in India to study its pornographic stone carvings depicting every known position of love. In order to have the stamina to test the positions, they were fed this eggplant dish: Slice an eggplant and cover with butter and minced chives on both sides. Brown the slices and cover with a spicy curry sauce.

The recipe (unspecific as it is) has been passed down from generation to generation, along with its reputation for making old men young again.

Most men get a stronger erection and feel more of a sensation when their bladder is full. However, some positions may be uncomfortable if it's very full.

> **NOTE:** Men with prostate problems should not practice this technique.

After much research, we've come up with a list of foods said to have aphrodisiacal effects. At the top of the list is, believe it or not, celery. Eat it every day, but keep in mind that it has diuretic properties, so don't overdo it. Of course we've all heard about eating oysters. They contain zinc and, like pumpkin seeds, are said to be wonderful for male genitalia. If you're going to eat oysters, be extremely careful to avoid contaminated sources.

The list continues with peaches, honey, parsley, cayenne pepper, bran cereals, and truffles. In fact, Napoleon credited truffles for his ability to sire a son.

▶ To improve sexual potency, do this yoga exercise twice a day, before breakfast and before bedtime. Sit on the floor with back straight, head up, and feet crossed in front of you. Tighten the muscles in the genital area, including the anus. Count to twenty, then relax and count to twenty again. Repeat the procedure five times in a row.

Sexual Desire

Doctor of Chinese medicine Maoshing Ni (Dr. Mao), author of *Secrets of Self-Healing* (Avery), explains, "In classical Chinese medicine, sexual desire is the function of the fire or yang energy of the kidney-adrenal network." But when diet, age, or lifestyle interferes with that energy, your libido can take a nosedive. Dr. Mao's remedies boost the kidney-adrenal fire by supporting hormonal function and align-

ing the mind and body to allow people to reconnect with their sexuality.

"Libido-enhancing foods are typically warming and pungent in nature and taste and can help motivate the yang or body's fire energy," writes Dr. Mao. His recommendations include garlic, onions, scallions, leeks, chives, ginger, cinnamon, fennel, turmeric, cayenne pepper, black pepper, and horseradish. Also helpful for a low libido: lentils, black beans, kidney beans, sesame seeds, walnuts, yams, sea cucumber, blueberries, raspberries, and cranberries, as well as organic shrimp, eggs, lamb, and chicken. Avoid dairy and raw or cold foods; they can cause dampness in the body, which decreases circulation in the sex organs.

Dr. Mao (www.askdrmao.com) shares a recipe that just may help rev up your sex drive.

LIBIDO SOUP

1 chopped onion
1 chopped leek
3 chopped chive stalks
10 slices fresh ginger root
1 teaspoon turmeric
1 teaspoon cayenne pepper
4 cups canned chicken stock

Combine all ingredients and boil for 30 minutes. Eat at least one bowl a day.

Garlic is said to stimulate sexual desire and the production of semen. Eat raw garlic in salads and use it in cooking and take garlic supplements daily. Then find a woman who doesn't mind the smell of garlic. By the way, is it a coincidence that the French and Italians have a steady diet of garlic and are said to be vigorous lovers?

Mint is supposed to restore sexual desire. Eat mint leaves, drink mint tea, or suck on peppermint Altoids. It's also good for eliminating garlic breath, making you more pleasant to be near.

Maca, an ancient herb from the jungles of Peru, is now used around the world for its sex-boosting powers. According to Susan M. Lark, M.D., author and lecturer, "Along with enhancing your libido, maca has also been used to normalize menstrual cycles and menopausal symptoms, help with vaginal dryness, increase energy, stamina, mental clarity, and regulate the endocrine and immune systems."

Maca is available at health food stores in capsules, powder, and liquid extract forms. Follow the dosage on the label.

Contrary to what we've been led to believe about cold showers, they might help stimulate sexual desire. Every day for about two months, take a cold shower or cold sitz bath and notice a rejuvenated you.

NOTE: If you have prostate problems, cold showers or baths should be avoided.

For instant sexual stimulation, use short applications of cold water, particularly on the nape of the neck.

In Japan, men are advised to firmly squeeze their testicles daily, once for as many years as they are old. We told this to a neighbor who is on in years. He said, "There goes my day!"

Heighten a Man's Pleasure

Touching a man's testicles before his orgasm is a wonderful way for a woman to greatly excite her lover. It also may hasten as well as heighten his orgasm.

NOTE: Touching the testicles just after orgasm is a no-no. It gives an unpleasant, almost painful sensation.

Sex and the Heart

It's a myth that sex is dangerous to the heart, according to Dr. Richard A. Stein, director of the heart exercise laboratory at the State University of New York Downstate Medical Center.

The stress to the heart is really very mild. The average heart rate increases to 115 to 120 beats per minute during intercourse—a muscle workload equal to walking up two flights of stairs.

WARNING: If a man is cheating on his mate, the heart rate and risk rise with the excitement and the danger of being caught.

FOR WOMEN ONLY

Sexual Desire

Lack of sexual desire often stems from a lack of communication between a woman and her man. Sex counseling may be the necessary remedy. Meanwhile, try one or more of the following suggestions.

❦ Licorice (the herb that's available at health food stores, not the candy) has female hormones in it. In France it might not be uncommon to see women drink licorice water, believing it may improve their love life. Powdered licorice is available at health food stores. Drink 1 teaspoon in 1 cup of water and get out the black lingerie.

NOTE: If you have high blood pressure, use the lingerie but not the licorice.

❦ As for the "Not tonight, honey" syndrome, eating a piece of halvah may awaken sexual desire. This Middle Eastern treat (available at gourmet food shops and health food stores) is made with sesame seeds and honey. The sesame seeds are high in magnesium and potassium. Honey has aspartic acid. All three substances have been known to help women overcome lack of lust.

❦ In Greek mythology, Anaxarete was cold to her suitors. How cold was she? She was so cold that Aphrodite, the goddess of love, turned her into a marble statue. That's cold!

Here is an antifreeze that might work even for Anaxarete. Boil 1 cup of finely minced chive leaves and roots (available at a greengrocer) with 2 cups of champagne. Then simmer until reduced to a thick cupful. Drink it unstrained. It's no wonder this syrup may work. Centuries later we learned that the syrup is rich in vitamin E (the love vitamin). Also, champagne has always been known to provoke passion. It was an often-used ingredient in Casanova's erotic cookery.

Ancient Teuton brides drank honey beer for thirty days after their wedding ceremony. It was said to make the bride more sexually responsive. The custom of honey beer for a month, poetically referred to as a "moon," is the source of the term *honeymoon.*

Rather than go through the big bother of preparing honey beer the way they did way back when, herbalists simplified it to a tea made from hops and honey.

Place 1 ounce of hops (available at health food stores) in a porcelain or Pyrex container. Pour 1 pint of just-boiled water over the hops, cover, and allow to stand for 15 minutes, then strain. Add a teaspoon of raw honey to a wineglass of the tea and drink it an hour before each meal. If you prefer warm hops and honey, heat the tea before drinking.

Honey has aspartic acid and vitamin E. Honey and hops contain traces of hormones. All of these ingredients are said to stimulate female sexuality. We'll drink to that!

Hundreds of years ago, witches wore necklaces of acorns to symbolize the fertile powers of nature. In some circles, it is still believed that by carrying an acorn you will attract and promote sexual relations, resulting in conception.

Orgasm Heightener

The ancient Japanese, masters of sensuality, invented Ben Wa balls. Later, in the eighteenth century French women referred to them as *pommes d'amour* ("love apples").

Doctors throughout the world recommend these brass (or gold-plated steel) balls that are placed in the vagina for their therapeutic value. They strengthen the bladder (which helps prevent incontinence) and help tighten the walls of the vagina, and the big bonus is they give women more control over the frequency and intensity of orgasms. They're also beneficial for women who are pregnant (they're said to make the birth process a little easier).

They are sold in stores that sell adult sex toys. If you Google "Ben Wa balls" you will find many sites, including www.healthy andactive.com, along with their toll-free number, 866-363-0578.

FOR COUPLES

Time for Love

Testosterone, the sexual-desire-stimulating hormone in men, is at its lowest level in the body at bedtime, 11:00 P.M. It's at its highest level at sunrise. No wonder you men may not want to make love at night before going to sleep. Try getting up with the roosters, brush your teeth, then do it and give yourselves something to crow about.

Tea for Two

Turkish women believe fenugreek tea makes them more attractive to men. Besides the sexual energy it may give them, the tea has a way of cleansing the system, sweetening the breath, and helping eliminate perspiration odors.

Men suffering from lack of desire and/or inability to perform have turned to fenugreek tea with success.

Many men with sexual problems lack vitamin A. Fenugreek contains an oil that's rich in vitamin A. Trimethylamine, another substance found in fenugreek and currently being tested on men, acts as a sex hormone in frogs. If you want to do your own testing, add 2 teaspoons of fenugreek seeds to 1 cup of just-boiled water. Let it steep for 5 minutes, stir, strain, and add honey and lemon to taste. Drink a cup a day, and don't be surprised if you get the urge to make love on a lily pad, or turn into a prince.

Sexy Clam Bake

Bake the meat of a dozen clams for about 2 hours at 400 degrees. When the clam meat is dark and hard, take it out of the oven, let it cool, and pulverize it to a powder, either in a blender or with a mortar and pestle. Take ½ teaspoon of the clam powder with water, 2 hours before bedtime, for one week. This Japanese folk remedy is supposed to restore sexual vitality.

Aphrodisiacs

We heard about a married couple whose idea of sexual compatibility is for both of them to get a headache at the same time.

They're the ones who asked us to include aphrodisiacs. The word itself means "any form of sexual stimulation." It was derived from the name of Aphrodite, the Greek goddess of love, who earned her title by having one husband and five lovers, including that handsome Greek guy Adonis. Enough about her!

Here are recipes for you and your mate that can add new vigor and uninhibited sensuality to your love life.

SENSATION STIRRER

To get in the mood, get in a warm bath to which you've added 2 drops of jasmine oil, 2 drops of ylang-ylang oil, and 8 drops of sandalwood oil. These essential oils are natural, organic substances that work in harmony with the natural forces of the body. Health food stores carry these "oils of olé."

In the interest of conserving water, bathe together.

PASSION FRUIT

Fruit beginning with the letter *p* are said to be especially good for increasing potency in men and enhancing sexual energy in women. The fruits we recommend are peaches, plums, pears, pineapple, papaya, and persimmon. If you have the same charming accent that my grandmother had, you can include the ever popular, potassium-rich "panana."

TONIC FOR HAPPY LOVERS

The English have a commercial preparation called Tonic for Happy Lovers. The recipe consists of combining 1 ounce of licorice root (the herb, not the candy) with 2 teaspoons of crushed fennel seeds (both available at health food stores) and 2 cups of water. Bring the mixture to a boil, lower the heat, cover, and simmer slowly for 20 minutes. After it has cooled, strain it and bottle it. Take 1 to 3 tablespoons twice a day.

NOTE: If you have high blood pressure, do not take licorice root.

POTION AND CHANT FOR ENDURING LOVE

Stir a pinch of ground coriander seeds into a glass of fine red wine while repeating this chant together:

Warm and caring heart
Let us never be apart.

Both of you sip the wine from the same glass, taking turns. When the wine is all gone, your love should be here to stay.

NATIVE AMERICAN PASSION PROMOTER

Add 2 tablespoons of unrefined oatmeal and ½ cup of raisins to 1 quart of water and bring it to a boil. Reduce heat, cover tightly, and simmer slowly for 45 minutes. Remove from heat and strain. Add the juice of 2 lemons and stir in honey to taste. Refrigerate the mixture. Drink 2 cups a day—one before breakfast and another cup an hour before bedtime. After doing this for a couple of days, don't be surprised if unbridled passion causes you to be late for work.

Oatmeal is rich in vitamin E. Is that where the phrase "sow wild oats" comes from?

A GEM OF A GEM

According to a gem therapist, wearing turquoise is said to increase its owner's sexual drive.

THE HONEYMOON PICK-ME-UP

This is an updated recipe of an ancient Druid formula. Sex therapists who prescribe it believe that taking it on a regular basis can generate a hearty sexual appetite.

Mix the following ingredients in a blender for several seconds: 2 level tablespoons of skim milk powder, water according to the skim milk instructions, ¼ teaspoon of powdered ginger, ⅛ teaspoon of powdered cinnamon, 2 tablespoons of raw honey, and a dash of lemon juice, plus any fresh fruit or pure fruit juice you care to add. It's a great snack before the games begin.

FERTILITY: INCREASING YOUR ODDS

If you're among the one in seven American couples having a tough time getting pregnant even though there's no explainable medical cause for not conceiving, continue reading, and be prepared to make changes in your diet.

New research from the world-famous Nurses' Health Study reveals that what you eat (or don't eat) can improve your fertility.

If you have *ovulatory infertility*—problems producing a monthly egg—the solution may be as simple as eliminating trans fats from your diet. That means you must forget about french fries, do away with doughnuts, and say no to most fast-food fare.

Start at the supermarket, reading each label before putting a food in your cart. If the ingredient list includes shortening, partially hydrogenated vegetable oil, or hydrogenated vegetable oil, the food contains trans fats.

Unless the label clearly states "no trans fats," you can expect to find them in margarine, crackers, candy, baked goods, snack foods, fried foods, salad dressings, and too many processed foods to mention. Just check the label before you buy anything. (You'll be healthier for it whether or not you want to get pregnant.)

Also, the results of several studies agree that women who exercise moderately, about 30 minutes a day, are less likely to experience ovulation-related infertility than women who don't exercise daily.

Okay, once you're frying with olive oil instead of margarine, taking a half-hour brisk walk every day, and producing a monthly egg, here are other steps to take to help you conceive:

■ Take a daily multivitamin.

■ Eat iron-rich foods—green leafy vegetables and fruit, but not red meat (iron from raw food is absorbed better than from supplements).

■ Eat beans, nuts, lentils, and other fertility-boosting plant protein.

■ Add whole grains such as oatmeal and barley to your daily diet.

■ Have a glass of whole milk or other full-fat dairy products every day (a small bowl of ice cream is fine every now and then).

■ Cut back on coffee and alcohol or eliminate them completely.

■ Eliminate sugared sodas.

For a comprehensive guide, consider getting a copy of *The Fertility Diet* (McGraw-Hill) by the groundbreaking fertility researchers Jorge Chavarro, M.D., Sc.D., and Walter C. Willett, M.D., Dr.P.H., in collaboration with Patrick J. Skerret.

SINUS PROBLEMS

The symptoms of a sinus attack are mostly the same as those that accompany a cold or seasonal allergies—stuffed or runny nose, headache, congestion. In fact, you may have a sinus infection along with a cold, allergies, or a headache. (Check the "Colds, Flu, Sore Throat, Etc.," "Allergies and Hay Fever," and "Headaches" chapters for remedies that can help relieve your symptoms.)

The most common causes of troublesome sinus conditions are weather changes, air-conditioning, or an overheated room. The cause of a sinus problem may be something right under a person's nose: the dust that collects in one's mustache.

Pay attention to the times a sinus attack starts and stops, where you are, and what you're doing or handling. Eventually, you should notice a pattern and can discover sinus triggers. Once that happens, you'll be able to prevent sinus attacks. Until then, we're hoping these remedies will help.

Slowly, cautiously, and gently, inhale the vapors of freshly grated horseradish (available at the supermarket and greengrocer). While you're at it, mix equal amounts of grated horseradish and lemon juice. Eat 1 teaspoon an hour before breakfast and at least an hour after dinner. It gives long-lasting relief to some sinus sufferers who are good about taking it every day consistently.

NOTEWORTHY: First there was the neti pot. Now there's Nasaline (available at pharmacies and health food stores), an easy and neat modern version of the self-irrigating saline rinsing system that helps decongest and drain blocked nasal passages. It may also help prevent sinus-related infections.

Crush 1 clove of garlic into ¼ cup of water. Sip up the garlicky water into an eyedropper. (Make sure no pieces of the clove get into the dropper.)

Dose: Use 10 drops of clear garlic water per nostril, three times a day, for three days. At the end of the three days, there should be a noticeable clearing up of the sinus infection.

SKIN

Skin is the largest organ of the body. The average adult has seventeen square feet of skin. Whether you're thick- or thin-skinned, it weighs about five pounds.

Five pounds of skin covering seventeen square feet of body surface . . . that's a lot of room for pimples, blackheads, blisters, blotches, sores, enlarged pores, scars, itches, rashes, ringworm, wrinkles, and more, lots more.

Someone named Anonymous once said, "Dermatology is the best specialty. The patient never dies—and never gets well." Mr. Anonymous said that before reading this chapter.

Gimme some skin, and we'll give you some remedies!

Be sure to check out the "Face Facts" and "Looking Your Best" sections at the end of the chapter.

ACNE

The following acne remedies may or may not produce dramatic results overnight. Select one and stay with it for at least two weeks. If there's no improvement by then, go on to another remedy.

▶ This South American remedy was given to us by noted herbalist Angela Harris, who has used it to clear up the face of many a teenager. Wash with a mild soap and warm water. Then apply a thin layer of extra-virgin, cold-pressed olive oil (the olive oil label *must* say "extra-virgin, cold-pressed"). Do not wash it off. Let the skin completely absorb the olive oil.

Do this three times a day. Angela's experience has been that the skin clears up within a week.

For maintenance, wash and oil once a day.

> **NOTE:** Always wash your face with warm or tepid water. Very hot or very cold water can cause the breaking of capillaries (those squiggly little blood vessels).

▶ Using a juice extractor, juice 1 medium cucumber. With a pastry brush, apply the cucumber juice to the trouble spots. Leave it on for at least 15 minutes, then wash it off with tepid water. Do this daily.

Wet a clean, white cloth or towel with your fresh, warm first urine of the day, and pat it on the acne areas. Your urine has antibodies that help heal the condition. Leave it on as long as possible, then rinse with tepid water.

If you have access to an infant's wet diaper, apply it to the affected areas in addition to or instead of your own urine. You should see amazing results within a short period of time. And we'll keep this remedy as our little secret.

Acne Scars

To help remove acne scars, combine 1 teaspoon of powdered nutmeg with 1 teaspoon of honey and apply it to the scarred area. After 20 minutes, wash it off with cool water. Do this twice a week, and hopefully within a couple of months you will see an improvement.

PIMPLES

For that occasional eruption, mix the juice of 2 garlic cloves (see "Preparation Guide") with an equal amount of distilled white vinegar, and dab it on the pimple every evening.

Mix 1 teaspoon of fresh lemon juice with 1 teaspoon of ground cinnamon and smear the mixture on the pimple. It should shrink the pimple quickly.

BLACKHEADS

Before going to bed, rub lemon juice over blackheads. Wait until morning to wash off the juice with cool water. Repeat the procedure several evenings in a row and you'll see a big improvement.

BOILS

A boil is a skin abscess that usually starts as a reddened, tender area and in time becomes firm and hard. Eventually, the center of the abscess softens and becomes filled with white blood cells (pus) that the body sends to fight the infection.

> **CAUTION:** If pain gets progressively worse, or if you see a red streak emanating from the boil, get professional medical attention *immediately*. Do not wait!

Mix 1 tablespoon of honey with 1 tablespoon of cod liver oil (Norwegian emulsified cod liver oil is nonsmelly) and glob it on the boil. Bind it with a sterile bandage.

Reapply the mixture and the bandage every 8 hours.

To draw out the waste material painlessly and quickly, add a little water to about 1 teaspoon of fenugreek powder, making it the consistency of paste. Put it on the boil and cover it with a sterile bandage. Change the dressing twice a day.

This Irish remedy requires 4 slices of bread and 1 cup of milk. Boil the bread and milk together until it's one big, gloppy mush. As soon as the mush is cool enough to handle, slop some of it on the boil and cover it with a sterile bandage. When the glop gets cold, replace it with warm glop. Keep dressing the boil until you've used up all 4 slices of bread. By then, the boil should have opened.

Gently peel off the delicate membrane of a hard-boiled egg (under the shell), wet it, and place it on the boil. It should draw pus out and relieve the inflammation.

When the Boil Breaks

The boil is at the brink of breaking when it turns red and the pain increases. When it finally does break, pus will be expelled, leaving a temporary opening in the skin. Almost magically, the pain will disappear.

Boil 1 cup of water and add 2 tablespoons of lemon juice. Let it cool. Clean and disinfect the area thoroughly with the lemon water. Cover with a sterile bandage. For the next few days, two or three times a day, remove the bandage and apply a warm, wet compress, leaving it on for 15 minutes. Dress the area with a fresh, sterile bandage after each wet compress.

ENLARGED PORES

So you have some enlarged pores. Think of it this way: in our seventeen square feet of skin, we have about 1 billion pores. Percentagewise, look how few are enlarged.

To help refine those pores, put ⅓ cup of almonds into a blender and pulverize them into a powder. Add enough water to the powder to give it the consistency of paste. Rub the mixture gently across the enlarged pores from your nose outward and upward. Leave it on your face for a half hour, then rinse it off with tepid water. As a final rinse, mix ¼ cup of cool water with ¼ cup of apple cider vinegar and splash it on to tighten the pores.

To get and maintain results, treat your skin to this almond rub a couple of times a week.

Papaya contains the enzyme papain, which is said to do wonderful things for the complexion. Wash your face and neck. Remove the meat of the papaya (eating it is optional and a smart thing to do—it's delicious and great for your digestion) and rub the inside of the papaya skin on your skin. It will dry, forming a see-through mask. After 15 minutes, wash it off with warm water. Along with removing dead skin and tightening the pores, it may also make some light freckles disappear.

Extra-Large Enlarged Pores

We're talking really big pores here. Every night for one week, or as long as one container of buttermilk lasts, wash your face, then soak a wad of absorbent cotton in buttermilk and dab it all over your face. Leave it on for 20 minutes as it dries and tightens the pores. When the 20 minutes is up, smile and experience a weird sensation. Then wash the dried buttermilk off with cool water. Repeat the procedure every night for a week. You should be pleased with the results.

DEAD SKIN CELLS

A friend with beautiful skin uses Miracle Whip salad dressing to remove dead skin cells. She puts it on her face and leaves it there for about 20 minutes. Then she washes it off with warm water, followed by cold water. She claims that no other mayonnaise works as well as Miracle Whip salad dressing. It not only removes dead skin cells, it also tightens her pores. Maybe that's where the "miracle" comes in.

ELBOWS, KNEES, FEET

Make a paste by combining salt and fresh lemon juice. Rub this abrasive mixture on rough and tough areas such as elbows, feet, and knees. Wash the paste off with cool water.

Take the skin from half a ripe avocado and rub the inside of it against the rough areas of your elbows and/or knees. Keep rubbing. Don't wash the area until bedtime.

Rest your elbows in grapefruit halves to get rid of alligator skin. Make yourself as comfortable as possible and keep your elbows in the inside of the citrus fruit halves for at least a half hour. Rinse clean with cool water.

BLOTCHY, SCALY SKIN

Gently wash your face with warm water, pat dry, then apply cod liver oil, castor oil, or liquid lecithin to clean skin. Leave it on as long as possible. Use cool water to wash it off. Repeat the procedure as often as possible throughout the day and night.

BODY SCRUB: EXFOLIATE AND MOISTURIZE

Prepare yourself for a treatment used at some of the world's most luxurious spas.

All you need is 2 cups of kosher (coarse) salt and 1 cup of coconut oil (or almond oil or olive oil).

Mix salt and oil together until it's the consistency of a thick paste. Take it with you into the bathtub or shower. Slowly and methodically, massage your body with it, starting with your feet and working your way up to your neck.

NOTE: Do not apply it to your face or to any part of your body that has sores or eruptions of any kind. The salt will irritate the skin, making it worse.

Once the "body scrub" is completed, rinse with warm water, but no soap. You want to slough off the dead surface skin cells, keep the moisture in, and feel tingly and clean.

BLISTERS

If you have a blister, do not open it. Put a Band-Aid on it and leave it alone to dry out by itself.

If you have a blister that broke, clean it by dabbing it with hydrogen peroxide or alcohol on a cotton ball. Then let the air get to it so it can dry out naturally. When you must cover it, put on a Band-Aid and then your sock or stocking.

Blister Prevention

If you are going to be walking a lot while breaking in new shoes, help your feet fend off blisters by applying petroleum jelly or any thick ointment to the areas of your feet where you'd expect blisters to happen.

MOLLUSCUM CONTAGIOSUM VIRUS

See the "Children's Health Challenges" chapter.

RINGWORM

Ringworm is a contagious fungus infection. The name comes from the reddish ring that usually appears on the scalp or skin. These sometimes itchy, scaly patches may blister and ooze. Ringworm seems mostly to affect the scalp, but it can also show up on the body (particularly the groin area), the feet (see "Athlete's Foot"), and the nails (see "Toenail Fungus").

A woman shared this remedy her family used whenever she or any of her siblings had ringworm. Mix blue fountain pen ink with cigar ashes and put the mixture on the fungus-infected area. The woman said she has never seen it fail. Within a few days, the ringworm completely disappears.

If this remedy is going to get you into the habit of smoking cigars, stick with the ringworm, or try the next remedy.

❧ Mince or grate garlic and mix it with an equal amount of petroleum jelly. Apply the mixture to the trouble spots and cover with gauze. Leave it that way overnight. Throughout the next day, puncture garlic softgels and rub the squished-out oil on the afflicted areas. Repeat the procedure the following night and day if necessary. The garlic should stop the itching and help heal the rash.

❧ There are two versions of this remedy, and both worked for the people who told us about them. Soak a few pennies in distilled white vinegar for a minute, then rub the pennies on the ringworm. Do this in the morning and in the evening until the ringworm disappears. Or dip a penny or two in vinegar and tape the pennies on top of the ringworm. Repeat the process every morning until the ringworm is gone.

Ringworm Prevention

Avoid contact with infected people and pets. Do not use items that an infected person may have used, including combs, brushes, bed linens, telephones, hats, stuffed animals, gym mats, and shower stalls.

BROWN SPOTS (AKA SUN SPOTS, LIVER SPOTS, AGE SPOTS, OR LENTIGOS)

The following remedies may not produce instant results. These brown spots, thought to be caused by exposure to the sun or maybe even a nutritional deficiency, took years to form. Give the remedy you use a few months to work. Then, if there's no change, try a different remedy.

❧ Grate an onion and squeeze it through cheesecloth so that you have 1 teaspoon of onion juice. Mix it with 2 teaspoons of vinegar and massage the brown spots with this liquid. Do it daily—twice a day if possible—until you no longer see spots in front of your eyes.

❧ This Israeli remedy calls for chickpeas. You may know them as garbanzo beans, ceci, or arbus. If you don't want to prepare them from scratch, buy canned chickpeas. Mash about 1/3 cup and add a little water. Smear the paste on the brown spots and leave it there till it dries and starts crumbling off. Then wash it off completely. Do this every evening.

FRECKLES

Freckles . . . they're adorable! Sure, that's easy for us to say. We don't have them. If you do and you want to lighten them, or maybe even get rid of a few of the freckles that came out during the summer, apply lemon juice, the juice of parsley, or the juice of watercress at night and wash it off in the morning before you go outdoors.

❧ An old folk remedy for freckles is to wash your face with warm beer. So if you really want to get rid of those little brown speckles, get the warm beer and hop to it. Repeated washings several days in a row may be necessary. Also, right after the treatment, apply a light film of castor oil on your skin to prevent irritation of sensitive facial tissue.

❧ If you're determined to do away with your freckles, bottle your own freckle remover. Get 4 medium-size dandelion leaves (pick them yourself, or buy them at the greengrocer), rinse them thoroughly, and tear them into small pieces. Combine the leaves with 5 tablespoons of castor oil in an enamel or glass pan. Over low heat, let the mixture simmer for 10 minutes. Turn off the heat, cover the pan, and let it steep for 3 hours. Strain the mixture into a bottle. (Be sure to label the bottle.)

Massage several drops of the oil on the freckled area and leave it on overnight. In the morning, wash your face with tepid water. Do this daily for at least a week and watch the spots disappear.

❧ If you're desperate to get rid of those freckles of yours and other remedies have not worked, you may want to try this one: Take a glass of your morning urine and mix it with 1 tablespoon of apple cider vinegar. Add a pinch of salt and let it stand for 24 hours. Next, put it on the freckles for a half hour, then rinse with cool water and follow it with a thin film of castor oil. To get results, you will most likely have to do this several times. (Are you sure you really don't want freckles?)

❧ If you wake up in the morning, look in the mirror, and see freckles you never had before, try cleaning the mirror.

SCARS

According to herbalist Angela Harris, you can fade a scar by applying a light film of extra-virgin, cold-pressed olive oil every day. Be consistent and be patient. The scar won't disappear overnight.

STRETCH MARKS

After a shower or bath, gently massage sesame oil—about a tablespoon—all over your stretch-marked areas. Eventually, pregnancy and weight-loss stretch marks may disappear. Meanwhile, make up your mind to love your body exactly the way it is.

HARD-TO-HEAL SORES AND LESIONS

CAUTION: If you have a nonhealing blemish, have it checked by a dermatologist before using any home remedies.

Put pure, undiluted Concord grape juice on a sterilized cotton puff or gauze pad and apply it to the sore, binding it in place with a bandage. Do not wash the sore. Just keep the grape juice on it, changing the dressing at least once in the morning and once at night. Be patient. It may take two to three weeks for the sore to heal.

Finger Sores

When you have one of those painful inflammations around the fingernail, soak it in hot water. Then heat a lemon in the oven, cut a narrow opening in the middle of the lemon, and sprinkle salt in it. Take the infected finger and stick it in the lemon. Within minutes, the pain should disappear as the healing starts.

Weeping Sores (Infections with Pus)

CAUTION: If infection persists, it is important to have a health professional look at it.

Place a piece of papaya pulp on a weeping sore. Keep it in place with a big Band-Aid. Change the dressing every 2 or 3 hours until it clears up.

A honey (raw honey if possible) poultice is disinfecting and healing. Keep it on for a few hours.

Apply a poultice of either raw grated carrots or cooked mashed carrots to stop the throbbing and draw out the infection.

PSORIASIS

A cabin at the shore and frequent dips in the surf, or a trip to the Dead Sea, seems to work wonders for psoriasis sufferers. Next best thing: Dissolve ½ cup of sea salt in 1 gallon of water. Soak the psoriasis patches in the salt water several times a day.

The foremost authority on healing herbs, Dr. James Duke, explains in *The*

Green Pharmacy, "Several plant oils are chemically similar to fish oils, which have a reputation for helping to relieve psoriasis. Flaxseed oil contains the beneficial compounds eicosapentaenoic acid and alpha-linolenic acid." Dr. Duke reviewed studies showing that taking 10 to 12 grams (5 to 6 teaspoons) of flaxseed oil daily can help treat psoriasis. Some people respond very well to this remedy. It's certainly worth a try.

▶ Add 1 teaspoon of sarsaparilla root (available at health food stores) to 1 cup of just-boiled water and let it steep for 15 minutes. If it's cool enough by then, strain and saturate a white washcloth in the liquid and apply it to the trouble spots. You may need more than one washcloth, depending on the extent of the condition. If it seems to agree with you, do it morning and night for a week and watch for an improvement.

▶ If you're willing to try anything to help clear up this condition, every evening pat garlic oil on the affected area by puncturing a garlic softgel and squishing out the oil. Not a pleasant thing to do, but hey, if it helps . . .

ECZEMA

We reported that eating raw potatoes—2 a day—may work miracles in clearing up eczema. Well, it did for a woman who wrote to us, saying that she was in Australia and going through a terrible time. Eczema on her face made her feel and look awful. She came across our book that included this remedy. She started eating raw potatoes and the pain disappeared within the week; within two weeks, the condition cleared up completely.

▶ Oolong tea (available at health food stores and most supermarkets) has worked like magic for some people who had been suffering with eczema for years. Drink 4 cups of oolong tea daily and stick with it, giving it a chance to work. The tea is good; the results could be even better.

▶ Morning and night, mix a few tablespoons of brewer's yeast with water, enough to form a paste that will cover the affected area. Gently apply it and leave it on until it dries out and crumbles off.

HIVES

Hives usually disappear almost as fast and as mysteriously as they appear. If yours are hanging on, combine 3 tablespoons of cornstarch and 1 tablespoon of distilled white vinegar. Mix well and apply the paste on the hives. That ought to teach 'em to hang around!

▸ Add 1 cup of baking soda to a bathtub of tepid water and soak in it for 20 minutes.

HEAT RASH (PRICKLY HEAT)

Make a soothing powder by browning ½ cup of all-purpose flour in the oven. When it's cool, apply it on the rash.

Cornstarch is also soothing to use. No need to brown it. Just apply it.

▸ Rub the prickly heat area with the inside of watermelon rind.

SHAVING RASH

Men, ever get a shaving rash, particularly on your neck? Women, all we need to say are two words: bikini area.

Puncture a vitamin E softgel, squish out the contents, and mix it with a dab of petroleum jelly. Then gently spread the mixture on the irritated skin.

POISON IVY, OAK, AND SUMAC

At least one of the three poison weeds—ivy, oak, and sumac—grows in just about every state in our country. Contact with any of these plants usually causes the same irritating blisters, itching, and discomfort. Chances are if you're allergic to one, you're allergic to all. It's estimated that as many as 10 million Americans are affected by these plants annually.

Poison Ivy, Oak, and Sumac Prevention

If you know what these plants look like, you may be able to avoid them. Check out http://poisonivy.aesir.com/view/pictures .html for lots of photos of poison ivy, oak, and sumac.

While you're at it, check out the photos of nature's poison ivy antidote, jewelweed: http://altnature.com/jewelweed.htm. If you do get poison ivy and you do find jewelweed, crush the leaves and stems to get the juice. Apply the juice on the rash every hour throughout the day.

Poison Ivy Test

The white paper test will tell you if that patch of plants you just brushed up against is poison ivy. Take hold of the plant in question with a piece of white paper. Smush the leaves, causing liquid from the plant to wet the paper. If it's poison ivy, the juice on the paper will turn black within 5 minutes.

The Second You Know You've Touched Poison Ivy

You can wash off the plant's urushiol (the irritating oil) if you put your exposed body parts under cold running water. You have a very short window of opportunity to do this—about 3 minutes—so just hope the poison ivy patch you stepped in is near a waterfall, faucet, or garden hose.

When you're going into poison ivy territory, take green tomatoes with you. If you think you stepped in the ivy, squeeze the green tomato juice on your skin. It may save you the anguish of having poison ivy.

Poison Ivy Rash Relief

■ As soon as the itching starts, dab the area with a combination of equal parts of distilled white vinegar and rubbing alcohol.

■ Apply ice-cold whole-milk compresses. If you don't have milk, just use ice cubes.

■ Mash a piece of white chalk and mix it in a pint of water. Dip a washcloth in the chalky mixture and apply it to the rash throughout the day.

■ Rub slices of lemon on the area to stop the itching and heal the rash.

When our copy editor gets a poison ivy rash, she stands under a hot shower—as hot as she can stand it without burning herself. The itching increases and then suddenly diminishes. It may be that the heat depletes the cells of histamine. Relief usually lasts 6 to 8 hours.

FYI: People who are very allergic to poison ivy may also react to mango skin, cashews, and ginkgo trees.

Also see the "Itching" chapter.

Doing Away with the Poison Ivy Plant

Never, *never* burn poison ivy! The plant's oil—urushiol—gets in the air and can be inhaled. That can be very harmful to lungs. Instead, while wearing gloves, uproot the plants and leave them on the ground to dry out in the sun. Or kill them with a solution of 3 pounds of salt in a gallon of soapy water. Spray, spray, spray the plants, and then spray them some more. Wash your garden tools thoroughly with the same solution.

Once you've gotten rid of the poison ivy and cleaned your tools, carefully take off your gloves, turn them inside out, and dispose of them. You may also want to dispose of your clothes. Poison ivy oil may not wash out completely and can stay active for years.

LOOKING YOUR BEST

You don't have to have a million-dollar extreme makeover to look good. Here are ways to care for your skin at home, easily, inexpensively, and effectively.

Lips

LIP LINES PREVENTION

The way you may prevent those little crinkly lines around the mouth is by exercising the jaw muscle. Luckily, the jaw muscle can work the longest of all the body's muscles without getting tired. So whistle, sing, and talk. Tongue twisters are like the aerobics of the mouth, especially ones with the "m," "b," and "p" sounds. Here are a couple to start with:

Pitter-patter, pitter-patter, rather than patter-pitter, patter-pitter.

Mother made neither brother mutter to father.

CHAPPED LIPS

If your lips are chapped a lot of the time, make an effort to avoid licking your lips. When your saliva evaporates, it leaves your lips dry.

Get a bottle of vitamin E softgels (available at pharmacies and health food stores), carefully puncture one with a pin or needle, squish out the oil on your finger, then gently massage it on your lips before going out in the cold, or right after you've come in. And remember, don't lick your lips!

NOTE: Don't mistake cracks in the skin at the corners of your mouth for chapped lips. See: "Cracked Lips," below.

Apply a thin film of glycerin (available at drugstores) to soften and protect your lips.

CRACKED LIPS

The cracks in the skin at the corners of your mouth are usually caused by a vitamin B_2 (riboflavin) deficiency. Take a B_2 supplement and the problem should clear up quickly. The best dietary sources of riboflavin include brewer's yeast, almonds, organ meats, whole grains, wheat germ, wild rice, mushrooms, soybeans, milk, yogurt, eggs, broccoli, Brussels sprouts, and spinach. Flours and cereals are often fortified with riboflavin.

LIP GLOSS

Prepare your own lip gloss quickly and easily. In a small glass bowl, blend 1 teaspoon of coconut oil (available at health food stores) with 1 teaspoon of petroleum jelly. Either zap it in the microwave for about a minute or melt it in a double boiler on the stove. Pour the mixture into a clean lip gloss container (available at drugstores) and let it cool completely before using it.

Coconut oil will help heal chapped lips by locking in moisture. If you don't like the taste of it, you can replace it with cinnamon oil.

Wrinkles
WRINKLE REMOVERS

We know a man who has so many wrinkles in his forehead, he has to screw his hat on. That's a lot of wrinkles. He can start to smooth them out by relaxing more, by not smoking (fact: smokers have far more wrinkles than nonsmokers), and by trying one or more of the following remedies.

Before bedtime, massage the lined areas of your neck and face with extra-virgin, cold-pressed olive oil. Start in the center of your neck and, using an upward and outward motion, get the oil into those dry areas. Work your way up to and include your forehead. Let the oil stay on overnight. In the morning, wash with tepid water and then cold water. You may want to add a few drops of your favorite herbal essence to the olive oil and pretend it costs $60 a bottle.

It took years to get the folds in your face; it will take time and persistence to unfold them.

The most popular wrinkle eraser remedy we found requires 1 teaspoon of honey and 2 tablespoons of heavy whipping cream. Mix them together vigorously. Dip your fingertips in the mixture and, with a gentle massaging action, apply it to the wrinkles, folds, lines, creases, crinkles, whatever. Leave it on for at least a half hour . . . the longer, the better. You'll feel it tighten on your face as it becomes a mask. When you're ready, splash it off with tepid water. By making this a daily ritual, you may become wrinkle-free.

Take an apple—green is best—wash it, core it, cut it into pieces, and put it in a blender (with the skin). Add a tablespoon of milk and puree it. Apply the puree all over your face, forehead, and neck, especially massaging it into the wrinkles. Relax with it on for as long as it takes to dry. Then rinse with tepid water and pat dry. Repeat the procedure three times a week. After the first week, you should see a difference in your skin tone and those fine lines should be fading.

If you prefer grapes over apples, crush a few green seedless grapes and smush them all over your face, forehead, and neck. After about 15 minutes, rinse with tepid water and pat dry.

If you run out of apples or grapes, give yourself a potato mask. Peel and grate 1 large or 2 small potatoes and apply the grated mush all over your face, forehead, and neck. Leave it on until it dries and you get that tightening feeling. Rinse with tepid water and pat dry.

WRINKLE PREVENTION

To reduce the tendency to wrinkle, mash a ripe banana and add a few drops of peanut oil. Apply it to your face and neck (remember, upward and outward), and leave it on for at least a half hour. Wash it off with tepid water. If you do this daily, or even every other day, it should make your skin softer and less likely to get lined.

WRINKLES AROUND THE EYES

Mix the white of an egg with enough sweet cream to make it glide on around your eye area. Let it stay on for at least a half hour—an hour would be twice as good. Wash it off with tepid water. The vitamins, proteins, enzymes, and unsaturated fatty acids—all that great stuff—should nourish the skin cells enough to smooth out the little crinkles around the eyes. Repeat the procedure often, at least four times a week.

EYE WRINKLE PREVENTION

Before bedtime, apply a light film of castor oil on the delicate area around the eyes to help prevent wrinkles.

Puffiness Under the Eyes

We saw a man with so much puffiness under his eyes, it looked like his nose was wearing a saddle.

One of the reasons for puffiness may be an excessive amount of salt in one's diet. Salt causes water retention and water retention causes puffiness. Become aware of the amount of salt in your food. According to some experts, the average American diet includes five times the tolerable upper limit of sodium. The current tolerable upper limit is less than 2,300 mg of sodium a day. That means about 1 teaspoon of table salt per day. Keeping to this upper limit can eliminate puffiness and benefit your overall health.

Eliminating dairy products from your diet may also help eliminate puffiness under the eyes.

When you want to look your best, set your clock an hour earlier than usual. Give yourself that extra time to depuff. Either that or sleep sitting up so the puffs don't get a chance to form under your eyes.

INSTANT, TEMPORARY EYE TUCK

This showbiz trick is fine for a photo session, but not for anything that lasts longer than 3 hours.

Take an egg white and beat it until

frothy. Then, with a fine eyeliner brush, paint the under-eye area. The secret of success here is to paint as thin and as even a layer of egg white as possible. As you allow it to dry, you'll notice how the area tightens. Use liquid makeup on top, and instead of rubbing it on, gently pat on the makeup.

As soon as you wash off the egg white, lubricate the area with castor oil to help undo the drying effects of the egg.

FACE FACTS

The first thing to ask yourself is what kind of skin you have—dry, oily, combination, or normal? If you're not sure, Heloise, the helpful hints lady, has a test you can take.

Wash your face with shaving cream. Rinse and lightly pat dry. Wait about 3 hours so that your skin can revert to its regular self. Then take cigarette papers or any other thin tissue paper and press pieces of it on your face. If it sticks, leaving an oily spot that's visible when you hold it up to the light, you've got oily skin. If it doesn't stick, your skin is dry. If it sticks but doesn't leave oily spots, you've got normal skin. If the paper sticks on some areas, leaving oily spots, and doesn't stick on other areas, you have combination skin.

As soon as you determine your skin type, read on for ways to take care of it.

General Rules for All Skin Types

■ Always use an upward and outward motion when doing anything to your face— washing it, a facial, applying or removing makeup.

■ Use tepid water to wash your face. Hot or cold water may break the small capillaries in your face.

■ Wash your face at least two times a day. Washing removes dead cells and keeps pores clean. The morning wash-up is necessary because of metabolic activity during the night. The night wash-up is necessary because of all the dirt that piles up during the day. Wash with a mild soap and a washcloth or cosmetic sponge, upward and outward. Now, onward . . .

■ The best time to apply a facial mask is at night, when you don't have to put on makeup for at least 6 hours afterward, and after you've taken a bath or shower, or after you've gently steamed your face so that the pores are open.

Caring for Oily Skin
MAKEUP REMOVER

Cleansers seem to be a problem for oily skin because of the high alcohol content of most makeup-removing astringents.

They're usually too harsh for delicate facial skin on a regular basis. Instead, use 1 teaspoon of powdered milk with enough warm water to give it a milky consistency. With cotton puffs, apply the liquid to your face and neck, gently rubbing it on. Once you've covered your entire face and neck, gently remove makeup and dirt with a tissue. Rinse and pat dry.

OILY SKIN MASK

Kitty litter has great absorbency and can be used for lots of things, including the purr-fect facial for oily skin. Be sure to get a natural litter that's 100 percent clay, no chemicals added. Mash 2 tablespoons of the litter with enough water—about 1 ounce—to make it a paste consistency. Apply it to your just-washed face, but not to the delicate area around your eyes. Leave it on for about 15 minutes. Rinse off with tepid water and pat dry.

Caring for Dry Skin
MAKEUP REMOVER

Instead of using soap and water, cleanse your face with whole milk. Warm 2 to 3 tablespoons of milk, pour it into a small jar, add ½ teaspoon of castor oil, and shake well. Wet a cotton pad with the mixture and start cleansing, using upward and outward strokes. This combination of milk and oil is said to take off more makeup and city dirt than the most expensive pro-fessional cleansing products on the market. And it does it naturally, not chemically. Complete the treatment by sealing in moisture with a thin layer of castor oil.

DRY SKIN MASK

Take the inside skin of a ripe avocado and massage your just-washed face and neck with it. Or mix equal amounts of avocado (about ¼ cup) with regular sour cream (not fat-free). Gently apply the mixture on the face and neck (but not on the delicate skin around the eyes), and leave it on for at least 15 minutes. Rinse with tepid water. When you can no longer see a trace of it, use your fingertips to gently work the invisible oil into your skin with an upward and outward sweep.

MOISTURIZER

Wet your clean face and smear on a glob of petroleum jelly. Keep adding water as you thin out the layer of jelly all over your face and neck until it's no longer greasy. This inexpensive treatment is used at expensive spas because it's an effective moisturizer.

Caring for Normal or Combination Skin
ONCE-A-MONTH CLEANSING MASK

Put 1 cup of uncooked oatmeal in a blender and powder it. Add 3 drops of almond oil (available at health food stores),

½ cup of skim milk, and 1 egg white. Blend it all together, then spread it on your face and neck (not on the delicate skin around your eyes), and let it stay there for a half hour. Rinse it off with tepid water and pat dry.

For All Skin Types
MAKEUP REMOVER OUT OF DESPERATION

Forget to bring makeup remover? Go to his fridge and take out the whipped sweet butter, or look around for vegetable shortening. Keep it on your eyes and face for at least 30 seconds so that it has a chance to sink in, making it easier to gently wipe off the makeup.

SKIN AWAKENER AND PROTECTOR

A cosmetologist described this treatment as "the simplest natural healer for tired skin, giving you the glow of fresh-faced youth."

Mix 1 tablespoon of apple cider vinegar with 1 tablespoon of just-boiled water. As soon as the liquid is cool enough, wet a cotton pad and apply it to the face and neck.

Use this treatment often, at least every other day. Some people keep a plastic plant mister filled with equal amounts of apple cider vinegar and water to spray their bodies after a shower or bath. It not only restores the acid mantle (pH balance) of your skin, it also removes soap residue and hard water deposits.

SUN-ABUSED SKIN

Soften that leathery look with this centuries-old beauty mask formula. Mix 2 tablespoons of raw honey with 2 tablespoons of flour. Add enough milk (2 to 3 tablespoons) to make it the consistency of toothpaste.

Be sure your face and neck are clean and your hair is out of the way. Smooth the paste on the face and neck. Stay clear of the delicate skin around the eyes. Leave the paste on for a half hour, rinse it off with tepid water, and pat dry.

Now you need a toner. In a juice extractor, juice 2 cucumbers, heat the juice to the boiling point, skim the froth off (if any), bottle the juice, and refrigerate it. Twice a day, use 1 teaspoon of juice to 2 teaspoons of water. Gently dab it on your face and neck and let it air-dry.

Now you need a moisturizer. Consider using a light film of extra-virgin, cold-pressed olive oil. Skin absorbs it quickly and it's surprisingly not greasy.

TOWELING-OFF TIP

Towels made of 100 percent cotton will dry you faster and more thoroughly than towels made of blended fibers.

MIRROR, MIRROR, IN THE BATHROOM

Clean the mirror with shaving cream and it will prevent it from fogging up for several weeks. If you didn't do the shaving cream bit, after a shower or bath carefully use a hair dryer to unfog the steamed-up mirror.

PLEASING TWEEZING

If you can't stand the pain of tweezing your eyebrows, numb the area first by putting an ice cube on for a few seconds.

If you don't need to go so far as to numb the area but just want to have an easy time of it, tweeze right after a warm shower. The hairs come out more willingly then.

SLEEP

Abraham Lincoln took a midnight walk to help him sleep.

Charles Dickens believed it was impossible to sleep if you crossed the magnetic forces between the North and South Poles. As a result, whenever Dickens traveled, he took a compass with him so he could sleep with his head facing north.

Benjamin Franklin believed in fresh-air baths in the nude as a sleep inducer. During the night, he would move from one bed to another because he also thought that cold sheets had a therapeutic effect on him. (At least that's what he told his wife. Is that when she told him to go fly a kite?)

Talk about sleeping around . . . Louis IV of France had 413 beds and slept in a different one every night.

Einstein slept 12 hours a night; Edison slept only 4 hours.

Mark Twain had a cure for insomnia: "Lie near the edge of the bed and you'll drop off."

According to Franklin P. Adams, "Insomniacs don't sleep because they worry about it and they worry about it because they don't sleep."

INSOMNIA

There are three basic types of insomnia: not being able to fall asleep within 30 to 45 minutes after you lie down to sleep (the average person falls asleep within 20 minutes); getting less than 5 or 6 hours of total sleep time; and staying awake more than 30 to 60 minutes during the night (usually after a pee break).

You know you *really* have insomnia if you can't sleep even when it's time to get up.

A popular folk remedy for insomnia is counting sheep. We heard about a garment manufacturer who had trouble sleeping. Not only did he count sheep, he sheared them, combed the wool, spun it into yarn, wove it into cloth, made it into suits, distributed them in town, watched as they didn't sell, had them returned, and lost thousands on the deal. That's why he had trouble sleeping in the first place.

Here are some other remedies to help him—and you—get a good night's sleep.

Food and Drink

Help prevent sleepless nights by eating salt-free dinners and eliminating all after-dinner snacks. Try it for a few nights in a row and see if it makes a difference in your night's sleep.

Chamomile is the classic sleepytime folk herb. Steep a tea bag or 1 teaspoon of loose chamomile in 1 cup of just-boiled water for about 7 minutes. If you use the loose herb, strain it. Drink the tea right before bedtime.

An hour before you go to bed, drink a glass of pure, warmed grapefruit juice. If you need it sweetened, use honey.

> **CAUTION:** If you're taking medication, check with your doctor or pharmacist about negative grapefruit-drug interaction.

A naturopath we met has had great success in treating severe insomniac patients with goat's milk. He recommends they drink 6 ounces before each meal and 6 ounces before bedtime. Within a week, he has seen patients go from 2 hours of sleep a night to 8 restful hours of sleep night after night. (Some supermarkets as well as health food stores sell goat's milk.)

Eat a handful of raw cashews near bedtime to help you calm down, forget your cares, fall asleep, and stay asleep. The magnesium in the nuts can be very soothing to one's nervous system.

If you're not nuts about nuts and you need some way of letting go of the pressures of the day so that they don't keep you up all night, consider this: For 10 minutes before going to bed, sit in a chair, where it's quiet, away from the TV, and think about the day you had and the day that's coming up. Spend the time—no more than 10 minutes—focused on summing up what you did and what you will do. You may want a pad and pen to write a to-do list. When the time is up, take a deep breath, feel a sense of accomplishment, and go to sleep.

A glass of elderberry juice at room temperature is thought of as a sleep inducer. You can get pure elderberry concentrate at health food stores. Just dilute it, drink it, and hit the hay.

Nutmeg can act as a sedative. Steep half of a crushed nutmeg (not more than that) in hot water for 10 minutes. Strain and drink the nutmeg tea half an hour before bedtime. If you don't like the taste of it, use nutmeg oil externally. Rub it on your forehead at bedtime.

Folk-remedy recipes always include warm milk before bedtime to promote restful sleep. The National Institute of Mental Health believes it works because warm milk contains tryptophan. Tryptophan is an essential amino acid that increases the amount of serotonin in the brain. Serotonin is a neurotransmitter that helps to send messages from brain to nerves and vice versa. The advantage of a tryptophan-induced sleep, compared to sleeping pills, is that you awaken at the normal time every day and do not feel sleepy or drugged. You may want to stack the deck and make it more palatable by adding a couple of the ingredients sug-

gested above—a little nutmeg and some honey.

It is most advisable, for purposes of good digestion and sleep, not to have eaten within 2 to 3 hours of bedtime. However, a remedy recommended by many cultures throughout the world as an effective cure for insomnia requires you to eat a finely chopped raw onion before going to bed. If this is repugnant to you, you may want to check out the onion remedy under "Bed Tricks" (below).

Mental Exercises

This Silva Mind Method process seems to be a real snoozer (and that's a good thing). Once you're in bed, completely relax. Lightly close your eyes. Now picture a blackboard. Take a piece of imaginary chalk and draw a circle. Within the circle, draw a square and put the number 99 in the square. Erase the number 99. Be careful you don't erase the sides of the square. Replace 99 with 98. Then erase 98 and replace it with 97, then 96, 95, 94, and so on. You should fall asleep long before you get bingo!

Take your mind off having to fall asleep. Give yourself an interesting but unimportant fantasy-type problem to solve. For instance: If you were to write your autobiography, what would be the title? Whom would you cast as you when it's made into a film? How will you spend $50 million when you win the lottery?

🜂 Worried about not being able to fall asleep? Okay, then, don't let yourself go to sleep. That's right, try to stay awake. Sleep specialists call this technique "paradoxical intent." When we were children and our father used it on us, we precociously called it "reverse psychology." So take the worry out of trying to go to sleep and try hard to stay awake. You'll be asleep in no time.

Bed Tricks

Do not go to bed until you're really sleepy, even if it means going to bed very late when you have to get up early the next morning. Nothing will happen to you if you get less than 8, 7, 6, or even 5 hours of sleep one night.

🜂 A drop in your temperature is a signal to your body that it's time to sleep. If you take a bath or do some exercise a few hours before going to bed, your temperature will rise, then fall, and you should have an easier time falling asleep.

🜂 Try using an extra pillow. It works for some people.

🜂 Tossing and turning acts as a signal to the body that you're ready to get up. Force

yourself to stay in one position. (Lying on your stomach is more relaxing than on your back.)

🜂 Get into bed. Before you lie down, breathe deeply six times. Count to one hundred, then breathe deeply another six times. Now lie down. Good night!

🜂 Macrobiotic leader Michio Kushi says that when you can't sleep, put a cut raw onion under your pillow. No, you don't *cry* yourself to sleep. There's something in the onion that scurries you off to dreamland.

We have another version of this remedy that's as effective and won't mess up your pillow or linens. Cut a yellow onion in chunks and place it in a glass jar. Put the cover on the jar and keep it on your night table. When you can't fall asleep, or when you wake up and can't fall back asleep, open the jar and take a deep whiff or two of the onion. Close the jar, lie back, think lovely thoughts, and within 15 minutes you should be zzzzzzz-ing.

Exercise

Exercise during the day. Get a real workout by taking a class or disciplining yourself at home by following a sensible exercise plan. *Do not exercise right before bedtime.*

🜂 This relaxation exercise is a lovely way to end the day. Light a candle. Turn off all of the lights in the room except for the candle. Sit in a comfortable position with feet and hands uncrossed. Stare at the lit candle while relaxing each part of your body, starting with the toes and working your way up. Include ankles, calves, knees, thighs, genital area, stomach, waist, midriff, rib cage, chest, fingers, wrists, elbows, arms, shoulders, neck, jaw, lips, cheeks, eyes, eyebrows, forehead, and the top of the head. Once your entire body is relaxed, blow out the candle and go to sleep.

◗ Guilt-free masturbation is a wonderful relaxant and sleep inducer.

◗ Totally satisfying sex is a great and fun sleep promoter. Unsatisfying sex can cause frustration that leads to insomnia. So (with apologies to Tennyson), is it better to have loved and lost sleep than never to have loved at all?

Acupressure

A Chinese acupressure practitioner suggests you press the center of the bottoms of your heels with your thumbs. Keep pressing as long as you can—at least 3 minutes—or until you doze off.

Pillow Sedative

According to the record (please don't ask us which one), King George III was plagued with insomnia until a physician prescribed a hop pillow. Hops have been known to have a tranquilizing effect on people. Lupulin, an active ingredient in hops, has been used to treat a variety of nervous disorders.

Buy or sew together a little muslin or fine white cotton bag. Fill it with hops and tack it to your pillow. Change the hops once a month.

It is believed by some that the hop pillow will be a more effective sedative if you spray it lightly with rubbing alcohol. (Check "Sources" for herb companies that sell hops.)

Supplement

Melatonin is a hormone that's produced by the pineal gland and is involved in regulating sleeping and waking cycles. Since bright lights lower melatonin levels, it is not a good idea to read or do anything that requires bright lights on at bedtime. To get ready for bed, stay in a dimly lit room for at least half an hour before hitting the pillow.

If the dim lights don't seem to do it for you, you may want to consider taking a melatonin supplement—liquid or tablets—available at health food stores. Start with the lowest dosage, but first check with your health care provider for the go-ahead.

Desperation Remedy

If you've reached the point where you're willing to try just about anything, then rub the soles of your feet and the nape of your neck with a peeled clove of garlic. It's been known to help people fall asleep when nothing else has worked.

NIGHTMARES

Twenty percent of sleep time is spent dreaming. Two out of every five dreams can be described as scary, frightening, or terrifying. Hopefully, one of these remedies will help sweeten your dreams.

▶ Right before going to sleep, soak your feet in warm water for 10 minutes. Then rub them thoroughly with half a lemon. Don't rinse them off, just pat them dry. Get into bed, take a few deep breaths, and have pleasant dreams.

▶ As you're dozing, program yourself by saying, "I'm going to have happy dreams." Chances are your subconscious will grant your request.

▶ This antinightmare advice comes from Switzerland. Eat a small evening meal a few hours before bedtime. When you go to bed, sleep on your right side with your right hand under your head.

▶ Before you go to sleep, drink thyme tea and be nightmare-free.

▶ Lightly sprinkle essence of anise (available at health food stores) on your pillow so that you inhale the scent as soon as you lie down. It is said to produce restful sleep, happy dreams, and a spotted pillowcase.

▶ Lettuce has lactucarium, a calming agent, and was used by the great Greek physician Galen to cure his own insomnia.

Boil 2 cups of water, then simmer the outside leaves of a head of lettuce for 15 minutes. Strain and drink the lettuce tea right before bedtime. It's supposed to ensure sweet dreams and is also good for cleansing the system. (You won't wake up because of a bad dream, but you may wake up to go to the bathroom.)

▶ A gem therapist said that wearing a diamond, in any setting, protects the wearer from nightmares. Is that how and why the engagement ring tradition came about? Hmmmmm.

SNORING (POSSIBLE SLEEP APNEA)

A friend told us he starts to snore as soon as he falls asleep. We asked if it bothers his wife. He said, "It not only bothers my wife, it bothers the whole congregation."

Actually, snoring is not a joking matter. Chronic snoring—that is, snoring every night and loudly—may be the start of a serious condition known as sleep apnea. *Apnea* is Greek for "without breath." During the night, the throat relaxes and closes, blocking the windpipe and making it difficult to breathe. After holding one's breath for an unnatural amount of time (anywhere from 10 seconds to over a minute), the snore comes as the person gasps for air. The person awakens each time it happens, and it can happen dozens and dozens of times during the night without the person realizing it. The interrupted sleep causes that person to be tired all day.

If you have this condition, it can be dangerous being behind the wheel of a car, operating heavy machinery, or just crossing a street. Aside from the daytime accident aspect, sleep apnea may lead to high blood pressure and other serious health challenges.

If you think that you or your mate has sleep apnea, ask your doctor to recommend a sleep specialist right away, or locate a sleep clinic in your area. (Go to www.mapquest.com and type in "sleep clinic.")

Meanwhile, snorers may minimize or completely eliminate their nighttime noise by following any or all of the appropriate suggestions:

■ If you smoke, stop! Let your smoker's inflamed, swollen throat tissues heal.

■ If you drink, don't! Alcoholic beverages relax the respiratory system muscles, making it harder to breathe and, in turn, promoting snoring.

■ If you're overweight, trim down! Fat deposits at the base of the tongue contribute to the blocking of an already clogged airway. Also, wait a couple of hours after you've eaten before going to sleep.

The results of a controlled study published by the *British Medical Journal* concluded that regular training of the upper airways by playing a didgeridoo reduces snoring in people with moderate obstructive sleep apnea syndrome, allowing them and their partners improved sleep quality, which in turn reduces daytime sleepiness.

The didgeridoo is a rhythm wind folk instrument, so you play beats instead of melodic songs. Learning the instrument is intuitive and you don't need any previous musical training. Even though it's a wind instrument, you don't use lung power. The didgeridoo is played with gently vibrating lips, voice, and tongue movement.

For more information, visit L.A. Outback at www.laoutback.net and see their large selection of beautiful, affordable, authentic Aboriginal didgeridoos. They also have instructional CDs and videos. If you're not online, call 800-519-1140 and speak with any of the company's caring and helpful people.

▶ Snoring can be caused by very dry air. If there's a lack of humidity in your bedroom and you use a radiator in cold weather, place a pan of water on it, or simply use a humidifier.

▶ Prevent the snorer from sleeping on his or her back, and chances are he or she won't snore. You can do this by putting a tennis ball in a sock and sewing the sock on the back of the snorer's pajama top or nightgown.

▶ Lightly tickle the snorer's throat and the snoring should stop. Of course, the laughing may keep you up.

SLEEPWALKING

A Russian professor who studied sleepwalkers recommended that a piece of wet carpeting be placed right by the sleepwalker's bed. In most cases, the sleepwalker awakens the second his or her feet step on the wet carpet.

SLEEP TALKING

The medical term for sleep talking is *somniloquy*. It's not unusual for people who suffer from sleep apnea to talk in their sleep. Sleep talking can also be triggered by anything that causes poor sleep cycles, such as stress, health challenges, and even eating a big, heavy meal right before bedtime.

Once the sleep talker is healed of any or all of the triggers above, chances are the sleep talking will stop. Meanwhile, if your mate is a somniloquist, according to folklore, if you take hold of his big toe, he will tell you anything you want to know.

SMOKING

Surely you know that smoking can cause, contribute to, or worsen backaches, bronchitis, cancer, cataracts, diverticulosis, emphysema, endometriosis, gum problems, hangovers, hardening of the arteries, heartburn, infertility, osteoporosis, phlebitis, sleep disorders including sleep apnea, sore throats, tinnitus, ulcers, and varicose veins. And that's just for starters.

Cigarette smoking has been linked to every serious disease. We'll spare you the statistics from the American Heart Association, the American Lung Association, and the American Cancer Society on the estimated number of Americans who die before they reach retirement age because of smoking.

All the talk about sickness and premature death doesn't seem to motivate all smokers—especially teenagers or young adults—to stop. Dr. James Duke, master herbalist, has a wake-up call. He likes to remind young smokers that the habit hits men in the penis and women in the face. "Smoking damages the blood vessels that supply the penis, so men who smoke have an increased risk of impotence. Smoking also damages the capillaries in women's faces, which is why women (and men) smokers develop wrinkles years before nonsmokers."

One more reason for young women to quit: According to the findings of a study conducted by Dr. Brian Rinker and his colleagues with patients at UK HealthCare Cosmetic Surgery Associates, smoking contributes to women's ptosis (the medical term for sagging of the breast). Dr. Rinker says, "Smoking breaks down a protein in the skin called elastin, which gives youthful skin its elastic appearance and supports the breast."

Ready to stop smoking? We hope the following suggestions will make it easier.

AN EBBING-OFF PLAN

Mix ½ teaspoon of cream of tartar (available in supermarket spice or baking sec-

tions) into 8 ounces of orange juice and drink it right before you go to bed.

In the morning (or during the night), when you urinate, you will wash out some of the nicotine that's causing your cigarette addiction. From now on, have an ongoing dialogue with yourself. Each time you reach for a cigarette, ask yourself if you absolutely must smoke it, or whether you can wait awhile. That conscious awareness of each cigarette should enable you to hold out for some time. By asking yourself about it each time you want to light up, chances are you'll be able to let go of the urge, and by the end of the day you'll have smoked fewer cigarettes than the day before.

If you're committed to this process and take the cream of tartar in orange juice every night without fail, in thirty days or less you could and should be addiction-free and off cigarettes completely.

To make the ebbing-off process easier and more pleasant, read through the sensible suggestions below that can answer your cigarette craving with a variety of healthful food, psychological, and acupressure replacements.

SUBMERGE THE URGE

Foods and Drinks

Dr. James Duke smoked three packs of unfiltered, king-size cigarettes daily, until the day he quit—cold turkey. That was close to four decades ago. According to Dr. Duke, carrots helped him quit. He would munch on raw carrots instead of puffing on a cigarette. "If cigarettes are cancer sticks," says Dr. Duke, "carrots are anti-cancer sticks." He explains that caro-tenoids, the chemical relatives of vitamin A, help prevent cancer, especially if the carotenoids come from carrots or other whole foods rather than from cap-sules. Carrots also help lower cholesterol levels.

Buy a package of baby carrots and munch on them throughout the day in place of smoking cigarettes.

In addition to carrots, unsalted, raw sunflower seeds are another wonderful food to eat in place of smoking a cigarette. Tobacco releases stored sugar (glycogen) from the liver, and it perks up one's brain. Sunflower seeds provide that same mental lift. Tobacco has a sedative effect that tends to calm a person down. Sunflower seeds also stabilize the nerves because they contain oils that are calming, and B-complex vitamins that help nourish the nervous system. (Maybe that's why base-ball players often eat them during a game.) Tobacco increases the output of adrenal gland hormones, which reduces the allergic reaction of smokers. Sun-flower seeds do the same.

Keep in mind that the seeds are fairly high in fat, so don't overdo it. Consider buying sunflower seeds with shells. The shelling process will slow down your con-sumption of the seeds.

Marjoram is closely related to oregano, and both herbs are in the mint family. Tea made from marjoram (available at health food stores) can help you be a former cig-arette smoker. The tea makes your throat very dry, and so smoking will not be nearly as pleasurable. Marjoram is naturally sweet; nothing needs to be added to it. Have a cup of tea when you would ordi-narily have your first cigarette of the day. Try half a cup after that whenever you have an uncontrollable urge to smoke.

To many smokers, the thought of smok-ing a cigarette after they've had a grape-fruit or grapefruit juice is unpleasant. If you feel that way, good!

CAUTION: Grapefruit and grapefruit products, tangelos, and Seville oranges are known to have potentially serious in-teractions with certain drugs. If you're taking any medication, be sure to check with your pharmacist or health care provider before eating or drinking these citrus fruits.

Nobel laureate professor of chemistry Dr. Linus Pauling said to eat an orange whenever you have the urge to smoke. The Outspan Organization in Britain conducted experiments, and the results were impressive. By the end of three weeks, the orange-eating cigarette smokers smoked 79 percent fewer cigarettes than they ordinarily would have; 20 percent stopped completely. It seems that eating citrus fruit has a kick that's similar to smoking a cigarette. Incidentally, the Outspan Organization recommends that when you take a piece of orange instead of smoking a cigarette, first suck the juice out and then eat the pulp.

If eating an orange isn't that convenient when you're out and about, carry a small bottle of citrus juice with you, and whenever you feel like lighting up, take a swig of the juice. Since each cigarette robs your body of between 25 and 100 mg of vitamin C, the juice will help replenish it as well as keep you from smoking.

After your next cigarette, replace the nicotine taste in your mouth by sucking on a clove (the kind used for preparing ham). It sort of numbs your tongue and will make the next cigarette taste terrible.

If you hate the taste and sensation of a clove, then suck on a cinnamon Altoid (or any other flavor). It will take away the taste of nicotine, and without the lingering nicotine taste, your desire for another cigarette should be greatly reduced.

Acupressure

Next time you crave a cigarette, massage the palm of your right hand for a count of ten, then massage the palm of your left hand for a count of ten. To complete this process, massage the skin between your thumb and index finger on your right hand, then on your left hand, both for the count of ten. If you still have a craving, start all over by massaging your right palm.

This exercise should help you feel calmer and help you let go of the need to light up.

Press the acupressure point in the middle of the breastbone, directly between your two nipples. Press it three times in a row, holding it for 12 seconds each time, and don't be surprised if the urge to smoke is gone.

Mind Trip

Make a list of all the reasons you want to quit. You may want to divide the list into short-term reasons, such as wanting to be more kissable, and long-term reasons, such as wanting to walk your daughter down the aisle at her wedding. Keep the list handy and refer to it each time you're about to give in and smoke.

A professor of behavioral medicine suggests that when the craving comes over you, pick up a pen instead of a cigarette and write a letter to loved ones, telling them why smoking is more important than they are. Apologize for having to have someone take care of you when you're no longer well enough to take care of yourself. Tell them how you choose to die and how you'll miss sharing in their happiness. Got the picture? These unfinished (we hope) letters may give you the strength to pass up a cigarette one more time, each time, until you no longer have the horrible craving to smoke.

Are we being cruel to you? Certainly no more cruel than you're being to yourself when you smoke.

DETOXIFYING YOUR SYSTEM

To help cleanse your system of nicotine, and to help prevent tumors from forming, take ½ teaspoon of red clover tincture (available at health food stores) three times a day. Drinking a cup of red clover tea once or twice a day may also help.

To help detoxify your liver, drink 2 cups of milk thistle seed tea before every meal. In case you're worried about gaining weight now that you're not going to be smoking, these 6 cups of tea before meals should help you cut down on the amount of food you eat.

Apricots are rich in beta-carotene, potassium, boron, iron, and silica. Not only do they help prevent cancer, they are also good for the heart, for promoting increased estrogen production in postmenopausal women, for preventing fatigue and infection, and for healthy skin, hair, and nails. Apricots are especially good for helping to minimize the long-term potential harm caused by nicotine. Start eating a few dried apricots a day and continue eating them even as a nonsmoker. Buy unsulfured dried apricots. Sulfur-based preservatives (sulfites) can produce allergic reactions, especially in asthmatics. Also, the long-term accumulation of sulfites can cause unhealthy conditions.

THE DREADED WITHDRAWAL PERIOD

There are steps you can take to make the withdrawal process as torture-free as possible:

■ During the worst time, the first week or two of withdrawal, push yourself to exercise—walk, swim, dance, bowl, play tennis, play Ping-Pong, clean your house, clean our house, do gardening, play with a yo-yo. *Keep moving. Keep active.* It will make you feel better. It will make the withdrawal time pass quicker. It will also help prevent weight gain, especially if you eat the foods we've recommended above. Incidentally, gaining 5 to 10 pounds because you stopped smoking is worth it when you consider the health risks of smoking.

■ Be kind to yourself and don't place temptation in your face. Do not frequent bars or other places where smoking is allowed. Hang out at places where smoking is *not* permitted: movie theaters, museums, the library, houses of worship, adult education courses at schools.

Take a break from friends who smoke. Once you kick the habit, you'll have to see if you can be in their company without giving in to temptation. Maybe by then, you will have set a great example and motivated them to quit, or you will have met and made new, nonsmoking friends. Check out www.meetup.com, a free service that helps you meet up with groups of people who share your interests. (It's not a meet-your-mate kind of thing.) Type in your zip code and your interest (e.g., quitting smoking, or nonsmokers) and take it from there.

■ Figure out how much money you'll save every week, every month, and every year by not smoking. Decide on exactly what you want to do with that money—special treats for yourself—and actually put that money away in a safe each time you *don't* buy a pack of cigarettes when you ordinarily would have.

■ For young smokers or anyone adept at text messaging: The astounding results of a study led by Anthony Rodgers at the University of Auckland, New Zealand, concluded that text messaging can double the quit rate in young smokers. Rodgers refers to the use of texting as "chewing gum for the fingers."

Set a quit date. Send a text message to your nearest and dearest, tell them when you plan to quit, and ask them to send you supportive messages on that day, and to keep sending messages of encouragement, plus jokes and messages on other distracting, unrelated topics during the days that follow the quit day. If you know any quitters, be sure to ask them to keep sending motivational and inspirational text messages to you.

Right before your quit day, go to www .backpackit.com, which as of this writing is a free service where you can write text messages to yourself for them to send to you at designated times. Be sure to include pat-on-the-back phrases, such as:

▓ Good for you!
▓ You're strong and you will succeed!
▓ Be proud of yourself!

Also include reasons why you're quitting, such as:

* I want to stop the damage caused by smoking.
* I want to look, smell, and feel better.
* I don't want to spend so much money on something that can kill me.

After you've quit, when a craving comes over you, pull up and reread your favorite messages of support, to help prevent you from ever lighting up again.

ONCE YOU QUIT . . .

A nicotine-dependency researcher reported that nicotine causes smokers to process caffeine two and a half times faster than nonsmokers. So once you quit smoking and the nicotine is washed out of your system, you'll need only about a third as much coffee to get the same buzz you got from drinking coffee while still smoking. The same is true when drinking alcoholic beverages. Take into consideration that you'll get drunk faster without nicotine in your body. Think of the additional money you'll be saving on coffee and booze. You may want to add it to your "treats" fund (suggested above)—the money that you save once you stop buying cigarettes.

CLEARING THE AIR

If cigarette smokers are at your home or office, and you (foolishly) allow them to smoke, place little saucers of distilled white vinegar around the room in inconspicuous spots. The vinegar will absorb the smell of tobacco smoke.

To keep workers alert, many offices in Japan circulate the scent of the essential oils of lemon, peppermint, or cypress through the air-conditioning system. The workers reported a beneficial side effect: The aromatherapy seemed to reduce the urge to smoke. If you want to look into this for your company or own office, start by visiting www.aromathyme.com or call 888-AROMA-99.

SPRAINS, STRAINS, MUSCLE PAINS

SPRAINS

According to Dr. Ray C. Wunderlich Jr. of the Wunderlich Center for Nutritional Medicine in St. Petersburg, Florida, as soon as you get a sprain, take large amounts of enzymes hourly, in the form of fresh vegetable juices and/or bromelain (an enzyme found in pineapple that has anti-inflammatory properties), papaya, and pancreatic supplements (available at health food stores). The sooner you start taking enzymes, the quicker the healing process. Then read on to decide what to do next.

❧ During the first 12 hours after the injury, starting as soon as possible, apply an ice pack to the area to reduce the swelling caused by the sprain. Leave the ice pack on for 20 minutes, then take it off for 20 minutes. Extend the 12 hours of cold compresses to 24 hours if it seems necessary. It would be wise to seek medical attention to make sure the sprain is nothing more than a sprain and not a fractured, chipped, or dislocated bone.

❧ An alternative to the above is to dunk the sprained area into a basin of very hot water. Keep the water hot—not scalding, just hot—by adding more hot water during this 10-minute soaking period. When the 10 minutes is up, transfer the sprained area to a basin of ice-cold water and keep it there for 5 minutes. Next, bind the area with a wet bandage and cover the wet one with a dry bandage.

❧ Reduce the swelling of a sprain by taking the peel of an orange and applying the white spongy side on the sprained area. Bind it in place with a bandage.

❧ Comfrey (also called knitbone) is getting more and more popular among professional athletes and their smart coaches. This herb helps speed up the healing process and relieves the pain of pulled tendons and ligaments, strains, sprains, broken bones, and tennis elbow.

Use a comfrey poultice (see "Preparation Guide") on the injured area, changing it every 2 to 3 hours.

If you can't find comfrey roots and leaves at your health food store, check our "Sources" pages for herb companies that carry comfrey.

Sprain or Muscle Pain Preparations

Add 1 tablespoon of cayenne pepper to 2 cups of apple cider vinegar in an enamel or glass saucepan, bring it to a slow boil, then take the pan off the heat and let the mixture cool. Bottle it and use it on sprains, pains, and sore muscles.

Recurrent-Sprain Prevention

This applies mostly to athletes and dancers who keep spraining the same weakened parts of their bodies. Before a warm-up session, saturate a washcloth with water that's as hot as it can be without you burning yourself, and apply it to your vulnerable area for 10 to 15 minutes. In other words, preheat the trouble spot before you work out.

MUSCLE PAIN (CHARLEY HORSE)

Grate fresh ginger and squeeze the grated ginger through cheesecloth, getting as much juice as you can. Measure the amount of ginger juice and add an equal amount of sesame oil. Mix it thoroughly and massage it on your painful parts.

▶ This remedy is said to be particularly effective for a charley horse (muscle pain and stiffness). Vigorously scrub 3 small lemons, 2 small oranges, and 1 small grapefruit. Cut up the 6 fruits and put them into a blender, peel and all. Add 1 teaspoon of cream of tartar (available in your supermarket spice section) and blend.

Store the mixture in a covered jar in the refrigerator. Take 2 tablespoons of the concoction with 2 tablespoons of water twice a day—first thing in the morning and right before bedtime.

> **CAUTION:** If you're taking medication, check with your doctor or pharmacist about negative grapefruit-drug interaction.

Baths

Prepare strong ginger tea by steeping 2 teaspoons of ground ginger or fresh grated ginger in 2 cups of just-boiled water for 10 minutes. Add the ginger tea to a bathful of warm water. Relax in the tub for 20 to 30 minutes. This ginger tea bath helps relieve muscle stiffness and soreness and is wonderful for one's circulation.

▶ Soak in a tub of "old faithful"—Epsom salts. Pour 3 cups of it in warm water. Stay in the water 20 to 30 minutes and your charley horse pain should start galloping away.

STINGS AND BITES

This chapter deals with stings and bites from bees, wasps, hornets, yellow jackets, mosquitoes, spiders, ticks, dogs, and snakes.

> **CAUTION:** If you have a history of an allergy to stinging insects, have a physician-prescribed emergency sting kit on hand at all times!

Everyone knows: To avoid disease from biting insects and animals, don't bite any insects or animals! If *they* bite *you*, read on for practical and effective suggestions.

BEE, WASP, HORNET, AND YELLOW JACKET STINGS

When an insect stings, its stinger usually remains in the skin as the insect flies away. However, if the insect stays attached to its stinger in the skin, flick it off with your thumb and forefinger. Do not squeeze the insect . . . not that anyone would want to do that.

Now then, remove the stinger, but do not use your fingers or tweezers. Those methods can pump more poison into the skin. Instead, gently and carefully scrape the stinger out with the tip of a sharp knife or the edge of a credit card.

If you're into the dramatic, once the stinger is removed, suck the stung area like they do in snakebite-in-the-desert movies. Spit out whatever poison comes out. Every little bit of venom extracted will help minimize the swelling.

To relieve the pain and keep down the swelling of a sting, apply any one of the following for a half hour, then alternate it with a half hour of ice on the stung area:

■ Pack on a clump of wet mud. It's one of the oldest and most practical remedies for stings. If you haven't already removed the stinger, peeling off the dry mud will help draw it out.

■ Apply a little of your own fresh urine. (Hey, if you're outdoors and there's none of this other stuff around, you do what you gotta do!)

■ Put on wet salt.

■ Spray on an antiperspirant or an antihistamine (e.g., Benadryl). They contain chemicals that can neutralize the insect's venom.

■ Apply a slice of raw onion.

■ Apply a slice of raw potato.

■ Smear toothpaste on the sting.

■ Dab on equal parts of distilled white vinegar and lemon juice every 5 minutes until the pain disappears.

■ Combine equal parts of water and ammonia, dip a cloth in the mixture, and apply to the stung area.

■ If you just happen to have horseradish root, grate it and put it on the sting.

■ Use unseasoned meat tenderizer—$\frac{1}{3}$ teaspoon dissolved in 1 teaspoon of water—and put it on the sting. One of the main ingredients in meat tenderizer is papain, an enzyme from papaya that relieves the pain and inflammation of a sting and lessens allergic reaction. Use meat tenderizer only if you are not allergic to MSG.

■ Squeeze out the oil from a vitamin E softgel onto the stung area.

■ Wet a clump of tobacco and apply it to the sting.

■ Put on a drop of honey, preferably from the hive of the bee that did the stinging. (That's not too likely unless you're the beekeeper.)

■ Make a paste with water and baking soda—about 1 teaspoon water to about 1 tablespoon baking soda—and smear it on the bitten area. It can help draw out the heat, reduce the redness, inhibit the swelling, and take the itch out of a bite.

■ An application of wheat germ oil helps soothe a sting.

Don't forget the half hour of ice on the stung area in between any of the other applications.

Throat Stings

Being stung in the throat (on the inside, not on the neck) is a revolting thought, and it seems impossible. It's a rare occurrence, but it can and has happened, especially when eating fresh fruit. If it should happen, quickly mix 2 teaspoons of salt in a glass of water, then gargle with it. Keep gargling. The salt water will draw out the poison and, most important, will stop the area from swelling.

MOSQUITO BITES

Prevention

Remember how when you were a child and got eaten up by mosquitoes, your mother would say, "That's because you're so sweet"? There may be something to it. Experiments were conducted with people who completely eliminated white sugar and alcoholic beverages from their diets, then were deliberately surrounded by mosquitoes and gnats. Not only were those people not so sweet, they were not bitten. The insects didn't even bother to land on them. Conclusion: If you're sugar-free, it's bye-bye mosquitoes, and gnuts to gnats!

◗ Mosquitoes have been known to stay away from people whose systems have a high amount of vitamin B_1 (thiamine). Before you go to a mosquito-infested area, eat foods that are rich in B_1: sunflower seeds, Brazil nuts, fish, and brewer's yeast (available at health food stores).

◗ Keep scented (citrosa) geraniums on porches and other places you like to sit. This kind of geranium has oils in the leaves that mosquitoes dislike . . . it's like the scent of citronella.

The problem is that you will need to release the oils by rubbing leaves and breaking open the tiny glands where the oils accumulate. You may be better off burning a citronella candle.

If you dread mosquito bites more than you mind smelling from garlic, have we got a remedy for you. Rub garlic over all your exposed body parts before reaching a mosquito-infested area. Mosquitoes will not come near you. They hate garlic. Garlic is to mosquitoes what kryptonite is to Superman.

Biologist Eldon L. Reeves of the University of California tested garlic extract on five species of mosquitoes. The garlic got 'em. Not one mosquito survived.

Rubbing fresh parsley on uncovered skin, or squeezing out the juice of an aloe vera leaf and rubbing it on your exposed areas, should also repel mosquitoes without you having to tolerate the pungent smell of the stinking rose (garlic).

Mosquitoes prefer warm over cold, light over dark, dirty over clean, adult over child, and male over female. So, what are your odds of being bitten by a mosquito?

Mosquito Bite Treatment

Once you've been bitten, treat the bite with your own saliva. Then apply any of the following:

- Wet soap

- Wet tobacco

- Wet mud

- Watered-down ammonia

- Combined equal amounts of distilled white vinegar and lemon juice

SPIDER BITES

Four types of spiders have bites that can be serious:

- The black widow spider has a black shiny body and a red or orange hourglass marking on the underside of its abdomen. It's found in warmer regions of every state except Alaska.

- The brown recluse spider is also called the fiddle-back spider because of the violin-shaped marking on its back. It's found mainly in southern and midwestern states.

- The hobo spider is brown with a herringbone-like pattern on the top of its abdomen. It's found in the Pacific Northwest.

- The yellow sac spider is light yellow with a slightly darker stripe on the upper middle of its abdomen. It's found throughout the country.

If you think the spider that bit you is any of the above, try to remain as calm as possible and immediately call your doctor, a hospital, and/or a poison information center. To reach your local poison center in the United States and its territories, call 800-222-1222 or go to www.aapcc.org.

If you can collect the spider, or any part of it, do so for identification purposes.

Until you get professional help, apply ice on the bite to help prevent swelling. A poultice of raw grated potato on the bite would also be good.

Take nutrients that have anti-inflammatory action: vitamin C with bioflavonoids, 500 to 1,000 mg every 2 hours for several days (cut back on the dosage if you get diarrhea); bromelain, 500 mg three or four times a day on an empty stomach; and/or quercetin, 250 to 300 mg one to three times a day. (All are available at vitamin and health food stores.)

TICKS

Ticks are not a pleasant thought, but here's a remarkable remedy. If a tick has embedded itself in your skin, take clear fingernail polish and drip 2 drops on the insect. It will release its grasp and back out. Just wipe it off your skin.

ANIMAL BITES

If you've been bitten by an unfamiliar dog or by a wild animal, see your doctor immediately, or go to the nearest hospital's emergency room. You may need a rabies vaccine.

Any animal bite, even from your own pet—dog, cat, hamster, guinea pig, ferret, parakeet—could be dangerous. If the bite breaks the skin, bacteria in their saliva can cause infection. Report this to your doctor immediately and follow the steps below:

■ Wash the bitten area thoroughly with soap and water.

■ Apply pressure to stop the bleeding.

■ Cover it loosely with a sterile bandage.

■ If it doesn't stop bleeding, or if it puffs up or is red and painful, go to the emergency room at the closest hospital. You may need a tetanus shot.

SNAKEBITE

If you're going camping or are placing yourself in a situation where there's a chance of being bitten by a snake, we recommend that you first find out which snakes are in that area, and keep an appropriate snakebite kit handy.

If you do get bitten and you've run out

of snakebite kit or don't have one, call for professional medical help immediately. If that's just not an option, make a poultice out of 2 crushed onions mixed with a few drops of kerosene and apply it to the bite. (What are your chances of having onions and kerosene plus cheesecloth for the poultice?) After a short time, it should draw out the poison, turning the poultice green. Or do *you* turn green and the poultice . . . never mind. If you're anywhere near civilization, forget the above and hightail it to a doctor!

▶ If someone has been bitten by a snake and there's a smoker among you, mix a wad of tobacco with saliva or water. Apply this tobacco paste directly on the bite. As soon as the paste dries, replace it with another wad of the paste. Meanwhile, get the person who's been bitten to a doctor!

Rattlesnake Bites

Don't get rattled. Wet some salt, put a hunk of it on the bite, then wrap the area with a wet-salt poultice. Don't stand around reading this. *Get to a doctor!*

RATTLESNAKE BITE PREVENTION

Our Amarillo friend Sweet Ol' Bill (S.O.B.) told us that when cowboys camp out under the stars, they put their lariat ropes in a circle on the ground and put their sleeping bags in the middle of it. It seems to be a known fact in the Texas panhandle that rattlesnakes will not crawl across a rope.

CAUTION: Do this at your own risk, and keep a snakebite kit handy.

STRESS, TENSION, ANXIETY

"We live in the midst of alarms; anxiety beclouds the future; we expect some new disaster with each newspaper we read." Bet you won't guess who said that. It was Abraham Lincoln.

Okay, so stress, tension, and anxiety are nothing new. What can be new is your approach, which can help you dissolve this unhappy state of edginess.

Something to keep in mind are the words of Catherine Pulsifer, editor of Words of Wisdom 4 U (www.wow4u.com); "How we perceive a situation and how we react to it is the basis of our stress. If you focus on the negative in any situation, you can expect high stress levels. However, if you try and see the good in the situation, your stress levels will greatly diminish."

It's a start. Continue by doing yourself a favor and making lifestyle changes.

Start by cutting down on your sugar intake. Excessive sugar can contribute to nervous anxiety and spurts of energy followed by extreme fatigue, leading to more nervous anxiety. Eliminate or go easy on caffeinated drinks, stop smoking, and avoid alcoholic beverages. They all contribute to nervous anxiety and unnerving highs and lows. Take them out of your life. They're helping to take the life out of you!

For cases of extreme stress and chronic anxiety, seek professional assistance to help pinpoint the cause.

Meanwhile, follow writer Carin Hartness' advice: "Give your stress wings and let it fly away." Here are some suggestions that may help you create those wings.

❧ Sweaty palms, indigestion, hyperventilating, stiff neck, backaches, ulcers, dry mouth, tics, and even canker sores can be caused by stress, tension and anxiety.

There are as many symptoms and outward manifestations as there are reasons for it. Throughout this book, we address physical health challenges. In this chapter, we address the problems that may be causing those challenges.

Sit with your feet up, sip a cup of herb tea, read through these pages, and select a few foods and techniques that can help you *relaaaaax*!

FOOD AND DRINK

Chop a large onion into very small tidbits and add a tablespoon of honey. It tastes better than it sounds. Eat half the mixture with lunch and the other half with dinner. Onion contains prostaglandin, which is reported to have a stress-relieving effect.

❧ If strawberries are around, eat a few as a dessert after each meal (without the cream and sugar and not dipped in chocolate). You may *feel* a difference (you won't be as edgy), and you may *see* a difference (they'll make your teeth whiter). Also, they have no fat and are low in carbs and calories. You should be feeling better already.

❧ Kombu (available at health food stores and Asian markets) is a seaweed. Kombu tea can be a potent nerve tonic. Add a 3-inch strip of kombu to 1 quart of water and boil it for 10 minutes. Drink ½ cup of the tea at a time, throughout the day.

❧ In addition to kombu, these teas may help:

■ Sage tea relieves the jitters. Drink 3 cups a day. A bonus: Sage tea helps strengthen one's brain and memory.

■ Peppermint tea has a wonderful way of relaxing the system and relieving moodiness. Drink it warm and strong.

■ Chamomile is soothing and calming, especially at the end of a hectic day.

ACUPRESSURE

Do you have some clothespins hanging around? Take a handful of them and clip them to the tips of your fingers, at the start of your nails of the left hand. Keep them there for 7 minutes. Then put those clothespins on the fingers of your right hand for another 7 minutes. Pressure exerted on nerve endings is known to relax the entire nervous system. If the clothespins are too tight and causing pain, be creative and think of something else you can use, such as big paper clips.

Do this fingertip-pinching bit first thing in the morning, and before, during, or right after a particularly tense situation.

This acupressure exercise can relieve life's pressure . . . without clothespins. For at least 5 minutes a day, massage the webbed area between the thumb and index finger of your left hand. Really get in there and knead it. It may hurt. That's all the more reason to keep at it. Gradually, the pain will decrease, and so will the tenseness and tightness in your chest and shoulders. Eventually, you should have no pain at all and you will notice a difference in your general level of relaxation and state of well-being.

YOGA BREATHING EXERCISE

Alternate-nostril breathing is a well-known yoga technique used to put people in a relaxed state with a feeling of inner peace.

Pay attention; it sounds more complex than it is. Place your right thumb against your right nostril. Place your right ring finger and right pinky against your left nostril. (This is not an exercise for anyone with a stuffed nose.) Inhale and slowly exhale through both nostrils. Now press your right nostril closed and slowly inhale deeply through your left nostril to a count of five. While your right nostril is still closed, press your left nostril closed. Holding the air in your lungs, count to five. Open your right nostril and exhale to a count of five. Inhale through your right nostril to a count of five. Close both nostrils and count to five. Exhale through the left nostril to a count of five. Keep repeating this pattern for—you guessed it—5 minutes. Do it in the morning when you start your day and at day's end.

Visualization

This visualization exercise is used by hypnotherapists and at many self-help seminars. Make sure you're not going to be disturbed by telephones, pagers, cell phones, doorbells, dogs, whistling teapots, and so on. Sit in a comfortable chair. Close your eyes. (Wait! Read this first, then close your eyes.) Once your eyes are closed, put all of your awareness in your toes. Feel as though nothing else exists but your toes. Completely relax the muscles in your toes. Slowly move up from your toes to your feet, ankles, calves, knees, thighs, genital area, hips, back, stomach, chest, shoulders, arms, hands, neck, jaw, mouth, cheeks, ears, eyes, and brow. Yes, even relax the muscles of your scalp.

Now that you're totally relaxed, take three slow, deep breaths, then slowly open your eyes. Now, you go, girl . . . or guy!

BATH

There's a reason Epsom salts, an ancient natural healer, are still popular—they work! Pour 2 cups of Epsom salts into a warm-water bath. Set aside a half hour for pure relaxation in the tub—no interruptions, just 30 minutes of stress-free fantasizing.

HERBAL SUPPLEMENT

Valerian root, the natural forerunner to Valium, comes in capsules, tablets, tinctures, and liquid extracts and is available at health food stores. (Follow the dosage on the label.) There's a time-release formula that helps you maintain a feeling of relaxation throughout the day. Some people take valerian an hour before bedtime to help them fall asleep. Be aware that valerian can act as a mild diuretic, causing you to need to go to the bathroom in the middle of the night.

CAUTION: Unlike Valium, this herb is not addictive, but it has been reported that some people who use valerian root for long periods of time may develop headaches, insomnia, or agitation.

BEDTIME RITUAL

Before going to bed, take pen and paper into the bathroom for some quiet time. Sit on the throne and write the names of all the people whom you are allowing to stress you out. Also write the situations that are causing you to feel stressed. Once that's completed, tear the piece of paper into strips. As you do that, acknowledge that in a year, none of these things will matter. Keep tearing the page into smaller and smaller pieces, with the understanding that if these things will not matter in a year, why should you allow yourself to be troubled by them now? It's totally up to you to take the angst out of situations, and not give people power over you in this way.

Once you come to that understanding, drop the tiny pieces of paper into the toilet, then flush it, and feel empowered. Now get a good night's sleep, and when you see the people whose names were on that paper, smile to yourself. As you successfully deal with and handle the situations on that paper, pat yourself on the back.

DECORATING ADVICE

Harried housewives, do not paint your kitchen yellow to cheer you up. According to color therapist Carlton Wagner, a yellow room contributes to stress and adds to feelings of anxiety. (Another reason not to use yellow: Our mom always said that it attracts bugs.)

If you are on edge, high-strung, and, generally speaking, a nervous wreck, surround yourself with calming colors. Green has a harmonizing effect, since it's the color of nature. Earth colors should make you feel better. Wear quiet blues and gentle grays. It helps more than we realize.

HIGH ANXIETY

Need to calm down in the middle of a crisis? When you're feeling as though you may jump out of your skin—you're stuck in traffic and late for an appointment, or waiting for news from someone close to you, or (fill in the blank)—this breathing exercise can help slow down your heart rate, lower your blood pressure, and make you feel in control. And you can do it even if there are people around.

Put your hand on your stomach, inhale slowly and deeply, and feel your hand moving as you bring the air into your stomach. Then exhale slowly, while feeling your hand moving again.

After a few minutes of this slow, deep breathing, you should feel calmer and better able to handle the situation at hand.

STAGE FRIGHT

For many people, their number one fear is public speaking, or stage fright. Lots of professional performers get a bad case of butterflies before the curtain goes up. If you've done your homework, know your subject, and are comfortable with your material, you can turn nervous energy into a winning combination of enthusiasm and passion.

Here are a couple of exercises that can help you do that.

Before "showtime," stand squarely in front of a wall. Put both of your palms on the wall with elbows bent slightly, have your right foot a step in front of the left one, bend both legs slightly at the knees, and push! push! push! the wall. This flexing of your diaphragm somehow dispels the butterflies.

Remind us to tell you about the time Lydia thought a TV studio wall was immovable and it turned out to be part of a set that was quite movable. (That's one show to which we probably won't be invited back.)

A minute before you're on, slowly take a deep breath. When no more air will fit into your lungs, hold it for a couple of seconds, then let the air out very fast, in one big whoosh. Do this two times in a row, and you should be ready to go out there in complete control.

NERVOUS TICS

From time to time Joan gets a tic around her eye. She feels as though she's winking at everyone. The tic-off switch that works like magic for Joan is vitamin B_6, 200 mg.

CAUTION: Do not take more than 300 mg of B_6 a day. It can be toxic.

A tic may be your body's way of telling you that you need more calcium, magnesium, or both. A good supplement can help you get the 1,200 mg of calcium and 350 mg of magnesium that you may need daily.

SUNBURN

SUNBURN PREVENTION

Sunscreen . . . use it!

Use sunscreen with an SPF (sun protection factor) of at least 30. Use it all year long, not just in the summer. In fact, during the day, don't leave home without it!

If you have any question about whether or not you can get sunburned, look at your shadow. If your shadow is shorter than your height, you can get sunburned. Don't be surprised to see that your shadow can be shorter than your height as late in the day as 4:00 P.M. The sun is strongest at about 1:00 P.M. daylight saving time. If you're going outdoors, be sure to use sunscreen for the six hours around then (10:00 A.M. till 4:00 P.M.).

Optimal Protection

Apply sunscreen a half hour before going outside, allowing it to sink in before you go out in the sun.

While you're enjoying the sunny outdoors, reapply sunscreen often, especially if you perspire and/or go swimming. Don't hesitate to slather it on. One ounce of sunscreen should cover the exposed skin of an average-size adult wearing a swimsuit. Yes, you'll probably use up a 4-ounce tube during a day at the beach. You're worth it, especially when you consider the cost of down-the-road skin problems.

> **CAUTION:** If you're on medication of some kind, ask your doctor or pharmacist about interactions with sunscreen.

Protecting Infants

Do not use sunscreen on infants six months or younger. The chemicals in it may be too harsh for their delicate skin.

Babies that young should never be exposed to the sun for any length of time. The melanin (pigment) in their skin will not offer them proper protection.

When you take a baby out, dress him or her in a tightly woven long-sleeved shirt, long pants, and a wide-brimmed hat.

SUNBURN REMEDIES

When you didn't heed the advice above and you've gotten more than you've basked for, use one of the remedies below

immediately. Also see "Sun-Abused Skin" in the "Skin" chapter.

> **NOTE:** Severe sunburns can be second-degree burns. If the skin is broken or blistering, treatment should include cold water followed by a dry, sterile dressing, and follow that with a dermatologist's appointment.

Fill a quart jar with equal parts of milk and ice and 2 tablespoons of salt. Soak a washcloth in the mixture and place it on the sunburned area. Leave it on for about 15 minutes. Repeat the procedure three, four, or more times throughout the day.

Steep 6 regular tea bags in a quart of just-boiled water. When the tea is strong and cool, drench a washcloth in the liquid and apply it to the sunburned area. Repeat the procedure until you get relief.

Spread yogurt or sour cream over the sunburned area. This is particularly effective when the face is badly sunburned. Leave it on for 20 minutes, then rinse off with lukewarm water. The yogurt or sour cream is said to take the heat out of the sunburn, and tighten pores as well.

Prepare a healing lotion by beating the white of an egg and mixing in 1 teaspoon of castor oil. Gently rub it on the sun-burned skin.

▶ Empty a package of powdered nonfat milk or a quart of fresh low-fat milk into a tub of warm water and spend the next half hour soaking in it, soothing your sunburn.

SUNBURN PAIN PREVENTION

One way to prevent a sunburn from hurting is by taking a warm—yes, warm—shower right after sunbathing. According to a homeopathic principle, the warm water desensitizes the skin.

Sunburned Eyes and Eyelids

Make a poultice (see "Preparaton Guide" chapter) of grated apples and rest it on your closed eyelids for a relaxing hour.

▶ Make a poultice from the lightly beaten white of an egg and apply it on your closed eyes, securing it in place with an Ace bandage. Leave it on overnight. There should be a big improvement the next morning.

Cottage cheese in place of egg white is also effective.

TEETH, GUMS, AND MOUTH

TEETH

The hardest thing in your body is the enamel on your teeth. Unlike sharks, who have at least forty sets of teeth in their lifetime, we adults get only one set of thirty-two permanent teeth, and we should do whatever we can to keep them. For starters, visit a dentist at least once a year for an examination and a cleaning.

Be true to your teeth, or they will be false to you!

Toothache

Home remedies can help ease the pain of a toothache and, in some cases, alleviate tooth problems caused by nervous tension and low-grade infections. Since it is difficult to know what is causing the toothaches, make an appointment to see your dentist as soon as possible. More important, have the dentist see you.

Meanwhile, when the pain of a toothache is driving you to extraction, here's how you may get relief until you get to the dentist for the drilling, filling, and billing.

DOWN IN THE MOUTH

Pack powdered milk in a painful cavity for temporary relief.

An old standard painkiller is cloves. You can buy oil of cloves at a health food store, or whole cloves at the supermarket. Put a few drops of the oil on a wad of cotton and place it directly on the aching tooth. The whole clove should be dipped in honey that's been heated. Then chew the clove, slowly rolling it around the problem tooth. That will release the essential oil from the clove and ease the pain.

Split open a fresh, ripe fig. Squeeze out the juice of the fruit onto your aching tooth. Put more fig juice on the tooth at 15-minute intervals until the pain stops or you run out of fig juice. This is an ancient Hindu remedy. It must really work. When was the last time you saw an ancient Hindu with a toothache?

If you love garlic, this one's for you. Place a just-peeled clove of garlic directly on the aching tooth. Keep it there for a minimum of an hour. (You may want to see "Bad Breath," below, for remedies.)

Prepare a cup of stronger-than-usual sage tea. If your teeth are not sensitive to heat, hold the hot tea in your mouth for 30 seconds, then swallow and take an-other mouthful. Keep doing this until you finish the cup of tea. By then the pain should have faded away.

Take 50 to 100 mg of niacin to relieve the pain of a toothache. Don't worry if you get the "niacin flush." The redness and tingling will disappear in a short while—along with the toothache.

EXTERNAL TOOTHACHE REMEDIES

Fill a basin or two plastic shoe boxes with hot water and soak your feet. After about 10 minutes, dry your feet thoroughly, then rub them vigorously with bran. No, this didn't get mixed into the wrong category. This is a Cherokee Indian remedy for a toothache.

Prepare a cup of chamomile tea and saturate a white washcloth in it. Wring it out, then apply it to the outside of your cheek or jaw, over the area of the toothache. As soon as the cloth gets cold, redip it and reapply it. This chamomile compress should draw out the pain before it's time to reheat the tea.

Whenever the subject of toothaches came up in our home, we would prompt our dad to tell the "pig fat" story. He would begin by telling us that when he was a teenager, he had dental work done on a Thursday. Late that night, there was swelling and pain from the work the dentist did. In those days, dentists were not in their offices on Friday, and the thought of waiting until Monday was out of the question because the pain was so severe. Friday morning, our grandmother went to the nonkosher butcher shop in the neighborhood and bought a piece of pig fat. She brought it into the house (something she had *never* done before, since she kept a strictly kosher home), heated it up, and put the melted fat on a white handkerchief, which she then placed on her son's cheek. Within a few minutes, the swelling went down and the pain vanished.

Right about now in the telling of this story, our dad would get up and demonstrate how he danced around the room, celebrating his freedom from pain. We loved the story and couldn't hear it enough.

Recently, we've come across another version of that toothache remedy. Take a tiny slice of pig fat, lightly sauté it, and place it between the gum and cheek, directly on the sore area. Keep it there for 15 minutes, or however long it takes for the pain to subside. The dance afterward is optional.

Saturate a slice of toast with rubbing alcohol, then sprinkle some black pepper on it. Apply it externally to the toothache side of the face, with the peppered side touching the face, and keep it there until the pain subsides.

A similar version of this remedy requires a cheek-size piece of paper from a brown paper bag, soaked in distilled white vinegar, then sprinkled on one side with black pepper. Place the peppered side on the side of the face with the toothache, secure it with an Ace bandage, and keep it there for at least an hour, unless the pain goes away sooner.

Roast half of an onion. Then, when it's cool enough to touch but still hot, place it on the pulse (the underside) of your wrist on the opposite side of the body from your troublesome tooth. Keep it in place with a handkerchief or Ace bandage. By the time the onion cools completely, the pain should be gone.

ACUPRESSURE

This works like magic for some people; we hope you will be one of them. If your toothache is on the right side, squeeze the index finger on your right hand, on each side of your fingernail. As you're squeezing your finger, rotate it clockwise, giving that index finger a rapid little massage.

If you have someone who can do it for you—preferably someone with strong hands—all the better.

Cavity Prevention

According to the National Institute of Dental Research, to avoid being "bored" to tears by the dentist, eat a little cube of cheddar, Monterey Jack, or Swiss cheese right after eating cavity-causing foods (mainly sweets and starches). It seems that cheese reduces bacterial acid production, which may cause decay.

꩜ Blackstrap molasses contains an ingredient that seems to inhibit tooth decay. Sunflower seeds are also supposed to inhibit tooth decay. Have a tablespoon of molasses in water and/or a handful of shelled, raw, unsalted sunflower seeds daily. Be sure to rinse thoroughly with water after the molasses.

꩜ Pomegranate juice has been getting lots of press, and just about all of it is good. It seems to be due to a Pace University biology professor, Milton Schiffenbauer, Ph.D., who designed an exploratory study that was conducted by his students, proving that pure pomegranate juice and pomegranate liquid extract (available at health food stores) are effective in fighting viruses and bacteria. The juice and the extract could significantly reduce microbes found in the mouth that commonly cause cavities.

NOTE: If you drink too much pomegranate juice (sorry, but we don't know how much too much would be for you), it can cause constipation.

CAUTION: If you are taking any prescription medication, especially to help bring down your cholesterol, do *not* have pomegranate juice or extract. It may interact with the medication, similar to the way grapefruit interacts. (It may not, but the jury is still out, and better safe than lawsuit.)

꩜ Drink a cup of black tea in between and at the start of your meals.

Researchers from the University of Illinois College of Dentistry headed by Dr. Christina Wu believe that the components of black tea help prevent the harmful plaque bacteria in the mouth from causing cavities and gum disease by killing or suppressing growth and acid production of those little buggers.

꩜ If you can't brush after every meal, kiss someone. Really, kiss someone. It starts the saliva flowing and helps prevent tooth decay.

Preparing for Dental Work

As soon as you know you're going to the dentist to have work done, start eating pineapple every day. Have fresh pineapple or a cup of canned pineapple in its own juice, and drink a cup of 100 percent pineapple juice. Continue the pineapple regimen for a few days after the dental work is completed. The enzymes in pineapple should help reduce pain and discomfort. They can also help speed the healing process.

▶ Take 10 mg of vitamin B$_1$ (thiamine) daily for a week before your dental work is scheduled to begin. You may find that the pain during and after dental procedures will be greatly reduced. There's a theory that the body's lack of thiamine might be what lets the pain become severe in the first place.

TOOTH EXTRACTIONS

To stop bleeding, dip a tea bag in just-boiled water, squeeze out the water, and allow it to cool. Then pack the tea bag down on the tooth socket and keep it there for 15 to 30 minutes.

To stop pain, mix 1 teaspoon of Epsom salts with 1 cup of hot water. Swish the mixture around in your mouth and spit it out. *Do not swallow it unless you need a laxative.*

One cup should do the trick. If the pain recurs, get out the Epsom salts and start swishing again.

▶ Another pain relief method involves applying ice to your hand instead of your mouth. Wrap an ice cube in gauze or cheesecloth. (We're hoping you'll figure this out before the ice melts.) When your thumb is up against the index finger, a meaty little tuft is formed where the fingers are joined. Acupuncturists call it the "hoku point." Spread your fingers and, with the ice cube, massage that tuft for 7 minutes. If your hand starts to feel numb, stop massaging with the ice and continue with just a finger massage. It should give you 15 to 30 minutes of pain relief. This is also effective when you have pain after root canal work.

Loose Teeth

Strengthen your teeth with parsley. Pour 1 quart of just-boiled water over 1 cup of chopped parsley. Let it stand for 15 minutes, then strain and refrigerate the parsley water. Drink 3 cups a day until that loose-teeth feeling goes away.

Plaque Remover

Plaque is a film of living and dead bacteria that grows on your teeth. If it's not removed, in about twelve days it becomes rock-hard calculus, more commonly called tartar. Not good. If you don't want this to happen, here are a couple of ways to remove plaque.

■ Dampen your dental floss and dip it in baking soda, then floss with it on a daily basis. It may help remove some of the plaque buildup.

■ Mix equal parts of cream of tartar (found in supermarket spice sections) and salt. Brush your teeth and massage your gums with the mixture, then rinse very thoroughly.

Teeth Whitener

Burn a piece of toast. Really char it. Pulverize the charred bread, mix it with about ½ teaspoon of honey, and brush your teeth with it. Rinse thoroughly, put on a pair of sunglasses, look in the mirror, and smile!

Cleaning Your Teeth

The proper way to clean your teeth is the way you do it right before going to your annual dental checkup.

◗ Cut 1 fresh strawberry (fresh strawberries only and at room temperature) in half and rub your teeth and gums with it. It may help remove stains and discoloration without harming the enamel. It may also strengthen sore gums. Leave the crushed strawberry on the teeth and gums for a few minutes. Then rinse thoroughly with warm water.

NOTEWORTHY: If you're like us, then you grew up hearing your mother threaten, "I'm going to wash your mouth out with soap!" If we knew then what we know now, we would have let her do it and then said, "Thank you."

Several years ago, after the very first time Joan brushed her teeth with tooth soap (Perfect Prescription Original Shreds Tooth Soap from Vitality Products, Inc.), her gums stopped bleeding. That made her an instant convert from regular fluoride toothpaste to little shreds of soap, made with pure and wholesome whole-food ingredients, and she's been using tooth soap ever since.

Recently, Joan switched to the *liquid* version (Perfect Prescription Liquid Tooth Soap). A few drops of the liquid and a wet toothbrush and you're foaming at the mouth in seconds. Then, after a couple of rinses, your teeth and gums look and feel wonderfully clean.

The only way to know if tooth soap—shreds or liquid—is for you is to try it. The company offers a 100% money-back guarantee.

While you're at it, you may also want to try Perfect Prescription Tooth Swish. One *swish* can help remineralize your teeth, neutralize acids, stimulate your gums, and freshen your breath. See www.toothsoap.com or call 888-648-7771.

Clean Your Toothbrush

Dissolve a tablespoon of baking soda in a glass of warm water and soak your toothbrush in it overnight. Rinse it in the morning and notice how clean it looks and feels.

Keep in mind that bacteria from your mouth nestle in the bristles of your toothbrush and can reinfect you when you have a cold sore, a cold, the flu, or a sore throat. Be sure to clean your toothbrush daily when you have symptoms of any of the aforementioned health challenges.

GUMS

Pyorrhea and Gingivitis

NOTE: Gum problems should be evaluated by a dentist.

In parts of Mexico, pyorrhea is treated by rubbing gums with the rattle from a rattlesnake. (We'd hate to think of how they do root canals.) Keep reading for more practical ways to care for your gums.

Brian R. Clement, director of Hippocrates Health Institute in West Palm Beach, Florida, reports that garlic is the first and foremost remedy for clearing up gum problems. He also warns that raw garlic can burn sensitive gums. It is for that reason the institute's professional staff mixes pectin with garlic before coating the gums with it. The garlic heals the infection, while the pectin keeps it from burning the gums. Suggest this line of defense to a New Age, holistic, or open-minded periodontist.

Take coenzyme Q_{10}, at least 15 mg twice a day. Also, open a co-Q_{10} capsule and use the powder in it for brushing your teeth and massaging your gums.

Each time you take a co-Q_{10}, also take 500 mg of vitamin C with bioflavonoids.

Brush your teeth and massage your gums with goldenseal tea (available at health food stores).

Myrrh (yes, one of the gifts brought by the wise men) is a shrub, and the gum from that shrub is an antiseptic and astringent used on bleeding or swollen gums to heal the infection that's causing the problem. Myrrh oil can be massaged directly on gums, or use myrrh powder on a soft-bristled toothbrush and gently brush your teeth at the gum line. Do it several times throughout each day until the condition clears up or you see a periodontist.

Prepare your own toothpaste by combining baking soda with 1 or 2 drops of hydrogen peroxide. Brush your teeth and massage your gums with it, using a soft, thin-bristled brush. This toothpaste is a strong, abrasive disinfectant. Stop using it as soon as your gums are better.

Bleeding Gums

Bleeding gums may be your body's way of saying you do not have a well-balanced diet. After checking with your dentist, you might consider seeking professional help from a vitamin therapist or nutritionist, to help you supplement your food intake with the vitamins and minerals you're lacking. Meanwhile, start by taking 500 mg of vitamin C twice a day. Since vitamin C passes through your system within 12 hours, it's more beneficial to take a smaller dose twice a day, with breakfast and with dinner, rather than one larger dose.

Gum Pain Relief

Until you get to a dentist for professional help, this rinse may relieve the pain. Dissolve 1 teaspoon of sea salt (available in health food stores) in 1 cup of hot water. When it's cool enough to drink, take a mouthful and swish it around for about 10 seconds, then spit it out. Repeat the process until you empty out the cup. If the pain hasn't subsided, do it again every hour until you have no more pain or can get to a dentist.

BAD BREATH (HALITOSIS)

While no one ever dies of bad breath, it sure can kill a relationship. For occasional bad breath, here are some refreshing remedies that are worth a try.

> **NOTE:** If your bad breath is chronic rather than occasional, it's important to find the cause. Check for sinusitis or indigestion, and see a dentist for a tooth and gum evaluation.

It is believed that some cases of bad breath are caused by the stomach's faulty production of hydrochloric acid. It is also believed that niacin can regulate and even cure the problem. Taking niacin is quite an experience. Some people temporarily turn brick red all over soon after taking it. To prevent this "niacin flush," take no more than 50 to 100 mg at any one time. Niacinamide promises the same benefits and none of the side effects. Take it for a couple of weeks. You will know whether or not it makes a difference breathwise.

Suck on a piece of cinnamon stick (available at your supermarket spice section) to sweeten your breath. It can also satisfy a craving for a sweet treat.

According to Boston University Dental School professor Richard H. Price, DMD, "An overabundance of odor-producing bacteria in your mouth, particularly on the back of your tongue, is the most common cause of bad breath."

Dr. Price suggests ways to get rid of the food debris on which the bacteria thrive. Be sure to brush your teeth (and any dental work) twice a day, floss daily, and brush or scrape your tongue first thing in the morning and last thing at night. He also says that sipping about eight 8-ounce glasses of water daily will keep your mouth moist. That's important because saliva helps wash away the food debris on which the noxious bacteria flourish.

Stand in front of a mirror and stick out your tongue. Does it look coated, particularly the back half of it? If it is coated, you need to brush it just as you brush your teeth. You do brush your teeth, right? A brushed tongue may eliminate bad breath. Use your toothbrush or buy a tongue scraper (available at pharmacies and health food stores) and clean your tongue after breakfast and at bedtime.

When leaving an Indian restaurant, have you ever noticed a bowl filled with seeds there for the taking? They are most likely anise. Suck on a few of those licorice-tasting seeds to sweeten your breath . . . especially after eating a meal with cumin.

No More Morning Dragon Breath

At bedtime, take a piece of myrrh the size of a pea and let it dissolve in your mouth. Since myrrh is an antiseptic and can destroy the germs that may cause the problem, you may awaken kissing-sweet.

Onion and Garlic Breath

Suck a lemon! It should make your onion or garlic breath disappear. Some people get better results when they add salt to the lemon, then suck it.

> **CAUTION:** Do not do this often—only in an emergency social situation. The strongly acidic lemon juice is not good for tooth enamel.

Chew a clove to sweeten your breath. People have been doing that for more than five thousand years.

Chew sprigs of parsley, especially after eating garlic. Take your choice: garlic breath or little pieces of green stuff between your teeth.

Mix ½ teaspoon of baking soda into a cup of water, then swish it around your mouth, one gulp at a time, and spit it out.

Do not swallow this mouthwash. By the time you've rinsed with the entire cup, your breath should be fresh.

🔸 If you're a coffee drinker, have a cup of strong coffee to remove all traces of onion from your breath. Of course, then you have coffee breath, which to some people is just as objectionable as onion breath. Eat an apple. That will get rid of the coffee breath. Hey, a better idea is to forget the coffee and just eat an apple.

Mouthwash

Stock up on mint, rosemary, and fennel seeds (available at herb and health food stores) and prepare an effective mouthwash. For a daily portion, use ⅓ teaspoon of each of the three dried herbs or seeds. Pour 1 cup of just-boiled water over the mint, rosemary, and fennel seeds, cover the cup, and let the mixture steep for 10 minutes, then strain it. At that point, it should be cool enough for you to rinse with. You might also want to swallow a little. It's wonderful for digestion, which may be causing the bad breath.

🔸 Prepare your own mouthwash by combining ¼ cup of apple cider vinegar with 2 cups of just-boiled water. Let it cool and store it in a jar in your medicine cabinet. Swish a mouthful of this antiseptic solution as you would commercial mouthwash, for about a minute, then spit. Then be sure to rinse with water to remove the acid.

DRY MOUTH

When it's time to make that all-important speech or pop that critical question, you want to seem calm and sound confident. That's hard to do when your mouth is dry. When this happens, do not drink cold beverages. Doing so may help your dry mouth, but it will tighten up your already tense throat. Also, stay away from drinks with milk or cream. They can create phlegm and more problems talking. Warm tea is your best bet. If there's none available, gently chew on your tongue. In less than 20 seconds, you'll manufacture all the saliva you'll need to end your dry mouth condition.

🔸 Mix 1 tablespoon of honey with ½ cup of warm water and swish and gargle with it for about 3 to 5 minutes. Then rinse away the sweetness with water. The levulose in honey increases the secretion of saliva, relieving dryness of the mouth and making it easier to swallow.

CANKER SORES

Canker sores are painful and annoying, and they can last for weeks. They are believed to be brought on by stress and have been linked to a deficiency of niacin. Take 50 to 100 mg of niacin daily. Don't be alarmed if you get a "flush" from the niacin, although it doesn't usually happen unless you take 125 mg or more. The redness and possible tingling and itching do not last long and are completely harmless. Anyway, a daily dose of niacin may speed the healing process and also prevent a recurrence of the sores.

Get an ear of corn, discard the kernels, and carefully burn a little piece of cob at a time. Apply the cob ashes to the canker sore 3 to 5 minutes a day. (Too bad this isn't a remedy for the toes. We'd have "cob on the corn.")

According to psychic healer Edgar Cayce, castor oil is soothing and promotes healing of canker sores. Dab the sore with it each time the pain reminds you it's there.

Several times throughout the day, put a glob of blackstrap molasses in your mouth on the canker sore. Molasses has extraordinary healing properties. Be sure to rinse thoroughly with water after using molasses.

Take a mouthful of sauerkraut juice (use fresh from the barrel or in a jar found at health food stores, rather than the cans found in supermarkets) and swish it over the canker sore for about a minute. Then either swallow the juice or spit it out. Do this four to six times throughout the day every day until the sore is gone. It may disappear in only a day or two.

Eating yogurt with active cultures may ease the condition faster than you can say *Lactobacillus acidophilus.* If you don't want to eat yogurt, take lactobacillus tablets or capsules as an effective treatment for canker sores. Make sure the yogurt and/or the supplements have live cultures. Follow the dosage recommendation on the label.

Until you're able to round up any of the above ingredients, dip a regular black or green tea bag in just-boiled water. Squeeze out most of the water. When it's cool to the touch, apply it to the canker sore for 3 minutes. It should help ease the pain.

COLD SORES (FEVER BLISTERS)

A cold sore or fever blister is an infection caused by the herpes simplex virus. This painful and less-than-attractive sore usually shows up on one's lip. The good news is that help is here.

When a cold sore is on its way you'll feel a peculiar tingling sensation. At the very first sign of that tingle, lightly paint *colorless* nail polish on the area where the cold sore is about to emerge. The nail polish prevents the sore from blossoming.

Television producer Cyndi Antoniak got this unique remedy from her dermatologist. Since Cyndi first used this remedy successfully some time ago, she has never had another flare-up and has not had to use it again. Incidentally, the polish peels off naturally within a short time.

▶ If you already have a cold sore, speed up the healing process by cutting a peeled clove of garlic in half and rubbing it on the sore. Not pleasant, but effective.

▶ Combine 1 tablespoon of apple cider vinegar with 3 tablespoons of honey (preferably raw honey, found at health food stores) and dab the sore with the mixture in the morning, in the late afternoon, and at night.

▶ Grind up a few walnuts and mix them with 1 teaspoon of cocoa butter. Apply this nutty butter salve to the sore twice a day. The sore should be gone in three or four days.

▶ Lysine may inhibit the growth of the herpes virus that causes cold sores. Take an L-lysine supplement with dinner. Also see the "Herpes" chapter for more useful information.

▶ This folk remedy came to us from several folks across the country. If they weren't grossed out by it, maybe you won't be, either. Ready? Use earwax (your own, of course) on your cold sore to help heal it.

ULCERS

While a small percentage of people get ulcers from continual use of aspirin and other painkillers, a recent incredible discovery was made about the main cause of ulcers. About 80 percent of all ulcers can be blamed on *Helicobacter pylori* bacteria. It is estimated that half the American adult population has *H. pylori* present but dormant in their stomachs.

Why do some people develop ulcers and others don't? Our commonsense guess is that emotional upsets, fatigue, nervous anxiety, chronic tension, and/or the inability to handle a high-pressure job or situation in a healthy way may devitalize the immune system, lowering one's resistance to *H. pylori*.

If you're a member of the "fret set," we can suggest remedies for the ulcer, but you have to remedy the cause. Change jobs, meditate, look into self-help seminars, or do whatever is appropriate to transform your specific problem into something positive and happily manageable.

Please don't try any of the following remedies without your doctor's approval and blessing. Call your doctor *now* to consult, or for an appointment, then continue reading.

DISPELLING DIET MYTHS

According to a report in *Practical Gastroenterology,* "Aside from its failure to promote healing of gastric ulceration, the bland diet has other shortcomings: It is not palatable, and it is too high in fat and too low in roughage."

We also learned that milk may not be the cure-all everyone thought it was. It may neutralize stomach acid at first, but because of its calcium content, it promotes the secretion of gastrin, a hormone that encourages the release of more acid. Steer clear of milk.

HEALING FOODS

A high-fiber diet is believed to be best for the treatment of ulcers and prevention of relapses.

With your doctor's permission, take 1 tablespoon of extra-virgin olive oil in the morning and 1 tablespoon in the evening. It may soothe and heal the mucous membrane that lines the stomach.

Barley and barley water are a soothing food and drink that help rebuild the stomach lining. See "Preparation Guide."

Research has substantiated the effectiveness of cabbage juice, a centuries-old folk remedy, for relief of ulcers. While today's pressured lifestyle is quite conducive to ulcers, we at least have modern machinery to help with the cure: a juice extractor.

Juice a cabbage and drink a cup of the juice right before each meal, then another cup before bedtime. Make sure the cabbage is fresh, not wilted. Also, drink the juice as soon as you prepare it. In other words, don't prepare it ahead of time and refrigerate it. It loses a lot of value that way. According to reports on test groups, pain symptoms and ulcers disappeared within two to three weeks after starting the cabbage juice regimen.

Cabbage is rich in the amino acid glutamine. Glutamine helps the healthy stomach cells regenerate and stimulates the production of mucin, a mucoprotein that protects the stomach lining.

Also, cabbage contains gefarnate, a substance that helps strengthen the stomach lining and replace cells. (It's used in antiulcer drugs.)

Stop reading and start juicing!

For the acute distress of ulcers (and gastritis), Dr. Ray C. Wunderlich Jr., of the Wunderlich Center for Nutritional Medicine in Florida, recommends lecithin granules, 1 heaping tablespoon as needed. Lecithin capsules are also good. Both are available at health food stores.

URINARY PROBLEMS

The urinary system includes the kidneys, bladder, ureters, and urethra.

Many of the remedies are helpful for more than one condition. Therefore, most of the bladder and kidney ailments (infections, stones, inflammation, etc.) are bunched together in this section.

We suggest you read them all in order to determine the most appropriate one(s) for your specific problem.

URINARY PROBLEMS IN GENERAL

Drink plenty of fluids, including 3 to 4 cups of parsley tea a day. If you have a juicer, 1 or 2 glasses of parsley juice daily should prove quite beneficial. Also, sprinkle fresh parsley on the foods you eat. You may start to see improvements any time from three days to three weeks.

NOTE: Urinary infections, kidney stones, gravel, and inflammation of the bladder and kidneys should all be diagnosed and evaluated by health professionals. Along with their recommendations are the following worth-a-try remedies that may ease your condition by toning and strengthening your bladder and kidneys.

Onions are a diuretic and will help to cleanse your system. (See "Diuretics," below.) Also, for kidney stimulation, apply a poultice (see "Preparation Guide") of grated or finely chopped onion to the kidney area—the small of the back.

According to the Native Americans, corn silk (the silky strands beneath the husk of corn) is a cure-all for urinary problems. The most desirable corn silk is from young corn, gathered before the silk turns brown. Take a handful of corn silk and steep it in 3 cups of just-boiled water for 5 minutes. Strain and drink the 3 cups throughout the day. Corn silk tea can be stored in a glass jar, *not* refrigerated. If you can't get corn silk, use corn silk extract (available at most health food stores). Add 10 to 15 drops of the extract to a cup of water.

◗ Lots of folk remedies include the use of apple cider vinegar to help flush the kidneys and to provide a natural acid. The dose most sources agree on is 1 teaspoon of apple cider vinegar for every 50 pounds you weigh, added to 6 ounces of water. So if you weigh 150 pounds, take 3 teaspoons of vinegar in 6 ounces of water. Drink it twice a day, before breakfast and before dinner. Keep it up for two days, then stop for four days. Continue this two-days-on/four-days-off cycle as long as you feel you need it.

◗ Aduki (or adzuki or azuki) beans, available at health food stores, are used in the Orient as food *and* medicine. They're excellent for treating kidney problems. Rinse a cupful of aduki beans. Combine the cup of beans with 5 cups of water and boil for 1 hour. Strain the aduki bean water into a jar. Drink ½ cup of aduki water at least a half hour before meals. Do this for two days—six meals. To prevent the aduki water from spoiling, keep the jar in the refrigerator, then warm the water before drinking.

◗ Pumpkin seeds are high in zinc and good for strengthening the bladder muscle. Eat a palmful of unprocessed, unsalted, shelled pumpkin seeds 3 times a day.

◗ Carrot tops (the green leaves) and celery tops (the leaves plus the top part of the stem) are tops for strengthening the kidneys and bladder. In the morning, cover a bunch of cleaned carrot tops with 12 ounces of just-boiled water and let them steep. Drink 4 ounces of the carrot-top water before each meal. After each meal, eat a handful of scrubbed celery tops. Within four to five weeks, there should be a noticeable and positive difference in the kidneys and bladder.

DIURETICS

To stimulate urination, try any of the following in moderation, using good common sense by listening to your body, especially when it tells you, "Enough is enough!"

■ Celery: cooked in chicken soup or raw in salads

■ Watercress: in soup or salads

■ Leek: mild diuretic in soup; much stronger when eaten raw (and a perfect basis for a cheap joke about urination)

- Cucumbers: raw

- Corn silk: tea (see "Urinary Problems in General," above)

- Onions: raw in salads, and/or rub your loins with sliced onions (yes, you read that correctly)

- Horseradish: grate ½ cup of horseradish, boil it with ½ cup of beer, and drink three times a day

- Watermelon: eat a piece first thing in the morning and do not eat other foods for at least 2 hours after eating watermelon or any other melon

KIDNEY STONES: PREVENTION

A high level of oxalate in the urine contributes to the formation of most (calcium) kidney stones. If this problem runs in your family, or if you've already gone through the agony of a kidney stone, chances are you'll need to take every precaution to help prevent it from happening to you.

- Completely eliminate, or at least greatly limit, your intake of foods and beverages that are high in oxalates, or that can produce oxalic acid. That includes caffeine (coffee, black tea, colas, cocoa, chocolate),

spinach, beets, pecans, peanuts, and green bell pepper.

Stick with foods that are rich in vitamin A, which can help discourage the formation of stones. They include apricots, pumpkin, sweet potatoes, squash, carrots, and cantaloupe.

For more extensive lists of foods high and low in oxalates, go to the Web site of the University of Pittsburgh Medical Center (http://patienteducation.upmc.com/Pdf/LowOxalateDiet.pdf), or go to your favorite search engine and simply type in "foods high in oxalates."

- Start your day by drinking a glass of (preferably distilled) water in which you squeeze the juice of a lemon. The citric acid and magnesium in the lemon may help prevent the formation of kidney stones.

FREQUENT URINATION

Cherry juice or cranberry juice (make sure they have no sugar or preservatives added) has been said to help regulate the problem of constantly having to urinate. Drink 3 to 4 glasses of cherry or cranberry juice—room temperature, *not* chilled—throughout the day.

Both juices are also known to help heal kidney and bladder infections.

NOTE: Persistent frequent urination may be a sign of a urinary tract infection or diabetes, and should be checked by a health professional.

INCONTINENCE

Incontinence should be diagnosed and evaluated by a health professional. Meanwhile, you might try directing the stream of water from an ordinary garden hose (or from a shower hose attachment) to the soles of the feet for up to 2 minutes. It has been known to reduce incontinence, particularly in older people. It also helps circulation in the feet.

Also see "Bladder Control" in the "Women's Health Challenges" chapter.

VARICOSE VEINS

KEEPING VARICOSE VEINS FROM GETTING WORSE

- *Never* sit with your legs crossed. In a relaxed way, keep your knees and ankles together and slightly slant your legs. It's graceful-looking and doesn't add to the congestion that promotes varicose veins.

- Keep your feet elevated as much as possible. It's ideal to elevate your legs at or above the level of your heart for 20 minutes a few times a day.

- Wear flats or very low heels, never high heels.

- If you're overweight, do your legs a favor and lose those extra pounds.

- Exercise. Just walking a half hour every day will help your circulation.

- At the end of each day, stand in a tub of cold water. After 2 or 3 minutes, dry your legs with a coarse towel, then walk around your home at a brisk pace for about 2 or 3 minutes.

IMPROVING THE CONDITION

Folk medicine practitioners throughout Europe have been known to recommend the application of apple cider vinegar to help shrink varicose veins.

Once in the morning and once in the evening, dip a generous piece of cheesecloth in apple cider vinegar, wring it out so that it doesn't drip, and wrap it around the affected area. Lie down with your legs raised and relax that way for at least a half hour.

After each apple cider vinegar wrap session, drink 2 teaspoons of the vinegar in a cup of warm water. The practitioners tell us that by the end of one month, the veins shrink enough for there to be a noticeable difference.

▶ The following supplements (found in health food and vitamin stores) can be extremely helpful.

> **CAUTION:** Be sure to check with your doctor and/or nutritionist before adding supplements to your daily course of therapy.

■ *Hawthorn berries.* Rich in antioxidant bioflavonoids, hawthorn berries have been used for centuries as a nutritive tonic for the heart and vascular system

■ *Butcher's broom.* The root of this European plant is rich in natural fatty acids, sterols, and phenolic compounds that help circulation, especially to the lower extremities.

■ *Horse chestnut.* This seed has an anti-inflammatory effect and also improves the tone of the veins, helping to prevent blood from pooling in the legs and feet. Horse chestnut extract is available at health food stores.

■ *Diosmin/hesperidin.* The combination of these powerful antioxidant bioflavonoids is said to strengthen vascular structures and encourage healthy blood flow in the legs.

WARTS

No matter how you feel about warts, they have a way of growing on you.

Verruca vulgaris is the medical term for common warts. They usually appear on the hands, feet, and face, and are believed to be caused by a virus.

For research purposes we tried to get warts. We kept touching frogs. It's a fallacy. You do not get a wart from touching a frog. (Incidentally, you do not get a prince from kissing one, either.)

The award for the most outrageous folk remedies goes to warts. We got a million of 'em—folk remedies, that is, not warts. We've left out the uggah-buggah type remedies where you have to bury things when there's a full moon, and we left in the more sensible, easy-to-do remedies that work.

If you have a wart, find the one that works for you.

▶ TV host Regis Philbin shared his teacher's wart-removal remedy with his audience: First thing in the morning, put your spittle on the wart. After doing this consistently for about ten days in a row, the wart will disappear.

This is in keeping with Philbin's teacher's remedy (above), but with an added element, raw cashews. Before going to bed, chew a cashew or two, mixing them with your saliva. Then put the thoroughly chewed nut on the wart and cover it with tape. Dress it the same way every night until the wart goes away. We're told it takes about three weeks. Then you can chew and swallow the rest of the cashews.

Crush a fresh fig until it has a mushy consistency and put it on the wart for a half hour. Do that every day, using a fresh fig each time, until the wart disappears.

Apply a used tea bag to the wart for 15 minutes a day. Within a week to ten days you should be wartless.

Pick some dandelions. Break the stems and put the juice that oozes out of the stems directly on the wart, once in the morning and once in the evening, five days in a row. That should do it!

Grate carrots and combine them with a teaspoon of olive oil. Put the mixture on the wart for a half hour twice a day every day until the wart is history.

Dab lemon juice on the wart, immediately followed by a raw chopped onion. Do that twice a day, for 15 minutes each time.

Every morning, squish out the contents of a vitamin E softgel and rub it vigorously on the wart. We've been told that this remedy is slower than most—it takes about a month—but what's the rush?

Put a fresh slice of raw potato on the wart and keep it in place with a bandage. Leave it on overnight. Take it off in the morning. Then repeat the procedure again at night. If you don't get rid of the wart in a week, replace the potato with a peeled half clove of garlic.

Dab on the healing juice of the aloe vera plant twice a day until the wart disappears.

Every day, apply a poultice of blackstrap molasses (see "Preparation Guide" chapter) and keep it on the wart as long as possible. Also eat a tablespoon of molasses daily. In about two weeks, the wart should drop off without leaving a trace.

We heard about a woman who applied regular white chalk to the wart every night. On the sixth night, the wart fell off. Of course she was able to chalk it up to experience.

In the morning and in the evening, rub the wart with one of the following:

- Radish
- Juice of marigold flowers
- Bacon rind
- Oil of cinnamon
- Wheat germ oil
- A thick paste made with baking soda and water

If you don't have the patience to tend to the wart on a daily basis, consider finding a competent, professional hypnotist. Warts can actually be hypnotized away.

Warts on the Hand

Hard-boil 2 eggs and save the water. As soon as it's cool, soak the hand with the wart in the water for 10 minutes. Do it daily until the wart disappears.

We have written testimony from a college student who had a recurring wart on her hand. Her doctor burned the wart off and it came back. Topical medication inflamed the wart, making it worse. As a last resort, the young woman soaked her hand in egg water, and, after two days, the wart was gone.

Genital Warts

Gently rub the inner side of pineapple skin on the affected parts. Repeat every morning and evening until the warts are gone . . . or the pineapple's gone.

Warts on the Body

If you have warts on your body, you may have too much lime in your system. One way to neutralize the excess lime is to drink a cup of chamomile tea (available at health food stores) two or three times a day.

PLANTAR WARTS

Plantar warts are the kind you find on the soles of the feet, usually in clusters. The wart starts as a little black dot. Don't pick at it; you'll only make it spread. Instead, rub castor oil on it every night until it disappears.

At bedtime, puncture 1 or 2 garlic softgels and squeeze out the oil on the plantar warts. Massage the oil on the entire area for a few minutes. Put a clean white sock on your foot and leave it on while you sleep. Do this every night for a week or two, until the warts fall off.

Rub aloe vera gel on the plantar warts at bedtime and again in the morning. Use aloe directly from a plant, or the 100 percent gel available at health food stores. (The aloe lotions have too many additives.)

You may want to apply a Dr. Scholl's

bagel-like round pad for cushioning, to help relieve the pressure and pain, and to keep the aloe from wiping off on your sheet.

Of all the plantar wart remedies we've read or heard about, the most popular, by far, is a cotton ball dipped in organic apple cider vinegar (available at health food stores) and placed on the plantar warts. Lots of people secure it in place with duct tape; some use an Ace bandage, or Band-Aids. Most people say to change the vinegar-soaked cotton ball 2 or 3 times a day. It seems to take a week to a month for the warts to up and leave. All agree that this treatment is painless. Many said that after trying a lot of remedies, this was the only one that worked.

healthfully help you shed those unwanted pounds.

So, put some motivational reminders on your refrigerator:

- Nothing stretches slacks like snacks!
- To indulge is to bulge!
- Those who love rich food and cook it, look it!
- A cookie in each hand is not a balanced diet!

And start to practice "girth control."

NOTE: As for diet pills, they can be very helpful. Twice a day, we suggest you spill them on the floor and pick them up one at a time. It's great exercise, especially for the waistline.

WEIGHT CONTROL

This weighty subject is close to our heart, hips, thighs, midriff, stomach, and every other place we can pinch an inch, or two, or ten.

Whether you've spent years yo-yoing your way through one diet after another and are heavier than ever or just need to lose a few pounds to look better in that bathing suit, here are suggestions to

AS IF YOU DIDN'T ALREADY KNOW . . . : BASIC REDUCING PRINCIPLES

Change your lifestyle habits gradually. (The key word is *gradually*.) Little by little, day by day, replace a couple of fattening foods with healthier choices. In doing so, you become very aware of what you're eating. That's a major step in improving your daily food intake and taking off the pounds without feeling as though you're punishing yourself.

Also, *gradually* start exercising. (Sorry! But we owe it to you to mention this.) Maybe walk briskly for 10 minutes the first few days, then 12 minutes, then 15 minutes, and keep going until you work your way up to doing a supervised exercise program that's appropriate for you.

You don't have to call it "exercise." Keep in mind that a day without sunshine is like a day without serotonin, a brain chemical that can allay hunger. Your body needs sunlight to make serotonin, so get out there every chance you get, and walk, play, skip. Enjoy yourself! And don't forget the sunscreen.

▸ Be happy if you lose up to 2 pounds a week. In terms of keeping the weight off permanently, losing no more than 2 pounds a week makes sense. If you lose more, your body thinks you're going to starve, and in an effort to protect you from dying of hunger, it will slow down your metabolism. A loss of 1 or 2 pounds a week adds up to a big difference in a matter of months.

▸ Whenever possible, eat your larger meals early rather than late in the day. This gives your body lots of time to digest and burn off the calories. Keep this appropriate saying in mind: "Eat like a king in the morning, a prince at noon, and a pauper in the evening." While it's not always prac-tical, at least aim for a big lunch and a small dinner as often as you can.

▸ Spice up bland low-calorie, low-carbohydrate foods. They will be much tastier, and you'll eat slower and be full more quickly. Also, spicy food will in-crease your metabolism a little, helping you burn more calories.

REV UP YOUR METABOLISM

Kelp is seaweed that's rich in minerals and vitamins, especially the B vitamin family. Its high iodine content helps activate a sluggish thyroid. Dried kelp can be eaten raw, or crumbled into soups and on sal-ads. Powdered kelp can also be used in place of salt. It has a salty, fishy taste that may take getting used to. If you really don't like the taste, there are kelp pills. Follow the recommended dosage on the label. (Kelp—dried, powdered, and pills—is available at health food stores.) If you eat too much kelp, it can have a laxative ef-fect.

Along with the thyroid boost, kelp may make your hair shinier.

▸ At England's Oxford Polytechnic Institute, a study showed that adding 1 teaspoon of hot-pepper sauce and 1 teaspoon of mus-tard to every meal raised one's metabolic rate by as much as 25 percent.

Do not eat within 3 hours of going to sleep. The body seems to store fat more easily at night, when the metabolism slows down.

ANCIENT SLIMMING HERBS

Each of the herbs we're going to mention here has several wonderful properties. The one they all have in common is the ability to help the user to be a loser . . . a weight loser.

Please know that these herbs do not give you license to start eating as though there's no tomorrow. They are tools that may help decrease the appetite and/or metabolize fat quickly, but they should be used in conjunction with a well-balanced, healthy eating plan. (Even though we know you know that, we feel obligated to mention it . . . more than once.)

You may want to taste each herb before deciding on the one to stick with for at least one month. The herbs are available in tea bags or loose at most health food stores.

To prepare, add 1 teaspoon of the dried, loose herb (or 1 tea bag) to 1 cup of just-boiled water. Cover and let it steep for 10 minutes. Strain and enjoy.

Drink 1 cup about half an hour before each meal and 1 cup at bedtime. It may take a month or more before you see results, especially if you hardly change your eating habits. To enjoy an appreciable weight difference, eliminate foods with sugar, salt, white flour, and unhealthy fats, and the following herbal teas will work wonders:

■ *Fennel seeds.* Fennel is known to metabolize and throw off fatty substances through the urine. Fennel is rich in vitamin A and is wonderful for the eyes. It also aids digestion.

■ *Cleavers.* Like fennel seeds, cleavers is known to somehow accelerate fat metabolism. It's also a natural diuretic and can help relieve constipation. You may want to combine cleavers with fennel seeds as your daily drink.

■ *Raspberry leaves.* As well as having a reputation as a reducing aid, raspberry leaf tea is said to help control diarrhea and nausea, help eliminate canker sores, and make pregnancy, delivery, and the postdelivery period easier.

■ *Yerba maté.* We've heard that South American medical authorities who have studied this herb have concluded that this popular beverage can improve one's memory, nourish the smooth tissues of the intestines, increase respiratory power, help prevent infection, and is a tonic to the brain, nerves, and spine, as well as an appetite suppressant and a digestive aid.

NOTE: Yerba maté contains caffeine (not as much as coffee). While it may act as a stimulant, it should not interfere with sleep.

■ *Horehound.* This Old World herb is a diuretic and is used in cases of indigestion, colds, coughs, and asthma. It is also reported to be an effective aid for weight reduction.

It probably took you a while to reach your current weight. And it may take you a while to lose it. Be patient with yourself and give the herbs time to do their stuff.

KILL THOSE CRAVINGS

We have a friend who's a light eater. As soon as it gets light, she eats. But seriously . . .

We told this friend about the grape juice remedy recommended by world-famous healer Edgar Cayce. Since starting this grape juice regimen, our friend's craving for desserts has almost disappeared, her eating patterns are gradually changing for the better, and she's fitting into clothes she hasn't worn in years.

Take 3 ounces of pure grape juice (no sugar, additives, or preservatives) mixed with 1 ounce of water half an hour before each meal and at bedtime. Drink the mixture slowly, taking from 5 to 10 minutes to down each 4-ounce glass.

Even though you know when enough is enough, there are times when it's hard to stop eating the foods you love, especially when they're right in front of you. If you're serious about controlling your weight, take a stick of mint-flavored gum and chew it. You will not find the food in front of you all that palatable with the taste of mint in your mouth. The gum will help save you from yourself at the buffet, or anytime food is readily available after you've had your fill.

This Chinese acupressure technique is said to diminish one's appetite. Whenever you're feeling hungry, squeeze your earlobes for one minute. If you can stand the pressure, clamp clothespins on your lobes and leave them there for those 60 seconds.

We wonder if women who wear clip-on earrings are generally slimmer than women who don't. Hmmmmm.

A woman we know dieted religiously. That means she wouldn't eat anything when she was in church. All kidding aside, she was out of control, desperate, and tired of all the fad diets. She looked in our "overweight remedies" file and decided to follow the apple cider vinegar plan.

First thing in the morning, drink 2 teaspoons of apple cider vinegar in a glass of water. Drink the same mixture before lunch and dinner, making 3 glasses of apple cider vinegar in water every day.

Within three months, the woman was no longer out of control or desperate. She felt that her days of binges were over and, thanks to the apple cider vinegar, she had the strength and willpower to stick to a balanced, healthy eating plan as the pounds slowly but surely came off.

▶ Lecithin is said to help break up and burn fatty deposits from stubborn bulges. It can also give you a full feeling after eating less than usual. The recommended daily dose is 1 to 2 tablespoons of lecithin granules.

▶ Color therapist Carlton Wagner claims that blue food is unappetizing. Put a blue lightbulb in the refrigerator and a blue spotlight in your dining area. Wagner points out that restaurants know all about people's response to the color blue with regard to food. When food is served on blue plates, customers eat less, saving the restaurants money on their all-you-can-eat "blue plate" offers.

▶ If you have a craving for fattening food, drink 10 ounces of water and wait a half hour. If you still have that craving, chances are you'll feel full from the water and will eat a lot less than usual. (More about beverages below. Keep reading.)

▶ If you crave pasta, check out low-carb options under "Pasta Possibilities" in the "Diabetes" chapter.

THE IMPACT OF BEVERAGES

A study reported in the *American Journal of Clinical Nutrition* showed that drinking water or juice before a meal, rather than beer, wine, or a cocktail, goes a long way with weight control. The imbibers consumed an average of 240 calories in the alcoholic beverage and wolfed down about 200 more calories in their meal. They also ate faster. It took them longer to feel full, but that didn't stop them. They continued eating past the point of feeling full. And all that because they had an alcoholic drink before their meal. Water, waiter, please!

If you're going to opt for juice instead of water, choose tomato juice rather than fruit juice. According to a scientific report, people who frequently drink soda (diet or sugar-sweetened) have higher hunger ratings than people who drink unsweetened or naturally sweet beverages. If you are a soda drinker, experiment by going off all soda for a week, then pay attention and see if your desire for food decreases.

SNACKS

Fruit is a great, easy-to-prepare, fibrous, health-giving sweet treat. We could fill a book naming each fruit, its nutritional values, and ways to prepare it. Instead, we suggest that you be adventurous and creative. Go to your greengrocer or any ethnic market and find exotic fruit to add to your repertoire. Be sure to clean fruit before you eat it. (See "Preparation Guide" for a do-it-yourself fruit and vegetable cleaner.)

▨ Ever think of having a sweet potato as a snack? Sweet potatoes are rich in potassium, vitamin A, folate, and vitamin C. They are easy to prepare, fat-free, and worth the 100 to 140 satisfying calories.

▨ When you crave something crunchy, get out the finger vegetables. Chomp on baby carrots, jicama, fennel sticks, strips of yellow and red bell pepper, and the old standby, celery. On a weekend morning, prepare a bowl of the cut-up vegetables. Keep them in ice water in your refrigerator, and reach for them whenever you need to nibble.

Gum Before a Snack Attack

A research study presented at the 2007 annual scientific meeting of the Obesity Society concluded that chewing gum before an afternoon snack helped reduce hunger, diminish cravings—especially for sweets; not as much for salty snacks—and promote fullness.

Not only did the study's participants eat 25 to 47 fewer calories at each snack time, the chewing gum also improved their mood by reducing anxiety and stress and increasing contentment and relaxation.

HIGH-PROTEIN LUNCH

If you have a high-protein lunch—fish, soy products, yogurt, eggs, turkey, chicken, red meat (if you must)—you may find yourself eating fewer calories for dinner. Two or three ounces of protein is said to trigger production of a hormone that cuts your appetite and leaves you feeling satisfied. Give it a try. Stay away from high-carbohydrate noon meals—pasta, rice, potatoes—and see if a portion of protein (along with veggies or salad—the good stuff) helps reduce your calorie intake at dinner.

FAT'S WHERE IT'S AT

"An unlikely hero in the battle of the bulge is in fact classified as a fat," says Jade Beutler, licensed health care practitioner and author of *Understanding Fats and Oils: Your Guide to Healing with Essential Fatty Acids* and *Flax for Life,* and a foremost authority on the many benefits of flaxseed oil. According to Beutler's research findings, flaxseed oil:

- Decreases cravings for fatty foods and sweets

- Stokes metabolic rate

- Creates satiety (feeling of fullness and satisfaction following a meal)

- Regulates blood sugar

- Regulates insulin levels

- Increases oxygen consumption

The ideal method of taking flaxseed oil for purposes of weight loss or maintenance is 1 to 2 tablespoons daily, in divided doses, taken with each meal.

EATING OUT TIPS

As soon as you're served food at a restaurant, ask for a doggy bag. Explain that you're into portion control and don't want to tempt yourself to finish everything on the plate.

If you are eating at a buffet, keep your used dish. In other words, don't let the busboy take your dish, allowing you to get a new one. If you see the used dish, it will be a constant reminder of the food you've already eaten.

Okay, so you're having pizza. Take paper napkins and blot the top of the slice. You'll take off up to a teaspoon of fat. Also, just have one slice, and round out your meal with a delicious little salad—lettuce, tomato, onion, and whatever other greens you have in the fridge, with a low-fat Italian dressing.

HOLIDAYS–THE TOUGH TIMES

- Eat healthy, nonfattening food right before you go to a holiday party.

- Forget about losing weight during the holidays. Settle for not gaining weight. Fill up on sweet potatoes, fruits, vegetables, white-meat turkey, whole-grain bread, and an occasional tiny portion of an obscenely fattening dessert.

- Drink designer water or sparkling water with a twist of lemon. A little wine is okay, if you must, but stay away from mixed drinks or liqueurs.

■ According to Alan Hirsch, M.D., director of the Smell and Taste Treatment and Research Foundation in Chicago, "People who are exposed to smells of food during the day eat less at night." Before going for that holiday meal, sniff around your kitchen cabinets and refrigerator.

> **NOTEWORTHY:** If friends haven't told you about Hungry Girl, then consider us your friends and listen up.
>
> For fun-to-read diet tips and tricks, guilt-free food finds, low-cal recipes, weight-losing inspiration, and much more, visit and subscribe to Lisa Lillien's Hungry Girl free daily newsletter at www.hungry-girl.com. While you're at it, you may want to pick up a copy of Lisa's entertaining book, not surprisingly called *Hungry Girl: Recipes and Survival Strategies for Guilt-Free Eating in the Real World* (St. Martin's).

DETERMINING YOUR WEIGHT-HEALTH PROFILE

Body mass index (BMI) is one of the most accurate ways to determine when extra pounds translate into health risks. BMI is a measure that takes into account a person's weight and height to gauge total body fat in adults.

According to the federal government guidelines, the definition of a healthy weight is a BMI of 24.9 or less. A BMI of 25 to 29.9 is considered overweight. People who fall into the BMI range of 25 to 34.9 and have a waist size of over 40 inches for men and 35 inches for women are considered to be at especially high risk for health problems.

BMI is reliable for most people between nineteen and seventy years of age, except for women who are pregnant or breast-feeding, competitive athletes, body builders, and chronically ill patients.

To use the table below, find your height in the column on the left. Move across to the number closest to your current weight. Scoot up to the top of the column and see the BMI number for that height and weight. Or let the Department of Health and Human Services figure it for you at www.nhlbisupport.com/bmi.

If your number is between 25 to 29.9, *now* is the time to do something about it. And you can. If you've read this far in this chapter, it seems to us, you really do want to do what it takes to take off those pounds. Do it, be proud of the results, and make the people who love you a lot happier.

BODY MASS INDEX CHART

BMI (kg/m²) Height (inches)	19	20	21	22	23	24	25	26	27	28	29	30	35	40
					Body Weight (pounds)									
58	91	96	100	105	110	115	119	124	129	134	138	143	167	191
59	94	99	104	109	114	119	124	128	133	138	143	148	173	198
60	97	102	107	112	118	123	128	133	138	143	148	153	179	204
61	100	106	111	116	122	127	132	137	143	148	153	158	185	211
62	104	109	115	120	126	131	136	142	147	153	158	164	191	218
63	107	113	118	124	130	135	141	146	152	158	163	169	197	225
64	110	116	122	128	134	140	145	151	157	163	169	174	204	232
65	114	120	126	132	138	144	150	156	162	168	174	180	210	240
66	118	124	130	136	142	148	155	161	167	173	179	186	216	247
67	121	127	134	140	146	153	159	166	172	178	185	191	223	255
68	125	131	138	144	151	158	164	171	177	184	190	197	230	262
69	128	135	142	149	155	162	169	176	182	189	196	203	236	270
70	132	139	146	153	160	167	174	181	188	195	202	207	243	278
71	136	143	150	157	165	172	179	186	193	200	208	215	250	286
72	140	147	154	162	169	177	184	191	199	206	213	221	258	294
73	144	151	159	166	174	182	189	197	204	212	219	227	265	302
74	148	155	163	171	179	186	194	202	210	218	225	233	272	311
75	152	160	168	176	184	192	200	208	216	224	232	240	279	319
76	156	164	172	180	189	197	205	213	221	230	238	246	287	328

NOTEWORTHY: If you want a scale that can measure body fat, weight, hydration, and muscle mass, then give you a holistic analysis, consider getting the HealthSmart Glass Electronic Body Fat Scale. Once you program in your personal data, the scale is able to suggest a course of action to help you meet your goals. It's helpful if you are technically inclined, or have a techie you can turn to for assistance. Visit www.ckbproducts .com for wholesale prices to the public and no minimum purchase, or call 888-CKB-BUYS for their catalog.

DIET PLANS

Okay, no more sabotaging yourself by buying a diet book, glancing at it, and going to the fridge to reward yourself for buying the book and glancing at it. Instead, take a realistic, practical approach to finding a book with a plan that suits your lifestyle and whose food is palatable. Then make up your mind that it will work for you, and do it!

Here are some books to consider.

■ *The South Beach Diet: The Delicious, Doctor-Designed, Foolproof Plan for Fast and Healthy Weight Loss* by Arthur Agatston, M.D. (Rodale). This is a reasonable, eat-almost-everything (including snacks and dessert) diet. It's easy to follow and stick to, especially since they have a selection of packaged foods at supermarkets.

■ *The Duke Diet: The World-Renowned Program for Healthy and Lasting Weight Loss* by Howard J. Eisenson, M.D., and Martin Binks, Ph.D. (Ballantine). The nutritional, exercise, and behavioral plans are simple and sensible. Read the book, follow the advice, adhere to the menu, and get results. Then think of the money you've saved on a stay at the famous Duke Diet and Fitness Center in North Carolina.

■ *The Perricone Weight-Loss Diet: A Simple 3-Part Plan to Lose the Fat, the Wrinkles, and the Years* by Nicholas Perricone, M.D. (Ballantine). This plan is for those serious about eating to get healthier, feel better, and lose weight in the process.

CELLULITE ELIMINATOR

Former model Maurine Klimt is getting older *and* better. Determined to get rid of cellulite, she started taking omega-3 fatty acids in the form of flaxseeds. Maurine grinds the seeds in a little coffee grinder, sprinkles 1 to 2 tablespoons on oatmeal, and then adds a touch of maple syrup. After eating the flaxseed-topped oatmeal daily for months, she reports the cellulite is no longer there. Although Maurine eats healthy and exercises, she credits the flaxseeds for the loss of cellulite.

FIRM THIGHS

Sonoma Mission Inn Spa and Country Club is graciously sharing its once-secret treatment for jiggly thighs. The key ingredient is rosemary. (No, that's not a personal trainer who gives you a workout.) Rosemary is an herb that stimulates circulation and drains impurities, leaving skin firmer and tighter. Mix 1 tablespoon of crushed dried rosemary (available at herb and health food stores) with 2 tablespoons of extra-virgin olive oil. Smooth the mixture over the thighs, wrap plastic wrap around them, and leave it on for 10 minutes. Then rinse the mixture off your thighs. Do this treatment at least once a week.

LEG SLIMMING

Every night, rest your feet as high on a wall as is comfortable while you're lying on the floor or in bed. Stay that way for about an hour. At most, your legs will slim down. At least, it will be good for your circulation.

EXERCISE THAT WON'T SEEM LIKE EXERCISE

Have you heard about the concept of 10,000 steps a day? It started in Japan about 40 years ago, when people combined their healthy diet with an all-day workout, taking 10,000 steps (equal to about 5 miles) throughout their waking hours.

The average American takes 2,300 to 4,000 steps daily (equal to about 1.5 to 2 miles).

Several university and institute researchers studied this exercise plan and agree that it's quite worthwhile. The 10,000 steps is equivalent to a steady 30-minute workout.

To make this part of your life, start by buying a pedometer. Strap it on you in the morning and take it off at bedtime. It will keep track of the number of steps you take each day. After a few days, you'll have a good idea of your average daily number. Thereafter, you need to make an effort to increase that number each day, until you get into a daily routine of 10,000 steps.

Here are some ways to step it up:

■ Whenever you're on a wireless phone, walk around the room as you talk.

■ Most TV commercials have music. Instead of channel-surfing during the commercial and letting your thumb get all the exercise, get up and dance to the music.

■ When you're doing household chores, don't look for shortcuts. Make separate trips when setting and clearing the table. Do the same for putting away laundry.

■ When you go supermarket shopping, don't be your usual organized self. Buy one item at a time in the sections you frequent, and keep going back and forth—reading labels for fat, calorie, carbohydrate, and sodium counts, and the list of ingredients, of course—until your cart is full and you're ready to walk to the checkout.

> **CAUTION:** With the next suggestions, keep safety in mind. Do these during the day, when there are lots of people around.

■ Forget elevators and escalators. Use the stairs.

■ Take the farthest parking spot possible from your destination.

■ Get off the train or bus a stop or two before your regular stop and walk the rest of the way.

■ Whenever you're kept waiting, if it's practical (like at an airport), use that time to pace up and back or down the hall.

See how creative you can be in finding ways to add steps to your days . . . and, ultimately, years to your life.

WOMEN'S HEALTH CHALLENGES

We've come a long way, baby! Today, we talk openly about menstruation, pregnancy, and menopause, not as sicknesses but as natural stages of life. (Although it does still come as a little surprise when we see TV commercials advertising sanitary napkins and a spokesperson wishes us a "good period.")

And good for you women who are questioning the male-dominated medical profession after hearing countless stories about hysterectomies, radical mastectomies, and other surgeries that are sometimes performed whether a woman needs them or not.

Knowledge is power. Television talk shows, telephone help lines, the Internet, bookstores, and libraries are filled with women's health information. We hope you are taking advantage of these sources so that you can intelligently and happily take responsibility for your own body, and make smart choices for professional medical care, that will result in your good health.

Meanwhile, here are home remedies—some whispered down from generation to generation—that may help whatever is bothering you.

ORGAN-SOOTHING MASSAGE (KNEADING YOUR NEEDS)

Gently but firmly massage the back of the leg around the ankle. Massaging that area can relax tension, stimulate circulation, and soothe all female organs.

PREMENSTRUAL SYNDROME

Premenstrual syndrome (PMS, also called PMT or premenstrual tension) is a collection of 150 separately identified physical, psychological, and emotional symptoms related to a woman's menstrual cycle. Fortunately, most women experience only a few symptoms a week or two before menstruating. The most common are water retention, bloating, breast tenderness and swelling, stress, anxiety, depression, mood swings, food cravings, fatigue, and acne flare-ups.

If you usually have some of these PMS symptoms, we suggest that you read all of the remedies here, as well as the ones below under "Menstruation." They're quite interchangeable and can be beneficial both before and during your period.

⬧ Chamomile tea (available at supermarkets and health food stores) is a superb tension reliever and nerve relaxer. As soon as you get that PMS feeling of anxiety, prepare a major mugful of tea and sip it throughout the day.

⬧ Increase your calcium intake. On a daily basis, it is a good idea to eat at least one portion each of two or three of these calcium-rich foods: leafy green veggies (collard greens, dandelion greens, kale, mustard greens, broccoli, turnip greens, watercress, parsley, endive); canned salmon, sardines, and anchovies; figs; and yogurt.

Minimize or completely eliminate caffeine and alcoholic beverages. They increase the amount of calcium lost in the urine.

Check with a nutritionist to help you determine the appropriate calcium supplement dosage for your age and weight.

⬧ Peppermint tea is soothing. It also helps digestion and rids you of that bloated feeling. Drink a cup of peppermint tea after (not during) your meal.

NOTE: If you are taking homeopathic or allopathic medicine, check with your health professional before drinking peppermint tea. Peppermint is a strong herb and may interfere with your medicine doing its job.

MENSTRUATION

Whether you call it your period, menses, falling off the roof, or even your aunt from Redbank, here are some worthwhile suggestions for that time of the month.

MENSTRUAL CRAMPS

Reduce your salt intake the week before you're expecting your period. It should cut down on the cramps and the bloating.

 Drink yarrow tea (available at health food and herb stores), a couple of cups a day. A screenwriter friend would miss up to three days a month of work because of period pains. We told her about yarrow tea, and it works like magic for her. She no longer has to take time off from her work to double over in pain.

The tea has an odd, not very good taste, but so what, as long as you get results.

 When it comes to menstrual cramps, how do naturalists spell relief? L-e-a-f-y g-r-e-e-n-s. Eat lots of dark green leaf lettuce (e.g., romaine), cabbage, and parsley before and during your period. To get the full benefit of all vegetables, eat them raw or steamed. Aside from helping reduce cramps, the leafy greens are diuretics and will relieve you of some bloat.

 When your menstrual pains drive you to drink, make that drink 1 ounce, or 2 ounces at most, of warm gin. Gin is prepared from a mash consisting of 85 percent corn, 12 percent malt, and 3 percent rye, and is distilled in the presence of juniper berries, coriander seeds, and other flavoring agents. The combination seems to quell the pain. Remember now, no more than 2 ounces of gin! You may get rid of the cramps, but you don't want to have to deal with a hangover.

Obviously, don't follow this remedy if you have or have had a drinking problem. If you do try this remedy, do *not* drive!

Menstrual Irregularities

On a daily basis, thoroughly chew and then swallow 1 tablespoon of sesame seeds. Or grind flaxseeds and sprinkle a tablespoon on your cereal, soup, or salad. Both have been known to regulate menstrual cycles.

Lightening Excessive Flow

 If your menstrual flow is excessive, the following remedies have been said to help. We also suggest you see your gynecologist for a checkup.

IMPORTANT NOTE: Hemorrhaging requires immediate medical attention! If you are not sure about the difference between excessive menstrual flow and hemorrhaging, do not take a chance. If you are bleeding profusely, get medical attention *now*!

When bleeding excessively, stay away from alcoholic beverages and hot, spicy foods, except for cayenne pepper.

Add ⅛ to ¼ teaspoon of cayenne pepper to 1 cup of warm water or your favorite herbal tea and drink it. Cayenne pepper is a powerful bleeding regulator.

To lighten an unusually heavy menstrual flow, drink yarrow tea, 2 or 3 cups a day until the period is over. If you read the remedies above, you know that yarrow also helps eliminate cramps.

Mix the juice of half a lemon into 1 cup of warm water. Drink it down slowly an hour before breakfast and an hour before dinner.

Throughout the day, sip cinnamon tea made with either a piece of cinnamon stick steeped in 1 cup of hot water, 4 drops of cinnamon bark tincture (available at health food stores) in 1 cup of warm water, ½ teaspoon of ground cinnamon dissolved in 1 cup of just-boiled water, or a cinnamon tea bag steeped in just-boiled water.

To help control profuse menstrual flow, take time for thyme tea. Steep 2 tablespoons of thyme in 2 cups of hot water. Let it stand for 10 minutes. Strain and drink the first cup of tea. Add an ice cube to the second cup of tea, then soak a washcloth in it, wring it out, and use it as a cold compress on your pelvic area. Do this in the morning and before dinner.

Excessive Menstrual Flow During Menopause

If you have excessive menstrual flow during menopause, mix 1 ounce of grated nutmeg in 1 pint of Jamaican rum. Take 1 teaspoon 3 times a day for the duration of your period. If you have a challenge with alcohol, do *not* use this remedy.

Bringing On Menstruation

NOTE: None of these remedies will work if you are pregnant or do not have a uterus.

To help bring on and regulate menstruation, eat and drink fresh beets and beet juice. Have about 3 cups of beets and juice each day past your due date until the flow begins.

A footbath in hot water has been said to help bring on a delayed menstrual period.

In a circular motion, massage below the outer and inner ankle of each foot, as well as the outer and inner wrist of each hand. If there is tenderness when you rub those areas, you're in the right place. Keep massaging until the tenderness is gone. Chances are your period will start within a day or two.

Ginger tea can stimulate the onset of menstruation. Put 4 or 5 quarter-size slices of fresh ginger in 1 cup of just-boiled water and let it steep for 10 minutes. Drink 3 to 4 cups of the tea throughout the day. It also helps ease menstrual cramps.

PREGNANCY

The fact that you're reading this book leads us to believe that you're into healthful alternatives to allopathic, or conventional, medical therapies. So, you should know that herbs are powerful and are to be taken only when recommended by totally reliable sources and bought from totally reliable sources, *after* you consult with your health care provider.

The American Pregnancy Association (www.americanpregnancy.org) shares their list of unsafe and safe herbs during pregnancy.

Herbs to *avoid* during pregnancy:

- Saw palmetto
- Goldenseal
- Dong quai
- Ephedra
- Yohimbe
- Pau d'arco
- Passionflower
- Black cohosh
- Blue cohosh
- Roman chamomile
- Pennyroyal

The following herbs have been rated "likely safe" or "possibly safe" for use during pregnancy:

- *Red raspberry leaf.* Rich in iron, this herb has helped tone the uterus, increase milk production, decrease nausea, and ease labor pains. (See "Quick Labor, Easy Delivery, Speedy Recovery," below.)

- *Peppermint leaf.* Helpful in relieving nausea/morning sickness and flatulence.

- *Ginger.* Helps relieve nausea and vomiting. (See "Morning Sickness," below.)

- *Slippery elm bark.* Used to help relieve nausea, heartburn, and vaginal irritations.

■ *Oats and oat straw.* Rich in calcium and magnesium, these help relieve anxiety, restlessness, and irritated skin.

Stretch Marks: Prevention

Start massaging coconut oil (available at health food stores) on your abdomen at least once a day, and continue even after delivery, to help prevent stretch marks or to make them disappear.

Absorption is more efficient when using warmed coconut oil. Put the amount you want to use—1 or 2 teaspoons—into a little container, then put that container into a bigger container with hot water. It doesn't take long for the oil to warm up. Remember to do it daily for the results you want.

Morning Sickness

If you are troubled by morning sickness, check with your obstetrician about taking 50 mg of vitamin B_6 and 50 mg of vitamin B_1 daily. Since garlic greatly increases the body's absorption of B_1, make an effort to eat garlic raw in salads and to cook with it. A daily garlic supplement would also be helpful.

◗ A doctor at Brigham Young University recommends 2 or 3 capsules of powdered ginger first thing in the morning to avoid morning sickness. If you don't have capsules, mix ½ teaspoon of powdered ginger in a cup of warm water and drink it. (This remedy is also effective for motion-sickness sufferers.) Or suck a piece of fresh ginger. It's strong, but you get used to it.

◗ This folk remedy is an oldie and a goodie. Mix ⅓ cup of lime juice and ⅛ teaspoon of cinnamon in ½ cup of warm water. Drink it as soon as you awaken. It's known to be quite effective.

◗ At bedtime, mix 1 tablespoon of apple cider vinegar and 1 tablespoon of honey in a glass of water. Drink it, go to bed, and wake up feeling fine.

Constipation

Keep a chair, stool, or carton in the bathroom so that you can rest your feet on it when you're on the toilet seat. Once your feet are on the same level as the seat, lean back and relax. To avoid hemorrhoids and varicose veins, do not strain, and do not hold your breath and squeeze. Do a crossword puzzle, read the gossip columns in the newspaper, or do whatever lets you relax long enough for nature to take its course.

Quick Labor, Easy Delivery, Speedy Recovery

Some studies have reported that using red raspberry leaf during pregnancy can reduce complications and the use of interventions during birth.

Many sources, including obstetricians, agree on raspberry leaf tea for the mother-to-be. What they don't agree on, according to the American Pregnancy Association (www.americanpregnancy.org), is whether this should be used throughout pregnancy or just in the second and third trimesters, so many health care providers remain cautious and only recommend using it after the first trimester.

The consensus is that pregnant women should drink 2 to 3 cups of raspberry leaf tea a day, starting at least six weeks before the expected birth. Ask your doctor about it.

Whenever you start drinking the tea, prepare it by adding 1 teaspoon of dried raspberry leaves (available at health food and herb stores) to 1 cup of just-boiled water. Let it steep for 5 minutes, strain, and drink.

If you're looking for the easy way out, you can probably find raspberry leaf tea bags at your supermarket or health food store.

BREAST-FEEDING

Great News to Give You a Lift

According to the findings of a study conducted by Dr. Brian Rinker and his colleagues with patients at UK HealthCare Cosmetic Surgery Associates, breast-feeding does not adversely affect breast shape. The results of their blessed breast study showed no difference in the degree of breast ptosis (the medical term for sagging of the breast) between the women who breast-fed and those who didn't.

There are other factors that do affect breast sagging, among them the number of pregnancies, smoking (another reason to stop), and, mostly, a woman's age (comedian Phyllis Diller, now in her nineties, says her bra size is "36 long").

Cradling Baby

The Talmud (ancient Hebrew writings) suggests that a woman who begins to nurse her child should start on the left side, as this is the source of all understanding.

Psychologist Lee Salk found that 83 percent of right-handed mothers and 78 percent of left-handed mothers held their babies on the left side.

Holding a baby on the left side frees up the baby's left ear to hear its mother's voice. Sounds that enter the left ear go to the right side of the brain, which processes tone, melody, and emotion.

Nutritious Food

Add lentil soup to your diet. Lentils are rich in calcium and other nutrients necessary for nursing mothers.

Increase Mother's Milk

■ In a pot, add 1 teaspoon of caraway seeds to 8 ounces of water and bring it to a boil, then let it simmer for 5 minutes. Turn off the heat. Once it's cool, strain it and drink it. Several cups of caraway seed tea a day may increase a mother's milk supply.

■ Peppermint tea is said to increase the supply of mother's milk, and it's also known to relieve nervous tension and improve digestion. Drink a couple of cups a day.

> **NOTE:** Peppermint is a strong herb and may interact with medication. Check with your doctor before taking it, especially if you are taking anything homeopathic.

■ Brewer's yeast (available at health food stores) may also help. Follow the directions on the label.

■ Stimulate milk secretion with a mixture of fennel seeds and barley water. Crush 2 tablespoons of fennel seeds (available in the supermarket's spice section) and simmer them in a quart of barley water (see "Preparation Guide") for 20 minutes. Let it cool and drink it throughout the day.

Cracked and/or Sore Nipples

When herbalist Angela Harris was nursing each of her nine children, between nursings she would moisten black tea bags (usually Lipton's orange pekoe) and apply them to her cracked or sore nipples. They relieved the pain and helped heal the cracking.

MASTITIS

Mastitis is an inflammation of the breast. The two common kinds are acute mastitis, involving bacterial infection, and chronic mastitis, often with no infection—just tenderness and pain.

In either case, this condition should be checked out by a health professional.

If you have a bacterial infection, chances are you will be treated with antibiotics. See "Antibiotics" in the "Healthful Hints" chapter.

To relieve the tenderness and pain of mastitis, place a cabbage leaf on your breast and let your bra hold it in place. According to herbalist Angela Harris, the cabbage draws out the toxins and the pain.

CYSTITIS

Cystitis is an inflammation of the bladder. The symptom is usually painful urination.

> **NOTE:** Persistent cystitis may require antibiotics prescribed by a doctor. If that is the case, be sure to replace the beneficial bacteria that the antibiotics destroy. See the explanation above under "Antibiotics" in the "Helpful Hints" chapter.

Meanwhile, here are remedies that may help alleviate or eliminate the condition.

Even some physicians now prescribe cranberry juice for cystitis. You can get juice that's sugarless with no added preservatives at most supermarkets (be sure to read the ingredients listed on the labels), or you can buy cranberry concentrate (which needs to be diluted) at health food stores, or use cranberry capsules and follow the dosage on the label.

If you're drinking the juice, have 8 ounces in the morning before breakfast and another 8 ounces in the late afternoon. Drink it at room temperature, not chilled.

Take a garlic supplement. Follow the dosage on the label. If you don't mind smelling like a salami, drink garlic tea throughout the day. Peel a couple of garlic cloves, then mash them into hot water and let them steep for 5 minutes. You can also prepare garlic tea with 1 teaspoon of garlic powder in a cup of hot water.

According to Native Americans, corn silk (the silky strands beneath the husk of corn) is a cure-all for urinary problems. The most desirable corn silk is from young corn, gathered before the silk turns brown. Take a handful of corn silk and steep it in 3 cups of just-boiled water for 5 minutes. Strain and drink the 3 cups throughout the day. Corn silk tea may be stored in a glass jar, not refrigerated. If you can't get corn silk, use corn silk extract (available at health food stores). Add 10 to 15 drops of the extract to 1 cup of hot water and drink 3 cups throughout the day.

Cystitis Prevention

Women who frequently get cystitis may lessen the number of attacks or stop them forever by passing water immediately *after* intercourse.

We've heard of folk remedies requiring the cystitis sufferer to take baths. Recently, we were told by a research scientist that baths may actually cause the *recurrence* of the condition. If you are a bath taker and have recurring bouts of cystitis, refrain from taking a bath for at least a month. Shower instead. You just may find you aren't troubled with cystitis anymore.

BLADDER CONTROL

Kegel exercises, which work the pubococcygeus muscle, can help you gain control over your bladder, strengthen your abdominal muscles, and enhance sexual activity.

Each time you urinate, start and stop as many times as possible. While squeezing the muscle that stops the flow of urine, pull in on the muscles of the abdomen. You can also do this when *not* urinating. Sit at your desk, in your car, at the movies—anyplace—and flex, release, flex, release.

For another suggestion, see "Orgasm Heightener" in the "For Women Only" section of the "Sex" chapter.

VAGINITIS (VAGINAL INFECTION)

There are a half dozen common types of vaginitis, with the most usual symptoms being itching, burning, and discharge. Most vaginitis is caused by bacteria or fungus, especially if you wear tight, noncotton underwear.

If you currently have a vaginal infection that's itching to be cured, place a poultice (see "Preparation Guide") of cottage cheese, farmer cheese, or yogurt with active cultures on a sanitary napkin and wear it. Change the poultice every 3 to 5 hours. Chances are the itching will stop rather quickly and the infection will be gone within a week or so. If it lasts longer, see your health care provider.

Vaginitis Prevention

If you are prone to vaginitis, there are simple and easy things to wear, do, and avoid to help curb the recurrence of this annoying condition.

■ Wear cotton panties to absorb moisture, since moisture encourages the growth of organisms. For that reason, stay away from moisture-retaining garments such as pantyhose, girdles, leotards, tights, and so on.

■ Take showers instead of baths. Baths can add to your problems when your vaginal area is exposed to bathwater impurities.

■ Do not use any chemical products such as feminine hygiene sprays. Also, avoid tampons and colored or scented toilet tissue.

■ Do not launder panties along with socks, stockings, or other undergarments. Wash panties separately with a mild soap or detergent and rinse them thoroughly.

MENOPAUSE

If you are getting hot flashes, it could mean one of two things: Either the paparazzi are following you or you're going through menopause. We have no remedy for the paparazzi, but we can report on a few recommendations that have been known to relieve some of the menopausal chaos.

Step into a tub that has 6 inches of cold water in it. Carefully walk back and forth for about 3 minutes. Be sure to have non-slip stick-ons on the floor of the tub. Step out, dry your feet thoroughly, put on a pair of walking shoes (socks are optional), and take a walk—even if it's just around your room—for another 3 minutes. It's sure to make you feel calmer and better.

Andrew Weil, M.D., the guru of integrative medicine, has an effective recommendation for hot flashes and other symptoms of menopause. It is a combination of three herbs (all readily available at herb and health food stores): dong quai, chaste tree (*Vitex angus-castus*), and damiana. Take 2 capsules or 1 dropper of each of these herbs (you can mix the 3 herbal extracts into a cup of warm water) once a day at noon. Continue this regimen until the hot flashes stop. Once they do, taper off gradually: Take half the dosage for a week, then half of that for another week.

NOTE: If you're on medication, do not take herbs unless you check with your health professional. Herbs are powerful and may prevent your medication from doing what it needs to do.

The estrogenic substances in black cohosh may relieve menopausal symptoms, including hot flashes and vaginal dryness. You'll find the herb in tincture form at health food stores. Follow the recommended dosage on the label.

NOTE: Again, if you're on medication, consult with a health care professional before taking herbs.

A Viennese gynecologist has reported positive results among his female patients treated with bee pollen. Bee pollen contains a combination of male and female hormones. It has been known to help some women do away with or at least minimize the frequency of the hot flashes.

Gradually work your way up to taking three 500 mg bee pollen pills daily, or the granule equivalent. Both are available at most health food stores.

Night Sweats

Sage is a source of plant estrogens and has been used for centuries as a safe and effective treatment for night sweats.

One hour before bedtime, prepare and drink sage tea. If you grow sage in your garden, pour a cup of just-boiled water over 10 large, fresh sage leaves; if not, use 1½ teaspoons of dried sage. Let it steep for about 5 minutes, then strain it, wait until it's cool, and drink it. (If you drink it while it's warm, it may cause you to perspire and have a hot flash.) You can add honey to make it more palatable.

Do this for three nights in a row, then every other night, then three times a week until you're no longer bothered by night sweats.

Heavy Flow During Menopause

If you have heavier-than-normal menstrual flow during menopause, see "Lightening Excessive Flow" in the "Menstruation" section, above.

REMEDIES
IN A CLASS BY
THEMSELVES

KISS-KISS

There was a Kiel Osculatory Research Center in Germany, where scientists were studying the act of kissing. One of their findings is that the morning "Good-bye, dear" kiss is the most important one of the day. It helps start the day with a positive attitude that leads to better work performance and an easier time coping with stress. According to the researchers, that morning send-off kiss on a daily basis could result in earning more money and living a longer, healthier life.

For those of you who work at home, there are other things you can do to live a longer, healthier life. Read on.

LIFE-ENHANCING WATER

According to Pindar (c. 522–443 B.C.), the great lyric poet of ancient Greece, "Water is the best of all things." He said that without even knowing about Real Willard Water (RWW).

We first learned about RWW in 1980, when it was featured on CBS-TV's *60 Minutes.* Our interest in it has recently resurfaced. After doing more research, we have a better understanding of it, and Real Willard Water is now part of our daily must-haves.

Keeping the explanation simple, when the catalyst micelle (a submicroscopic aggregation of molecules) is added to water, it alters the molecular structure of the water. As a frame of reference for changing an element's molecular structure, think of how carbon can morph into a diamond, or into a graphite pencil.

Once the molecular structure of water is changed, the "altered" water, or Real

Willard Water (named for Dr. John W. Willard Sr., the inventor of the process), takes on unusual properties, including:

- Increasing absorption of nutrients

- Increasing elimination of toxins and wastes

- Acting as an extraordinary antioxidant, scavenging free radicals

- Reducing swelling

- Balancing the body's pH by raising alkalinity

- Helping heal skin conditions

The company's unsolicited testimonies claim that RWW has benefited a wide range of ailments, including dry eye syndrome, eczema, bronchitis, skin cancer, diabetes, twitching, high blood pressure, arthritis, intestinal problems, and the list goes on.

Check it out at Nutrition Coalition's Web site, www.willardswater.com, or have your questions answered by Willard Water experts Kolleen and Charlie Sunde at 800-447-4793.

CAUTION: There are companies selling Willard Water who may be messing with it—diluting it, mixing in additives, bottling it improperly—and offering a low price for an ineffective product.

Nutrition Coalition guarantees that you are getting the Real Willard Water, made and bottled at the Willard manufacturing plant in its full concentration, just as Dr. Willard made it and patented it.

LONGEVITY

In ancient Babylonian, Egyptian, Persian, and Chinese texts, one folk food is considered to be the secret ambrosia of youth, the formula for glowing health, the magic key to longevity. This folk food is bee pollen.

Take 1 tablespoon of bee pollen every day, and when you're a healthy 101-year-old who looks 70, you'll know it works.

HIGH-QUALITY ENERGY AND BALANCE AND MORE . . . MUCH MORE

NOTEWORTHY: Instead of telling you why table salt may not be good for you, we choose to tell you why the Original Himalayan Crystal Salt may be great for you.

Every metabolic function of the body relies on the presence of salt. The higher the quality of the salt you consume, the better your body should function.

The Original Himalayan Crystal Salt, PSYMPHONY, from American BlueGreen LLC, is said to be the highest grade of natural salt, containing all 84 ional minerals and trace elements that help keep your body in balance. While Ed Leach from American BlueGreen is the one saying that, there is research and a report of a human clinical trial that reinforce his assurance.

Here is a partial list of possible benefits from Original Himalayan Crystal Salt:

■ Promotes a healthy pH balance in cells, particularly brain cells

■ Promotes blood sugar health and helps to reduce the signs of aging

■ Promotes bone strength

■ Supports the libido

■ Naturally promotes and regulates sleep

■ In conjunction with water, is essential for the regulation of blood pressure. The thinking is that salt may be a contributing cause of high blood pressure. Original Himalayan Crystal Salt stones, in conjunction with water, make a supersalty solution called Sole. Drinking it daily is said to regulate and stabilize blood pressure.

This 250-year-old salt is mined from a pristine ecosystem in the Himalayan Mountains, and is available in several forms: fine granulated (for your salt shaker), coarse granulated (for cooking), crystal salt stones (used to prepare Sole, a drink taken before breakfast), and bath crystals.

To learn more about how Original Himalayan Crystal Salt could help bring your body into harmony, visit www.himalayan crystalsalt.com or call 877-224-4872.

To learn a lot more about the healing power of nature, read *Water and Salt: The Essence of Life* by Barbara Hendel, M.D., and Peter Ferreira (available through the same Web site).

YAWNING

Do not stifle a yawn. Yawning restores the equilibrium between the air pressure in the middle ear and that of the outside atmosphere, giving you a feeling of relief. And you thought you were just bored.

IMMUNE SYSTEM STRENGTHENER

We've all heard that confession is good for the soul. According to Dr. James W. Pennebaker, professor of psychology at the University of Texas and author of *Opening Up: The Healing Power of Expressing Emotions* (Guilford), "When we inhibit feelings and thoughts, our breathing and heartbeat speed up, putting an extra strain on our autonomic nervous system." By writing about the stresses in your life, you release pent-up emotions, freeing the immune system to do its real job, that of guarding the body against unwanted invaders. After following Dr. Pennebaker's formula exactly as directed, you should feel lighter, happier, and may experience better health during the next six months than you have during the last six months.

DR. PENNEBAKER'S PROCESS

1. Find a quiet place where you can be alone for 20 minutes.

2. Write down a confession of what's bothering you. Be as specific as you can.

3. Don't worry about spelling or grammar. Just write continuously for the entire 20 minutes.

4. Keep going, even if it feels awkward. Letting go takes practice. If you reach a mental block, repeat your words.

5. After four days of writing, you should be ready to throw the paper away and enjoy your newly recharged immune system.

6. Feel free to repeat the exercise anytime something stressful comes up. Regular release will keep your immune system strong.

HARMONY BY NAPPING

I t is said that a nap—a warm little cup of sleep—during the day can do wonders for balancing emotions and attitudes and, in general, harmonizing one's system without interference from the conscious mind.

Presidents Truman, Kennedy, Johnson, and Clinton were well-known nappers. Add to that prestigious list of productive people who were caught napping (so to speak) on a daily basis: Eleanor Roosevelt, John D. Rockefeller, Thomas Edison, Winston Churchill, and (wouldn't you know) Napoleon.

SINGING

O ur on-in-years aunt had Alzheimer's. One Thanksgiving we were with her at our cousin's home. Not only didn't she know who we were, but she didn't recognize our cousins, who were her own daughters.

At the end of the evening, Aunt Minnie stood at the door, waiting for her caretaker, and we stood with her. Desperate to make small talk, we asked if she remembered how the family used to get together. As an example, one of us mentioned an old Yiddish folksong and started singing it. Much to our surprise (shock was more like it), Aunt Minnie got happy and started singing along. She remembered every word and more choruses of the song than we knew. As you can imagine, we didn't stop there. During the next hour, whichever song titles we could dredge up from our memory, Aunt Minnie sang. It was astounding—a songfest at one unforgettable Thanksgiving.

We have since learned that lots of research is going on in this area. One of the findings is that music has the ability to access words in some people who have lost the capacity to speak: They can sing when they hear the melody played.

Studies show that singing, either in a chorus or solo, has tremendous benefits. It can enhance your immune system and your feeling of well-being, reduce your feelings of pain, increase lung capacity, give you more energy, and improve posture.

Seniors who sing, particularly in a chorus, reported fewer doctor visits, fewer eyesight problems, less incidence of depression, less need for medication, and fewer falls and other injuries.

Sing! And not just in the shower. Find a chorus in your area and ask to join. If you need to be coaxed out of your shell, sign up for singing lessons, in a group or one-on-one. Check your local music store for sing-along tapes, CDs, or DVDs. If you're on the Internet, search and you will find many sites with music and lyrics for a sing-along.

HAVE A GOOD CRY

Emotional tears have a higher protein content than onion-produced tears. A researcher at the St. Paul–Ramsey Medical Center accounts for that difference as nature's way of releasing chemical substances (the protein) created during an emotional or stressful situation. In turn, the release of those chemical substances allows the negative feelings to flow out, letting a sense of well-being return.

According to Dr. Margaret Crepeau of Marquette University, people who suppress tears are more vulnerable to disease. In fact, suppressing any kind of feeling seems to take its toll on one's system. Face your feelings and let 'em out!

INVIGORATING, STRENGTHENING, AND CLEANSING TONIC

NOTEWORTHY: Fifth-generation herb doctor Catfish Gray, known as "Man of the Woods," gathered herbs and roots from the Appalachian Mountains around his home in West Virginia to use for his revitalizing, system-cleansing, health-enhancing tonic. After decades of preparing and distributing his legendary tonic, Catfish agreed to share the formula with the Penn Herb Company.

Catfish Bitters are available in tea and capsule forms, and both contain eighteen herbs—ginseng, wild cherry bark, black cohosh, burdock, pipsissewa, queen-of-the-meadow root, red clover, yellow dock, sarsaparilla, spikenard, yarrow, goldenseal root, bloodroot, comfrey leaves, lobelia, peppermint, Solomon seal, slippery elm—for their special qualities such as blood purifying, organ detoxifying, lymphatic cleansing, restoring natural immune resistance, and boosting physical and mental performance.

If you're in Philadelphia, visit Penn Herb's store at 603 North 2nd Street, or check out Catfish Bitters at www .pennherb.com, or phone 800-523-9971.

CLAUSTROPHOBIA

If you dread being in a closed space, carry a green apple with you. Then when you step into an elevator or go on a subway train, you can expand your perception of the space's size by taking a bite of the apple and, more important, taking a whiff of it. According to Alan R. Hirsch, M.D., neurological director of the Smell and Taste Treatment and Research Foundation, the scent of green apples makes spaces seem larger. The same holds true for the smell of cucumbers.

If you have claustrophobic tendencies, you'll want to stay away from the smell of barbecued meat, which makes spaces seem more closed in.

GIVE HEALING ORDERS

A Johns Hopkins Hospital survey concluded that three out of four ailments stemmed from emotional factors. It makes sense: Crises in our lives cause emotional reactions that cause biochemical changes that disrupt the body's harmony, weaken immunity, and upset hormone production.

We do it to ourselves; we can undo it!

Relax every part of your body (follow the visualization exercise in the "Stress, Tension, Anxiety" chapter). Once you're completely relaxed, order your body to heal itself. Actually give your body commands out loud. Be direct, clear, and positive. Picture your specific problem. (There's no right or wrong; it's all up to your own imagination.) Once you have a clear picture of your problem, see it healing. Envision pain flying out of your pores; picture the condition breaking up and disintegrating. Say and see whatever seems appropriate to rid yourself of your particular health challenge.

End this daily session by looking in the mirror and repeating a dozen times, "Wellness is mine," and mean it!

HEALTHFUL HINTS, FUN FACTS, AND FOOD FOR THOUGHT

break down, it doesn't mean that your body *will* definitely absorb it; it means that your body *can* absorb it.

HEALTHFUL HINTS

TEST YOUR PILLS

According to chemist Larry Royce, the vitamins, minerals, and other supplements you may be taking may be passing right through your body without doing you a bit of good.

There's a simple test that can tell you whether or not your body has a chance of absorbing the ingredients in the pills you're taking.

Put the pill or capsule that you want to test in ½ cup of distilled white vinegar. A small pill should disintegrate within a half hour, a big pill within an hour. If a pill is *enteric-coated* (check the label for those words), it may take more than an hour to disintegrate.

The vinegar represents your stomach acids. If it doesn't break down the pill, chances are your stomach acids won't, either. If the pill doesn't break down, your body cannot absorb it. If the pill does

TAKING PILLS

■ Take pills standing up, and keep standing for about 2 minutes afterward. Taking them with at least ½ cup of water while standing will give the pills a chance to move swiftly along, instead of staying in your esophagus, where they may disintegrate and cause nausea or heartburn.

■ According to Dr. Stephen Paul of Temple University's School of Pharmacy, a multivitamin that includes the fat-soluble vitamins A, D, and E should be taken with the largest meal of the day. That is when the greatest amount of fat is available in the stomach to aid the absorption of the vitamins.

■ The water-soluble vitamins—C and B-complex—should be taken during a meal or a half hour before the meal. The vitamins help start the biochemical process that breaks down food, making it available to use for energy and tissue building.

■ If you take large doses of vitamin C, take it in small amounts throughout the day. Your body will use more of it that way, and you will help prevent urinary-tract irritation.

NOTE: Never take megadoses of any vitamins, minerals, or herbs unless you do so under the close supervision of a health professional.

ANTIBIOTICS: SETTING THE RECORD STRAIGHT

Each year doctors write 100 million antibiotic prescriptions for their patients. It is estimated that half of the prescribed antibiotics are unnecessary.

Antibiotics work only on *bacterial* infections, not *viral* infections. That means if you have the flu (a viral infection), the antibiotic will be useless. If you have strep throat, a sinus infection, pneumonia, or a severe skin infection, an antibiotic prescription is appropriate.

Antibiotics have no discretion. They destroy the good as well as the bad bacteria. Replace the beneficial bacteria with *Lactobacillus acidophilus*. You can do that by

eating yogurt—make sure the container says it contains live (active) cultures of *L. acidophilus*—by drinking acidophilus milk, or by taking an acidophilus supplement (available at vitamin and health food stores).

Whether you take a supplement, drink milk, or eat yogurt (fat-free is fine as long as it says it contains *L. acidophilus*), do it 2 hours *after* taking an antibiotic, making sure that it's also at least 2 hours *before* you have to take another dose of the antibiotic. Allow that amount of time before and after the antibiotic so that the acidophilus doesn't interfere with the work of the antibiotic.

Keep consuming acidophilus in some form for at least a couple of weeks after you stop taking an antibiotic. It will help normalize the bacterial balance in the intestines, getting your digestive system working properly again.

We're hoping that this information makes you a more informed patient who doesn't insist on an antibiotic—whether you need it or not.

MEDICINE EXPIRATION DATES

Over-the-counter products in their original, unopened packaging may last two years or more beyond the listed expiration date if they are kept in cool, dry areas (not in bathroom cabinets, exposed to heat and humidity).

Prescription medications, bottled by the pharmacist, may not last as long as medication in commercially sealed containers. Pay closer attention to their expiration dates. If you have any doubt about the effectiveness of the medication once it is past its expiration date, call and ask the pharmacist, or just get a new refill. Do not practice false economy when it comes to medication.

STORING PILLS

Do not store pills in kitchen cabinets or the bathroom medicine cabinet. It gets hot and humid when you cook in the kitchen and when you shower or bathe in the bathroom. Medication and supplements may lose potency in hot and humid places. Diabetic testing strips can become inaccurate due to heat and humidity. Store all pills and strips in a dark, cool place—a linen closet, a dining-room hutch, a bedroom armoire—and be sure they're unreachable by children and pets.

ARE YOU ABSORBING YOUR NUTRIENTS?

To best evaluate his patients' state of health, and to help them practice preventive medicine, Ray C. Wunderlich Jr., M.D. (www.wunderlichcenter.com) asks the most important question of all: "Does your bowel movement mark the toilet bowl?" Stools that adhere to the surface of the toilet bowl, leaving a mark, indicate faulty digestive capacity, usually of fat.

"No matter if one's diet is the best in the world, if not processed properly and absorbed," as Dr. Wunderlich poetically puts it, "one may feed the privy without being privy to nutrients that are being lost to that porcelain banquet."

MICROWAVING TO SAVE VITAMINS

Fewer vitamins are destroyed when you prepare food in a microwave. Prevent food from burning by adding a small amount of water—as little as possible to retain as many of the food's nutrients as possible. Also, cover foods (with glass, not plastic) while microwaving in order to reduce the zapping time and keep in more of the nutrients.

ITEMS YOUR PHARMACY SHOULD HAVE (BUT USUALLY DOESN'T)

NOTEWORTHY: Apothecary Products was founded in 1975 by a registered pharmacist whose innovative product lines are aimed at making life easier for both the pharmacist and the people they serve.

Since then, they have become the leading pharmacy supplier in the United States, and it's no wonder. Wait till you see their products. They have a huge variety of pill/supplement cases, including our favorite—a roomy, four-times-a-day weekly pill organizer (perfect for all the supplements we take). They also have foot care products, medical-alert jewelry, diabetic specialty products, ear care and pet care products, and so much more.

The company is constantly developing new products, and their beautifully designed, user-friendly Web site is one of the best places to find out about exciting new developments. Visit www.ezy dose.com, phone 800-328-2742 (general questions) or 888-770-8767 (place an order).

NEED A DROPPER FOR EYES, EARS, OR NOSE?

If you need a dropper *now* for any of your orifices and don't have one, you can im-provise with a straw. (Of course, you have to have a straw.) Dunk the straw in the liquid, then close off the top of the straw with your finger. A 2-inch piece of plastic straw will yield about 15 drops of liquid.

DO-IT-YOURSELF ICE PACK AND HOT-WATER BOTTLE

In an emergency situation, if an ice pack or hot water bottle or bag isn't available, ad-lib with one of the following:

■ Use an empty laundry detergent container filled with hot water as a hot water bottle; fill it with ice-cold water and use it as an ice pack.

■ If you want a flexible ice pack, use a package of frozen veggies, or dunk a towel in cold water, wring it out, and place it on aluminum foil in the freezer. Before it freezes stiff, take it out and mold it around the bruised or injured part of the body.

TAKING YOUR PULSE

■ Place the tips of your index, second, and third fingers on the inside of your other wrist, below the base of your thumb. Or place the tips of your index and second fingers on the base of your neck, on either side of your windpipe.

- Press your fingers lightly until you feel the pulsing beneath your fingers. You may have to move your fingers around a little, up or down, until you feel the pulsing.

- Use a watch or a clock with a second hand to count the beats.

> **NOTEWORTHY**: Instead of taking your pulse the old-fashioned way, you may want to consider buying a digital pulse watch, the kind runners use. Visit www.ckbproducts.com for wholesale prices to the public and no minimum purchase, or call 888-CKB-BUYS for their catalog.

SELECTING A DOCTOR

Of course you know to check a doctor's credentials, either through the HMO to which he or she belongs or on the Internet. Google "check doctors credentials" and you'll have a choice of free and pay Web sites that offer their services.

When shopping around for a doctor, you may want to take into consideration the doctor's age. Most desirable is a doctor who is close to your age so that he or she will have a better understanding of what you are going through and how best to test and treat you. It also helps if the doctor is the same sex as you. Can a man know what it's like to menstruate? Can a woman know what premature or delayed ejaculation feels like? (While it's something to consider, this is not to say that a younger or older physician of the opposite sex will not be a great caregiver.)

CLEANING STUFFED TOYS

The much-loved stuffed toys in your home are home to dust mites. Those dust mites can trigger allergic reactions such as asthma attacks. To kill those mighty mites, simply put each stuffed critter in a plastic bag and leave it in the freezer for 24 hours once a week. Explain to your child that the stuffed toy joined the cast of *Holiday on Ice* and it's showtime every Sunday, or whenever.

NATURAL AIR-POLLUTION CLEANERS

Your tax dollars have paid for National Aeronautics and Space Administration (NASA) research, and now you can benefit by it.

NASA's scientists discovered that several common houseplants can dramatically reduce toxic chemical levels in homes and offices. If you don't think your home or office is polluted, rethink it. There's benzene (found in inks, oils, paints, plastics, rubber, detergents, dyes, and gasoline); formaldehyde (found in foam insulation, particleboard, pressed-wood products, most cleaning agents, and paper products treated with resins, including facial tissues and paper towels); and trichloroethylene (TCE, which is found in dry-cleaning processes, printing inks, paints, lacquers, varnishes, and adhesives). Now you know, and now you can do something about it.

Here are low-cost, attractive solutions in the form of hardy, easy-to-find, easy-to-grow household plants:

■ Spider plant (*Chlorophytim comosum "Vittatum"*)—very easy to grow in indirect or bright diffuse light (soft light that's spread out rather than direct). Provide good drainage.

■ Peace lily (*Spathiphyllum* spp.)—very easy to grow in low-light locations.

■ Chinese evergreen (*Aglaonema modestum "Silver Queen"*)—very easy to grow in low-light locations. Remove overgrown shoots to encourage new growth, and keep the plant bushy.

■ Weeping fig (*Ficus benjamina*)—requires a little special attention. Indirect or bright diffuse light is best.

■ Golden pothos (*Epipremnum aureum*)—very easy to grow in indirect or bright diffuse light.

Moderately moist soil is preferred by all of these plants.

NASA recommends placing fifteen to eighteen plants in an 1,800-square-foot home. In a small to average-size room, one plant ought to do it, especially if it's a place where air circulates.

After the plants are in place, you, your colleagues at work, and/or members of your household may find that sore throats, headaches, irritated eyes, and stuffy noses have cleared up.

WHEN YA GOTTA GO . . .

In a public bathroom, use the first stall—the one closest to the door. Studies show that it's used the least and therefore has the lowest level of bacteria.

Also, once you've done what you came to do, stand up, then flush. That way, you will protect your bottom from the fine spray of water that may contain contagious bacteria from people who used the facility before you. That bacteria can be the cause of intestinal bugs, even hepatitis.

STOP BLAMING YOURSELF

If you misplace something—your glasses, keys, purse, whatever—do what young people do: Put it off on someone else. "Who moved my glasses?" "Who took my keys?" It sure beats thinking, "Uh-oh, a senior moment. I'm getting old." That kind of thinking will make you feel and behave like an old fart. (Hey, they say it on TV. Why can't we say it here?)

Think and talk like young people and you'll stay younger longer. You may even find your glasses faster and get your keys back from whoever took them!

FUN FACTS

COMING TO YOUR SENSES

The average pair of eyes can distinguish nearly 8 million differences in color.

The average pair of ears can discriminate among more than 300,000 tones.

The average nose can recognize 10,000 different odors.

There are 1,300 nerve endings per square inch in each average fingertip; the only parts of the body more sensitive to touch are the lips, the tongue, and the tip of the nose.

That covers four of our five senses. As for the fifth sense, everyone knows, there's no accounting for taste! Well, that's not exactly true. There are five basic accountable tastes: sweet, sour, bitter, salty, and umami (such as the savory taste of monosodium glutamate).

One's sense of smell plays a major part in discerning taste. If you hold your nose and close your eyes, you probably could not taste the difference between grated apple, potato, or onion. While still holding your nose, you probably couldn't differentiate between coffee or tea. Just for the record, what we consider taste is more accurately *flavor,* which is a combination of taste, smell, texture, and temperature.

FOOD FOR THOUGHT

BANANAS: THE SECRET OF STRINGLESSNESS

Save yourself the trouble of having to de-string a banana. Simply do what monkeys do: peel the banana from the bottom up. No strings attached.

BANANAS: SLOW DOWN THE RIPENING

Do not leave bananas in a bunch. Take them apart at the stem and they will not ripen as quickly.

BELL PEPPERS BY THE BUMPS

We found this fascinating but could not confirm it with any vegetable authority. So, for whatever it's worth: Bell peppers with three bumps (known in agricultural circles as *lobes*) on the bottom are sweeter and better eaten raw. Peppers with four bumps on the bottom are firmer and better to use for cooking.

EAT THE DECORATIONS

At a restaurant, the food that's served is most often artistically garnished to make it look good. Instead of moving the garnish to the side of the plate, eat the garnish, especially if it's green. It's probably the healthiest part of the meal.

SALBA

By the time you read this, we're hoping you already know all about Salba and are taking advantage of its many extraordinary qualities. If not, we're happy you're here reading this now, and please continue.

What Is Salba?

Salba is a nutrient-packed, ancient seed, *Salvia hispanica*, in the mint family. This little seed is now grown in Peru's ideal climate and environment, under strictly controlled conditions . . . the finest conditions on the planet.

Unlike any other grain, Salba has undergone intense, long-term human nutritional studies. Salba makes health and medical claims that no other grain can. (It is the only grain that has a medical patent pending. You can read about it in the "Diabetes" chapter.)

We would be remiss if we didn't acknowledge, with gratitude, Vladimir Vuksan, professor of endocrinology and nutritional sciences, Faculty of Medicine, University of Toronto. Dr. Vuksan is responsible for recent research that resulted in bringing to light the incredible nutritional value of this miraculous seed and its many health-giving gifts.

Salba's Superpowers

Mitch Propster, founder and CEO of Core Naturals, bills Salba as "nature's perfect whole food," and William "Rally" Ralston, managing partner of Salba Smart Natural Products, talks with awe about Salba and "the power of a single grain." True, both companies are selling the product, but they're selling it because *they* are so sold on it. We think you will be too after learning about all that Salba has to offer.

Gram for gram:

■ Salba has eight times more omega-3 fatty acids than salmon. In fact, omega-3 fatty acids are found more abundantly in Salba than in any other naturally occurring source known.

- Salba has four times more fiber than flaxseed.

- Salba has six times more calcium than whole milk.

- Salba has seven times more vitamin C than an orange.

- Salba has three times more antioxidants than fresh blueberries.

- Salba has three times more iron than spinach.

- Salba has fifteen times more magnesium than broccoli.

As if all of that weren't enough, Salba also has folate, B vitamins, potassium, zinc, selenium, and vitamin A. Salba is gluten-free and kosher.

How to Eat Salba

Salba seeds can be eaten whole or ground. Both have the same benefits.

Salba doesn't have a discernible flavor, and so it can be mixed into cereal, yogurt, salads (it makes them crunchy), sauces, smoothies, and burgers. You can also bake with it—up to 25 percent of the flour used in any recipe can be replaced with ground Salba. Also, Salba gel (a simple mixture of

Salba seeds in water, described in "Preparation Guide") can be used in place of eggs.

Once you start using Salba, you'll find that you can add it to just about any food you prepare without altering the taste of the dish.

Typical Dosage

For adults, 2 level tablespoons daily; for children, up to 1 tablespoon daily.

Since it is rich in fiber, you may have to be near a bathroom the first time or two that you take any appreciable amount. It has a cleansing effect, and that's a very good thing.

NOTEWORTHY: There are two Salba companies that we can wholeheartedly recommend for their integrity in terms of their quality products, starting with the highest grade of organic Salba and continuing with organically grown ingredients in their bars, chips, salsa, and other foods containing Salba:

- Core Natural Products, www.salbausa.com, phone 888-895-3603
- Salba Smart Natural Products LLC, www.salbasmart.com, phone 303-298-3833

Where to Buy Salba

As of this writing, all forms of Salba are available online (see above for two fine sources) and at health food stores (if it hasn't reached your local store yet, request it). Who knows—by now word may have gotten around and you may be able to find it at your supermarket.

STOCKING STUFFERS

When you bring onions and potatoes home from the store, put them in the cut-off leg of old pantyhose and keep them in a cool place. The hose allows the air to circulate around them. They will keep better and longer that way.

MOLD ON FOOD

It's not a good thing. While it probably won't kill you, it can make you sick. If you see mold on any kind of food, do not give it the smell test to see if it has gone bad. Just a whiff of the mold spores can trigger an allergic or respiratory reaction. Get rid of soft foods or drinks that have even a hint of mold. If hard foods, such as Swiss cheese, have mold, you can lop off the moldy part (play it safe and discard an inch all around the mold) and salvage the rest.

HERB AND SPICE STORAGE

When exposed to heat, as from the kitchen stove, spices and herbs lose their potency and their colors fade. While the refrigerator is ideal, it's impractical. Second best is to store herbs and spices in a cool, dry area.

SWEET AND SALTY SUBSTITUTES

When substituting honey for sugar in a recipe, use ½ cup of honey for every 1 cup of sugar. Honey has about 65 calories per teaspoon; sugar has 45 calories per teaspoon. Since honey is twice as sweet as sugar, use only half as much honey as sugar and save calories.

If salt is a no-no, use a spritz of lemon juice instead to help provide the kick that salt gives food.

SOURCES

For years we have known and dealt with most of the companies and services listed here. The few with whom we have not had a personal relationship have come highly recommended by people we trust. Even so, before you place your order, find out about guarantees, return policies, and whatever else you need to know to make you a happy shopper.

If you prefer shopping from a catalog in hand, rather than scrolling through pages on the computer, call and ask if a paper catalog is available. There are some super catalogs among these companies—for example, Magellan's (for travelers), UPCO (for pet owners), and Gaiam (great gift items). Some companies also offer free online newsletter subscriptions.

We're not being specific with regard to the companies that offer catalogs or newsletters because everything changes so quickly, including addresses, telephone numbers, and Web sites. At the time of publication, the contact information below was accurate. Hopefully it still is.

HERBAL PRODUCTS AND MORE

San Francisco Herb Company
250 14th Street
San Francisco, CA 94103
Phone: 800-227-4530
415-861-7174
www.sfherb.com

Penn Herb Co. Ltd.
10601 Decatur Road, Suite 2
Philadelphia, PA 19154
Phone: 800-523-9971
www.pennherb.com

Indiana Botanic Gardens
3401 West 37th Avenue
Hobart, IN 46342
Phone: 800-644-8327
www.botanicchoice.com

Herbally Grounded, LLC
4441 W. Charleston
Las Vegas, NV 89102
Phone: 866-676-1410
www.herballygrounded.com

**Great American Natural Products and
Old Amish Herbal Remedies**
4121 16th Street North
St. Peterburg, FL 33703
Phone: 800-323-4372
727-521-4372
www.greatamerican.biz
www.herbal-shops.com

Flower Power Herbs and Roots, Inc.
406 East 9th Street
New York, NY 10009
Phone: 212-982-6664
(Free in-store herbal consultations)
www.flowerpower.net

Blessed Herbs
109 Barre Plains Road
Oakham, MA 01068
Phone: 800-489-HERB (4372)
www.blessedherbs.com

Atlantic Spice Company
2 Shore Road
North Truro, MA 02652
Phone: 800-316-7965
508-487-6100
www.atlanticspice.com

VITAMINS, NUTRITIONAL SUPPLEMENTS, AND MORE

Swanson Health Products
P.O. Box 6003
Fargo, ND 58108
Phone: 800-437-4148
www.swansonvitamins.com

Nutrition Coalition, Inc.
Box 3001
Fargo, ND 58108
Phone: 800-447-4793
218-236-9783
(Willard Water and more)
www.nutritioncoalition.com
www.willardswater.com

Life Extension Foundation
P.O. Box 407189
Ft. Lauderdale, FL 33340
Phone: 800-544-4440
www.lef.org

Freeda Vitamins
47-25 34th Street, 3rd floor
Long Island City, NY 11101
Phone: 800-777-3737
(Kosher certified, 100 percent vegetarian,
sugar-free, salt-free, yeast-free, gluten-
free, lactose-free)
www.freedavitamins.com

BEE PRODUCTS AND MORE

C.C. Pollen Co.
3627 East Indian School Road, Suite 209
Phoenix, AZ 85018
Phone: 800-875-0096
602-957-0096
www.ccpollen.com

NATURAL FOODS AND MORE

Jaffe Bros. Natural Foods, Inc.
28560 Lilac Road
Valley Center, CA 92082
Phone: 760-749-1133
www.organicfruitsandnuts.com

Gold Mine Natural Foods Co.
7805 Arjons Drive
San Diego, CA 92126
Phone: 800-475-FOOD (3663)
www.goldminenaturalfoods.com

Barlean's Organic Oils LLC
4936 Lake Terrell Road
Ferndale, WA 98248
Phone: 800-445-3529
www.barleans.com

GEMS, NEW AGE PRODUCTS, AND GIFTS

Pacific Spirit
1334 Pacific Avenue
Forest Grove, OR 97116
Phone: 800-634-9057
www.mystictrader.com

Gemisphere
2812 NW Thurman Street
Portland, OR 97210
Phone: 800-727-8877
www.gemisphere.com

Crystal Way
2335 Market Street
San Francisco, CA 94114
Phone: 415-861-6511
www.crystalway.com

PET FOOD AND PRODUCTS

Halo Purely for Pets
12400 Race Track Road
Tampa, FL 33626
Phone: 800-426-4256
www.halopets.com

Harbingers of a New Age
717 East Missoula Avenue
Troy, MT 59935
Phone: 406-295-4944
www.vegepet.com

UPCO
P.O. Box 969
St. Joseph, MO 64502-0969
Phone: 800-254-UPCO (8726)
816-233-8800
www.upco.com

HEALTH-RELATED PRODUCTS

Apothecary Products
11750 12th Avenue South
Burnsville, MN 55337-1295
Phone: 800-328-2742
www.ezydose.com

Gaiam—A Lifestyle Company
360 Interlocken Blvd., Suite 300
Broomfield, CO 80021
Phone: 877-989-6321
www.gaiam.com

HEALTH-RELATED TRAVEL PRODUCTS

Magellan's (Essentials for the Traveler)
110 West Sola Street
Santa Barbara, CA 93101
Phone: 800-962-4943
(Worthwhile travel tips and advice on Web site)
www.magellans.com

HEALTH EQUIPMENT AND MORE

ReBuilder Medical, Inc.
636 Treeline Drive
Charles Town, WV 25414
Phone: 866-724-2202
www.rebuildermedical.com

CKB Products Wholesale
8212 Chancellor Row
Dallas, TX 75247
Phone: 888-CKB-BUYS (252-2897)
www.ckbproducts.com

Acme Equipment
1032 Concert Avenue
Spring Hill, FL 34609
Phone: 800-882-0157
(Equipment replacement parts available,
from kitchen appliances to complex
hydraulic needs)
www.acmeequipment.com

AROMATHERAPY, FLOWER ESSENCES, AND MORE

Flower Essence Services
Box 1769
Nevada City, CA 95959
Phone: 800-548-0075
(Flower essence therapy products)
www.fesflowers.com

Aroma Vera
5310 Beethoven Street
Los Angeles, CA 90066
Phone: 800-669-9514
www.aromavera.com

Aroma Thyme
3553 St. Albans Road
Cleveland, OH 44121
Phone: 888-AROMA-99 (276-6299)
www.aromathyme.com

SERVICES

World Research Foundation (WRF)
41 Bell Rock Plaza
Sedona, AZ 86351
Phone in Arizona: 928-284-3300
Los Angeles office: 310-827-0070
www.wrf.org

For a very reasonable fee, cofounders Steve Ross and LaVerne Boeckmann will do a search (which includes 5,000 international medical journals) and provide information on the newest holistic, alternative, complementary, and allopathic medicine, ranging from ancient to current traditional techniques and healing therapies to the latest technologies.

Also for sale are tapes and videos on specific ailments and rare or little-known (extraordinary) therapies.

The foundation's library in Sedona has more than 20,000 books, periodicals, and research reports and is available to the public free of charge.

When you visit the Web site, click on "Books," which will turn into "Info Packets," and you will then be able to click on the A-to-Z selection for the ailment you want to research.

American Board of Medical Specialties
1007 Church Street, Suite 404
Evanston, IL 60201
Phone verification: 866-ASK-ABMS
(275-2267)
Phone: 847-491-9091
www.abms.org

The ABMS is an organization of twenty-four approved medical specialty boards. It offers a toll-free number where you can confirm that a specialist is exactly that. Just provide the doctor's name, and the ABMS will verify at no charge whether the doctor is listed in his or her specialty.

Consumer Information Catalog (CIC)
Phone: 888-8-PUEBLO (878-3256)
www.pueblo.gsa.gov

The CIC lists more than two hundred free and low-cost publications from Uncle Sam on everything from saving money, staying healthy, and getting federal benefits to buying a home and handling consumer complaints. To get your free copy of the catalog, call or visit the Web site. Also on the Web site, you can read, print out, or download any CIC publication for free.

INDEX

ABOUT THE AUTHORS

JOAN WILEN and LYDIA WILEN are energetic health investigators who have helped enlighten millions with their amazing "cures in the kitchen" through their numerous books, media tours, and frequent appearances on national and local television shows, including *The Today Show*, *CBS This Morning*, and *Good Day New York*. They have also been guests on hundreds of radio shows.

The Wilens have conducted frequent lectures and workshops, and have had articles written by and about them for major magazines and newspapers, including *Cosmopolitan*, *The New York Times*, and *Parade*. They also had a weekly, celebrity-driven full-page feature in the *New York Daily News Sunday Magazine* for two years, and three rotating features in *New York Newsday*. They currently contribute to the *Bottom Line/Personal* newsletter and live in New York City.